RURAL HEALTH NURSING

Barriers and Benefits

Laurie Anne Ferguson
DNP, APRN, ANP-BC, FNP-C, CPNP, FNAP, FAANP
Founding Dean and Professor
Emory & Henry College School of Nursing
Marion, Virginia

Kenneth Lowrance
DNP, APRN, CNS, FNP-BC, CNE, FAANP
Professor of Professional Practice, Retired
Texas Christian University
Harris College of Nursing and Health Sciences
Fort Worth, Texas

DEStech Publications, Inc.

Rural Health Nursing

DEStech Publications, Inc.
439 North Duke Street
Lancaster, Pennsylvania 17602 U.S.A.

Printed in the United States of America
10 9 8 7 6 5 4 3 2 1

Main entry under title:
Rural Health Nursing: Barriers and Benefits

A DEStech Publications book
Bibliography: p.
Includes index p. 313

Library of Congress Control Number: 2022931128
ISBN No. 978-1-60595-157-7

Table of Contents

Foreword

Rural populations have long been underserved, especially in terms of access to and receipt of appropriate healthcare. The economic downturn of recent years in many communities has led to the closure of many acute care hospitals thereby enhancing this disparity in rural areas. Despite this, rural health experiences and careers are increasingly becoming an opportunity for nurses of all levels of educational preparation to provide health promotion and care for people in these communities. Identifying and implementing options for these individuals, families, and communities to access a health provider and treatment options provides more opportunities for rural health nurses.

Rural areas may have minimal to no access to healthcare providers and facilities compared to urban areas, thus causing many rural individuals to go without healthcare or at the least, to face profound barriers to access quality, cost-efficient care. Underinsured and uninsured individuals struggle to sustain a quality of life with little to no health care options. In small communities where everyone knows each other, the presence of social stigma, and the challenge to maintain confidentiality and privacy are other obstacles which may expose individuals to embarrassment when seeking care for issues of mental illness, alcohol or drug dependency, and abuse. The issues of privacy related to such issues need to be prioritized to avoid barriers in receiving or delaying critical treatment.

An exciting yet challenging specialty for the nursing profession, rural health careers encompass the many challenges with distance, transportation, deficiency in health literacy, and inadequate or no health insurance coverage. However, advances in technology have enabled the use of telehealth to facilitate individuals' access to health care providers who may be many miles away, but who can provide the needed treatments and care needed. Every level of nursing has a potential role in rural health care delivery ranging from the nursing assistant to the doctoral-prepared nurse to help meet the needs of this deserving population. Challenges abound, but who better to meet these than a nurse? The rural setting provides a setting for abundant opportunities for innovation, quality improvement, research, and implementation of evidence-based practice.

Geographical isolation and decreased access to care is only part of the challenge. As nurses, we are faced with many challenges including those with acculturation. Acculturation exists when an individual is exposed to dissimilar groups or cultures. A personal story illustrates this concept of a nurse's lack of familiarity with some of the cultures within the region. Growing up surrounded by rolling hills and farmlands may not provide the experience of living or working on a farm. The lack of familiarity with the dialect and nomenclature of the farming culture was revealed during a triage in the emergency department in a rural setting.

The call came in, and the ER staff prepared for an incoming trauma from a farming accident involving a bush hog. The nurse was unprepared and disturbed by the devastating trauma that a boar/hog could inflict upon a person. The nurse learned quickly that a bush hog was not the type of wild boar but rather a farming implement used to mow and clear brush! During the triage, the young nurse was unable to make sense as to why a person would choose to remove a jammed branch from a running mower blade. After years of living in the rural farmlands and using a bush hog, it was more understandable. After watching farmers on their tractors with lights leading their path as they worked the fields late into the night and into the early morning hours covering hundreds of acres, hour after hour, it was easier to understand why such quick decisions might be made. The intent was not to be unsafe, but due to distress, exhaustion, and other stressors experienced by the farmer. Through assimilation with the rural farming culture, the nurse now has a better understanding. Knowledge is power.

Rural Health Nursing: Barriers and Benefits discusses a wide range of topics and issues to enhance nurses' rural health knowledge and understanding. Rural Health nursing should be embedded in nursing curricula or as a stand-alone course, especially in the Advanced Practice Nursing programs. Nurses have a crucial role in the care provision for rural communities. Rural Health Nursing: Barriers and Benefits provides a thorough and exciting educational means to guide nurses in thinking beyond just bedside hospital nursing. The nurse in the rural setting uses a sophisticated skill set that encompasses far more than nursing skills to address the challenges and opportunities in the rural setting. As nurses, we must advocate and be the voice for those who are faced with barriers in rural settings to access appropriate quality care whether it be face-to-face or by the use of advanced technologies such as telehealth.

This book brings to life the barriers and benefits of practice in the rural setting, but most of all, the professional and personal gratification of working and applying theory and practice in this setting.

Saundra R. Farmer DNP, MSN, RN
Founding Chair Department of
Nursing/BSN Program Director

Teressa M. Wexler, EdD/ET, MSN, RN, CHSE
Clinical Assistant Professor
Emory & Henry College
School of Nursing

Preface

Our passion for improving healthcare in rural areas fueled our desire to gather some of the world's experts on rural nursing to provide a comprehensive discussion on the issues, challenges, and rewards of working in rural communities. None of us imagined a worldwide COVID-19 pandemic in 2020, which would highlight nurses and other healthcare workers as frontline heroes and expose deficits in our healthcare system, particularly for rural areas and First Nations People. COVID-19 changed our daily lives and "business as usual" by expanding virtual interactions and telehealth. Digital connectivity challenges aside, telehealth has received greater support and implementation due to the pandemic and provides one bridge for rural populations to access care including access to specialists. The subsequent result is this text which provides information on issues, policies and systems, and a lengthy discussion of challenges in American Indian and Alaska Natives people in the United States. It is our desire to provide a wide-ranging reference of rural health issues as well as to highlight the unique rewards of rural health nursing practice. This has been a labor of love and we hope it provides invaluable insights.

LAURIE ANNE FERGUSON
KENNETH LOWRANCE

List of Contributors

Editors

Laurie Anne Ferguson, DNP, APRN, ANP-BC, FNP-C, CPNP, FNAP, FAANP
Founding Dean of Nursing, Emory & Henry College, Emory, VA

Kenneth W. Lowrance, DNP, APRN, CNS, FNP-BC, NEA-BC, NEA, FAANP
Professor of Professional Practice, Texas Christian University, Fort Worth, TX

Contributors

Vicki Brooks, DNP, APRN, FNP-BC
Assistant Professor of Professional Practice, Family Nurse Practitioner Program Coordinator, Texas Christian University, Fort Worth, TX

Angeline Bushy, PhD, RN, FAAN
Professor, University of Central Florida, Orlando, FL

Dennis J. Cheek, PhD, RN, FAHA
Abell-Hanger Professor of Gerontological Nursing, Texas Christian University, Fort Worth, TX

Jill Cochran, PhD, APRN, C-FNP, FAANP
Associate Professor, West Virginia School of Osteopathic Medicine, Lewisburg, WV

Monica Daniels-Mika, MRCP, MS
Centennial Area Health Education Center

Joy Elwell, DNP, FNP-BC, APRN, CNE, FAAN, FAANP
Professor and Director DNP Program, University of Connecticut, Storrs, CT

Wendy Fletcher, DNP, APRN, FNP-BC, FAANP
Managing Partner, The CheráWen Group, LLC
Co-Owner/APRN, Main Street Medical Associates (Morehead, KY)

Dwain Harris, MHA
National Health Education Center

Loretta Heuer, PhD, RN, FAAN
Professor/School of Nursing, North Dakota State University, Grand Forks, ND

Barbara Jackson, PhD, RN
President, Faculty Council Chair, PhD in Health Professions Education Program Director of Assessment and Accreditation; Associate Professor, Lansing School of Nursing and Clinical Sciences, Bellarmine University, Louisville, KY

Holly Jeffreys, DNP APRN FNP-BC
Founder & CEO Panhandle Family Care LLC, Panhandle, TX;
West Texas A&M University, Department Head Nursing & Associate Professor, West Texas A&M University, Canyon, TX

Ruth McCaffrey, DNP, APRN, FNP-BC, GNP-BC, FAAN, FAANP
Emeritus Professor, Florida Atlantic University, Boca Raton, FL

Kathleen T. McCoy, DNSc PMHNP-BC PMHCNS-BC FNP-BC FAANP
Associate Professor, University of South Alabama, Mobile AL

Tammy L. McKamie, MSN, RN, OCN, ACGN
Advanced Clinical Genetics Nurse; CHRISTUS St. Michael W. Temple Webber Cancer Treatment Center, Texarkana, TX

Rhoda Owens, PhD, RN
Assistant Professor, University of North Dakota, Grand Forks, ND

Julianne Sanguins, PhD, RN
Research Program Manager, Health & Wellness Department, Manitoba Metis Federation; Assistant Professor, Department of Community Health Sciences, University of Manitoba; Adjunct Scientist, Manitoba Centre for Health Policy, University of Manitob, Winnipeg MB Canada

Audrey Snyder, PhD, RN, FAAN
University of North Carolina Greensboro

Misty L. Wilkie, PhD, RN, FAAN
(Turtle Mountain Chippewa) Associate Professor & Niganawenimaanaanig Program Director, Bemidji State University

Steven Zucker, D.M.D., MEd
Nova Southeastern University

CHAPTER 1

Rural Health Theory

Rhoda Owens

Objectives:

1. Describe the development of rural nursing theory and its importance to rural healthcare and nursing practice.
2. Discuss characteristics of rural nurses and rural healthcare and the implications for practice.
3. Analyze rural nursing theory and its use in rural nursing and advanced nursing practice to deliver patient care at multiple types of rural facilities and communities.
4. Explain the opportunities and rewards for nurses working in a rural setting.

Discussion Questions:

1. Discuss how the first rural nursing theory has changed over the years. What are the implications for advanced practice nursing?
2. Describe how you perceive "rural advanced practice nursing" as similar and/or different from "urban advanced practice nursing." How could a new advanced practice nurse from an urban area integrate successfully into rural practice and a rural community?
3. Explain the opportunities and rewards a nurse and/or advanced practice nurse could encounter while working in a rural setting.
4. Analyze possible challenges and barriers a rural advanced practice nurse could encounter at a rural healthcare facility and community while planning and providing patient care. Identify some common rural population characteristics. How could the nurse incorporate this knowledge to better promote access to safe quality care and good patient outcomes?

INTRODUCTION

Rural nursing theory has provided a basis for rural healthcare practice and research. The theory has been revised throughout the years due to changes in the healthcare system, policy, rural populations, and new research findings. Working in a rural setting confronts rural nurses including advanced practice nurses with several barriers and challenges. Yet working in rural areas can be rewarding and provide nurses with several opportunities. It is important that all nurses working at various rural healthcare settings be prepared to practice in rural communities. When compared to urban healthcare settings, practicing as a nurse in a rural healthcare setting requires a unique set of knowledge, skills, and competencies. All rural nurses must acquire rural specific practice knowledge and skills to provide better access to care and deliver safe, quality, patient-centered care leading to positive patient outcomes. Rural nurses must be able to meet the existing challenges and eliminate barriers as much as possible while providing patient care. Leaders at rural healthcare facilities and nursing education programs must prepare and support all rural nurses as they enter practice and continue to work in rural communities. This preparation and support have been shown to increase recruitment, work satisfaction, and retention for rural nurses that will contribute to the efforts in meeting the healthcare needs and access for rural and vulnerable populations.

HISTORY OF RURAL NURSING THEORY

It is important for all nurses to have knowledge on the beginnings of rural nursing theory. Rural healthcare and rural nursing theory have also changed over the years based on new research and rural nursing practice experiences, and changes in the healthcare system, policy, and rural populations. All rural nurses must use this knowledge to guide their delivery of patient care at multiple types of rural health facilities and communities.

Rural nursing theory had its beginnings in the research completed by Long and Weinert (1989), nurse researchers at Montana State University College of Nursing. Long and Weinert (1989) completed qualitative and quantitative descriptive research on the experiences of sparsely rural Montana populations. Prior to the publication of this research, it was believed that nursing care of rural and urban populations were similar. Through their research, a descriptive middle-range theory emerged that contains three theoretical statements and concepts that support differences between rural and urban nursing practice. Similar to other past and current rural nursing researchers, Long and Weinert (1989) believe that one cannot apply the same theories to both rural and urban nursing. As compared to urban nursing, rural nursing is unique because of the rural population's health perceptions, characteristics, lifestyles, and the nurse's role as a generalist in clinical practice. As compared to the urban population, rural residents have different characteristics and lifestyles that rural nurses must understand in order to provide safe quality patient-centered care. This middle-range theory provides a foundation and framework for present and future research and rural nursing practice. Similar to other nursing theories, Long and Weinert's (1989) theory is also based on the nursing principles of person, nurse, environment, and health. Since the release of this first rural nursing theory, several researchers have confirmed or revised portions of the theory based on their research findings and literature reviews.

Long and Weinert's (1989) rural nursing theory defines rural nursing as, "the provision of healthcare by professional nurses to persons living in sparsely populated areas" (p. 114) and contains three theoretical statements and several key concepts. The first statement (theoretical statement #1) is that, "Rural dwellers define health as the ability to work, be productive and do usual tasks" (p. 120). Over the years through additional research in rural health and review of the literature, nurse researchers have added to Long and Weinert's (1989) first theoretical statement. Researchers discovered that rural residents further define health as holistic (Lee and McDonagh, 2018) which adds to their desire to work and be productive. In addition, Lee and Winters (2004) found that rural residents, who work in service jobs, must be able to function by being physically, mentally, and emotionally fit.

Through a review of the literature, the most recently revised theoretical statement #1 of Long and Weinert's (1989) theory was revised using a more holistic perspective. Lee and McDonagh (2018) revised theoretical statement #1 as, "Rural residents define health as being able to do what they want to do; it is a way of life, and a state of mind; there is a goal of maintaining balance in all aspects of their lives" (p. 52). Older rural residents and those with ties to extractive industries are more likely to define health in a functional manner—to work, to be productive, and to do usual tasks (Lee and McDonagh, 2018). Younger rural residents have become more focused on health promotion and illness prevention due to increased internet and media exposure emphasizing health promotion and preventive practices (de la Rue and Coulson, 2003). Furthermore, rural providers have increased their overall focus on patient education and preventive care further contributing to this trend (de la Rue and Coulson, 2003). Rural nurses must use this knowledge of how rural residents define and perceive health as they plan, implement, and evaluate patient-centered care. Rural nurses must now use a holistic perspective that includes mental, physical, social, and spiritual aspects while caring for rural populations. In addition, rural nurses must focus more on health promotion and prevention. Rural residents' health perceptions influence their motivation to seek health promotion and illness treatment that could affect their health outcomes (Lee and McDonagh, 2018).

The second theoretical statement in Long and Weinert's (1989) original theory relates to the "insider" and "outsider" phenomenon. "Rural dwellers are self-reliant and resist accepting help or services from those seen as 'outsiders' or from agencies seen as national or regional welfare programs" (Long and Weinert, 1989, p. 120). In addition, "Help, including needed healthcare, is usually sought through an informal rather than a formal system" (Long and Weinert, 1989, p. 120). For example, individuals are more likely to seek healthcare advice from whom they personally know such as close relatives, neighbors, or friends in their communities before traveling to outside health care facilities.

Based on a literature search, Lee and McDonagh (2018) have revised Long and Weinert's (1989) second theoretical statement. The most recent revisions of this second statement are, "Rural residents are self-reliant and make decisions to seek care for illness, sickness, or injury depending on their self-assessment of their severity of their present health condition and of the resources needed and available" (Lee and McDonagh, 2018, p. 52). In addition, Lee and McDonagh (2018) added, "Rural residents with infants and children experiencing illness, sickness, or injury will seek care more quickly than for themselves" (p. 52). In other words, adults view infant and children's healthcare needs as more important than their own healthcare needs. The impact of available internet and social media also influence rural population's healthcare-seeking behavior (Lee and McDonagh, 2018). Rural residents are now more likely to search available internet or social media for healthcare advice. Travel distance to a healthcare facility could also affect their decisions on where to seek formal system care and advice with their healthcare needs. Still, rather than immediately seeking information from healthcare professionals, rural persons are more likely to seek out health information from family, friends, neighbors, and other sources such as the media, popular magazines, books, and the internet. However, rural residents have become more willing to seek out information from "outsiders" and healthcare professionals when they believe it is necessary (Lee and McDonagh, 2018). It is important for rural nurses to keep this in mind as they care for rural populations.

Lastly, the third theoretical statement in Long and Weinert's (1989) original theory is, "Health care providers in rural areas must deal with a lack of anonymity and much greater role diffusion than providers in urban or suburban settings" (p. 120). The main concepts included in this statement include a *lack of anonymity* and *role diffusion* (Long and Weinert, 1989). Research and literature continue to support this statement. Rural nurses must also be able to cope with a sense of isolation from professional peers and other resources. When compared to urban nurses, rural nurses more often work alone or with only a few nurses at a particular healthcare setting, leading to these feelings of isolation (Bushy, 2012; Winters and Lee, 2018).

Because of the smaller population numbers and community, it may be difficult for the rural nurse to maintain personal and professional boundaries, leading to feelings of role diffusion and lack of anonymity. There are fewer nurses and healthcare facilities. For example, the nurse may have a patient who is a neighbor, a schoolteacher for his or her child, and attend the same church. The nurse and patient may be friends. These relationships can lead to confidentiality and privacy issues. Often while attending various community events a rural nurse will be asked healthcare advice from community members she or he cares for at a clinic, hospital, or other healthcare setting. As a result, all rural nurses generally interact with patients and their families in a variety of social and community roles leading to a lack of anonymity and role diffusion. It is a challenge for rural nurses to maintain privacy, confidentiality, and personal and professional boundaries in rural communities (Bushy, 2012; Winters and Lee, 2018). Rural nurses must be able to adapt to these feelings of role diffusion and lack of anonymity as it is a part of living and working at a rural community.

Rural nurses must be aware that rural population's demographics and health issues differ from those of urban populations. As compared to urban populations, rural populations are more elderly and have less healthcare insurance, and purchase medications that are more expensive. Rural populations experience more occupational health hazards and issues. In addition, they suffer more diseases that are chronic and an increased prevalence of problem behaviors, such as smoking, obesity, and lack of exercise (Molinari and Monserud, 2008). Rural nurses must take these factors into account as they plan, provide, and evaluate patient-centered care in rural communities.

CHARACTERISTICS OF RURAL NURSES

Knowledge of rural health theory is essential for all nurses to appreciate the similarities and differences between rural and urban nurse characteristics. Adequate understanding of this knowledge could help the nurse adapt to rural nursing practice and community life. Rural nursing practice is distinctive in it nature and scope when compared to urban nursing practice (Bushy, 2012; Long and Weinert, 1989; Scharff, 2018). Rural nursing theory provides nurses a foundation to apply rural nursing clinical knowledge and practice skills essential for providing rural residents with safe quality patient-centered care.

Both rural and urban nurses can fill the generalist role; however, the definitions differ because of their practice environments and challenges. Rural generalists are nurses who practice in multiple clinical areas who care for diverse patients. The role of a rural generalist requires a nurse to obtain certain knowledge, skills, and competencies to care for patients across the lifespan with a variety of acute and chronic conditions (Bushy, 2012; Winters and Lee, 2018). Rural nurses must acquire advance clinical knowledge no matter if they work in hospital, private, clinic, or community health practice (Long and Weinert, 1989; Molinari and Monserud, 2009; Scharff, 2018; Winters and Lee, 2018). Their scope of practice broadens and expands. Generally, they have quite a bit of autonomy in their practices (Bae, 2016; Bushy, 2012; Winters and Lee, 2018). For example, in a rural hospital setting a nurse during a single shift may care for medical, surgical, pediatric, obstetric, and emergency room patients. In contrast, urban generalists are often new to the nursing profession and practice medical-surgical nursing (Winters and Lee, 2018). These new nurses graduate as generalists from their programs. As they continue in their careers they may choose to specialize in such areas as critical care, surgery, obstetrics, pediatrics, etc. Generally, rural generalists are experienced nurses who have greater independence and autonomy, practice at a smaller rural facility, and care for patients with ages ranging from birth to death who have a wide variety of acute and chronic health issues. Rural nurses embrace the independence, variety, and autonomy they experience (Scharff, 2018; Winters and Lee, 2018).

Researchers discovered several rural nurse demographic characteristics that encourage nurses to practice at rural healthcare settings. Rural nurses prefer the rural lifestyle and most are born and raised in a rural community. They choose to live and work in rural communities due to their rural birthplace, location of family, social relationships, relocation with a spouse, and the rural facility is in close proximity to their homes. In addition, most are passionate about providing rural populations with quality care and access to healthcare (Molinari, Jaiswal, and Hollinger-Forrest, 2011; Owens, 2018; Winters and Lee, 2018).

Another challenging characteristic for rural nursing is providing quality care to patients with limited resources. They work in small healthcare facilities with limited medical equipment and specialists. Often there is a lack of other interprofessional team members to refer patients and collaborate with on patient care needs. Patients may need to travel many miles to seek referrals, specialty care, and further medical tests causing a lack of access to quality medical care. Patients may not be able to afford the costs of medical care and/or traveling to larger cities for additional care not offered at the rural facility. Rural nurses must be knowledgeable about available rural community resources and processes for making patient referrals to larger facilities that will support and facilitate continuity of care (Scharff, 2018; Winters and Lee, 2018).

Rural nurses must successfully cope with a lack of anonymity since they know everyone who works at the rural facility (providers, nurses, etc.) and most of their patients and families (Long and Weinert, 1989; Scharff, 2018). A nurse's personal and professional boundaries often overlap and diffuse with each other. This can be difficult for some nurses. For example, it is common for a nurse to care for a patient, know the patient as a neighbor, and attend similar community events with the patient. When nurses begin practice in a rural community, they are perceived as an "outsider", "new", or "new-comer", and not always trusted by rural individuals (Long and Weinert, 1989; Scharff, 2018). However, through time the nurses become an "insider", "old", or "old-timer" and gain the trust of community members (Long and Weinert, 1989; Scharff, 2018). The time to make the transition between these terms appears to vary among rural nurses and communities. Generally, nurses are considered "new" for about two years and after three to five years they progress towards "old" and further acceptance as they become more known and competent (Scharff, 2018). Nurses who have practiced in the community 10 years or greater are considered "seasoned" and eventually perceived as an "old-timer" which may take 20 or more years (Scharff, 2018). Research has found that rural nurses who are very skillful, flexible, and socially likeable reach the "old-timer" status sooner than nurses who lack one of those characteristics (Scharff, 2018). It is important for rural nurses to become involved in their community events to help them adjust to the rural environment. Overall, it is important to note that rural nurses are highly respected, valued, trusted, viewed as prestigious, and considered role models in the community. Their rural community residents view them as providing valuable healthcare service access (Bushy, 2012; Scharff, 2018; Winters and Lee, 2018).

As compared to urban nurses, rural nurses must take more self-responsibility for ongoing education and professional development. Because of their facility size and geographic location, rural nurses may have less opportunity to attend conferences and other professional development opportunities. Rural healthcare facilities may have fewer funds to assist nurses with professional development opportunities. However, the topics and content offered in the out-of-town conferences may not be always applicable to rural nursing practice. Most rural nurses rely on each other for additional skill and knowledge development. In addition, rural nurses seek knowledge by reading nursing journals, webinars, online sources, websites, and textbooks (Owens, 2018; Scharff, 2018).

Rural nurses generally have unique interpersonal relationships with whom they work at their rural healthcare facilities, such as other interprofessional team members (providers, nurses, pharmacists, radiology technicians, nursing assistants, administrative assistants, etc.). In addition, they develop close relationships with their patients and families that can be very rewarding. These relationships help promote work satisfaction (Owens, 2018; Scharff, 2018). Rural nurses provide long-term care for patients and their families. Many rural residents have a cultural expectation of being taken care of by someone they know. Rural residents often report they believe care in rural facilities is of better quality, more personable, and less rushed than that experienced in more urban healthcare facilities (Scharff, 2018). This also has a positive influence on rural nurses. They describe the workflow as slower paced and at times, their roles overlap with other interprofessional team members' roles. The nurses have an opportunity to get to know other workers on a personal level. These personal relationships can occur at urban healthcare facilities, but rural nurses are more likely to be personally acquainted with other workers and therefore expected to have more interpersonal exchange (Bushy, 2012; Scharff, 2018). However, in smaller healthcare facilities some rural nurses work with few other professionals, leading to feelings of isolation.

ADVANCED PRACTICE NURSING AT RURAL COMMUNITIES

Similar to other nursing practice licensure levels, advanced practice nursing differs in rural settings as compared to urban settings. Little research has actually been completed with rural advanced practice nurses. However, it does make sense that in order to provide safe, quality, patient-centered care, advanced practice nurses must also acquire knowledge on rural health, rural nursing theory, rural populations, and apply it to their practices. Their scope of practice, and required skills, knowledge, and competencies are different from other rural nurses. Researchers recommend that rural advanced practice nurses receive specialized rural education content and clinical training that prepare them to address the healthcare needs, barriers, and disparities of rural populations.

Living and providing healthcare in rural communities presents certain challenges to advanced practice nurses. Providers may enter rural health care practice not properly trained to navigate the barriers for rural living and health care challenges. This lack of training can lead to feelings of burnout and high turnover, affecting their successful ability to provide healthcare (Chipp *et al.*, 2010). Chipp *et al.* (2010) explored the experiences of various rural providers, including advanced practice nurses, as well as required knowledge and skills, and lessons learned while practicing in rural communities. First, providers must be able to establish and build community relationships to obtain the trust of community members. These dual relationships blur personal and professional boundaries. Many times an advanced practice nurse is the sole medical provider in a rural community. Providers must establish some type of limit setting so that they have time to rest, recuperate, and avoid being on call 24 hours a day (Chipp *et al.*, 2010). Second, providers must be equipped to deal with rural lifestyle challenges and self-care practices. They become generalists and must be aware of the rural community's culture and diversity. Since many times rural advanced practice nurses practice alone or with a few other providers, they must be prepared for the feelings of isolation that they may experience. Community involvement and interaction are key to preventing isolation (Chipp *et al.*, 2010). For rural advanced practice nurses, practicing as a generalist with autonomy can result in a rewarding career since they practice in their full scope of practice. Lastly, living and working in a rural community can also be very rewarding. These rewards for rural providers include natural beauty, access to outdoor activities, slower pace of life, fewer people, limited urbanization, and satisfaction with the healthcare service they provide rural communities (Chipp *et al.*, 2010).

Hauenstein *et al.* (2014) developed a model, *The Transformational Nursing Leadership in Rural Health Care* model, a descriptive health services model that provides a basis for educational content and clinical experiences that support advanced practice nursing at rural settings. In this model, advanced practice nurses interact with rural community healthcare facilities in promoting health, preventing illness, and managing chronic health diseases (Hauenstein *et al.*, 2014). The advanced practice nurses use local community resources and recognize the importance of family and community relationships, rural culture, and social values that are critical to successfully providing care (Hauenstein *et al.*, 2014). Lastly, the model recognizes rural population barriers to seeking healthcare such as lower income, education, stoicism, and travel distance and other environmental barriers (Hauenstein *et al.*, 2014).

Since working at a rural healthcare facility can be different from working at an urban healthcare facility, advanced practice nurses must transition to their unique role and professional identity. Completing this process can also be challenging and rewarding and promote advanced practice nurses' work satisfaction. Rural nursing at all practice levels requires personal and professional adaptation to develop the rural nurse identity (Scharff, 2018). Researchers discovered that role transition and change in professional identity begin for nurse practitioners while they are enrolled in their nurse practitioner education programs and continue into the postgraduate period of practice, however these nurse practitioners did not practice in rural areas (Heitz, Steiner, and Burman, 2004; Steiner, McLaughlin, Hyde, Brown, and Burman, 2008). This process is often challenging and difficult. Similar to other nurses, nurse practitioners while transitioning have reported experiencing stress, anxiety, isolation, inadequacy, role ambiguity, and being overwhelmed leading to feelings of incompetence and work dissatisfaction (Barnes, 2015; Poronsky, 2012). When individuals develop the attitudes, behaviors, and learn the knowledge and skills related to the roles and responsibilities of a profession, they experience successful role transitions to their new professional identities (Owens, 2018; Johnson, Corwin, Wilson, and Young, 2012; Trede, Macklin, and Bridges, 2012). Furthermore, individuals experience increased work satisfaction and are more likely to stay at their places of employment if they successfully transition to their new professional identities (Owens, 2018; Sabanciogullari and Dogan, 2015; Trede, Macklin, and Bridges, 2012). As a result, healthcare facility leaders should be encouraged to have support systems in place to help rural advanced practice nurses complete their role transitions and professional identity developments in a variety of rural healthcare settings and communities.

Rural advanced practice nurses can develop feelings of connectedness versus disconnectedness while practicing at rural healthcare settings. Conger and Plager (2008) completed a qualitative study with 30 advanced practice master's nursing graduates who had been in practice for at least one year since graduation. Participants expressed feelings of connectedness in the rural remote areas when they experienced four aspects of the environment: development of support networks, relationships with large urban medical centers, availability of electronic communications, and connections within the rural community (Conger and Plager, 2008). When one or more of these four environmental factors were absent in their practices, the participants experienced feelings of disconnectedness. When the nurses experienced feelings of connectedness they were likely to stay in the rural community as compared to those who felt disconnected. It is important that advanced practice nursing students receive preparation in rural nursing theory and experience clinical practicums in rural and remote areas to help them be successful in their rural practices. In addition, leaders in nursing education programs and rural practice settings must emphasize environmental factors that lead to a sense of connectedness (Conger and Plager, 2008).

Rural advanced practice nurses need to develop support networks. New graduates should continue relationships with their former classmates by regularly communicating with them. Other sources of support that need to be sought out by advanced practice nurses include other nurses, mentors, providers, and other interprofessional team members working in the same healthcare facility (Conger and Plager, 2008). In addition, rural advanced practice nurses must establish strong relationships with urban facility center providers as these individuals provide an opportunity to discuss complex patient care situations and a referral source when the medical needs of their patients are too great for rural facilities (Conger and Plager, 2008). Rural advanced practice nurses desire communication on the results of completed tests on their patients at the urban facilities. This can be accomplished by either planned telephone or face-to-face communication. Advanced practice nurses experience frustration and feelings of disconnectedness when they lacked these supportive networks and relationships (Conger and Plager, 2008).

Finally, a feeling of connectedness can result through electronic means (Conger and Plager, 2008). One example is the use of telecommunication equipment such as telemedicine. Rural advanced practice nurses can use telemedicine to communicate a patient's assessments, diagnosis, and treatment for consultations and referrals with urban providers and specialists. In addition, use of the internet for communication and continuing education is helpful. Advanced practice nurses experience fewer feelings of isolation and loneliness with the use of electronic methods in their communication efforts. Those advanced practice nurses who lack dependable internet service feel more disconnected (Conger and Plager, 2008).

Research has important implications for leaders at rural healthcare facilities and nursing education programs. Supportive programs must be developed and implemented that enhance rural healthcare provider training to live in rural communities and practice at rural healthcare facilities. These programs have the potential to promote recruitment and maintain a rural provider workforce that can meet the healthcare needs in rural communities.

Adult learning and role transition theory could be utilized to help guide the rural advanced practice nurse's transition to rural clinical practice and provide safe, quality, patient-centered care. A role can be defined as "a character assigned or assumed; a socially expected behavior pattern determined by an individual's status in a particular society, or a function or part performed especially in a particular operation or process" (Meleis, 1975, p. 265). Role transition can be defined as "a change in an individual's self-identity within a certain context that occurs through the development of new knowledge and skills, as well as a change in behavior, role relationships, interactions, expectations, and abilities" (Meleis, 1975, p. 266). Since a nurse practitioner must acquire and implement unique knowledge and skills related to rural nursing theory, he or she needs to complete a role transition to a new self-identity (Owens, 2018).

Illeris' Transformative Learning and Identity theory (Illeris, 2014) is an example of an adult learning theory that can be used to understand the rural advanced practice nurse's transition into rural clinical practice and a new professional identity as a rural provider. Illeris (2014) believes that an individual's identity develops and/or changes through transformative learning. An individual's identity is developed by his or her experiences, self-perceptions, and perceptions of others. Illeris' (2014) theory contains three dimensions of learning that occur in some setting in society. The first dimension is *content* or what is actually learned. The second dimension is *incentive*, which involves an individual's reason or motivation to learn something. Lastly, *interaction* is the third dimension. Similar to other adult learning theories, Illeris (2014) believes that an individual has prior learning experiences in life and that new learning adds to these prior learning experiences. The individual links the new knowledge to already developed attitudes, skills, knowledge, competencies, and abilities (Illeris, 2014). Change in the individual's *identity* is the result of the interaction of the content, incentive, and interactions experienced by the individual in some type of social setting. Lastly, the change in identity and learning are specific to the social situation (Illeris, 2014). Through this transformative learning process, an advanced practice nurse changes his or her professional identity to a rural provider of patient-centered care.

Little research has explored rural nurse practitioners and their identity formation and role transition to clinical practice. Using Illeris' (2014) Transformative Learning and Identity and Meleis' (1975) theories, Owens (2018) through a qualitative study explored rural nurse practitioners' perceptions of their role transition experiences while transitioning their first year of practice to their rural family nurse practitioner primary care positions. In addition, Owens (2018) examined if and how new rural family nurse practitioners developed their new professional identities. This study took place with 10 participants working at 10 different rural healthcare facilities in three different Midwestern states.

Based on study findings, Owens (2018) proposes a new model: *The Rural Nurse Practitioner Transition and Professional Identity Model* (see Figure 1.1). Please note that central to the model is that the nurse practitioners as adult learners were self-directed active learners of new skills, knowledge, and roles

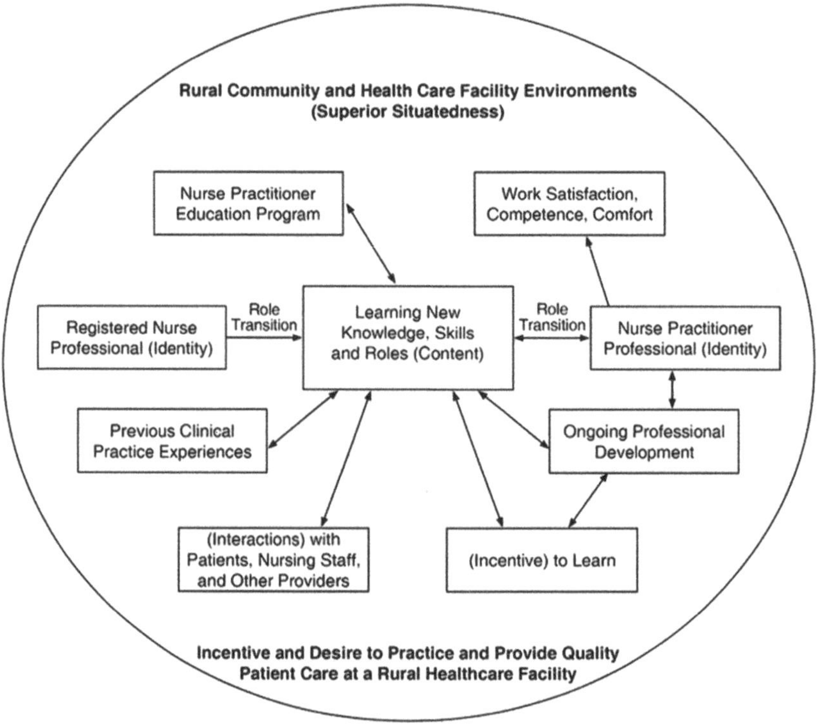

FIGURE 1.1. *Rural Nurse Practitioner and Professional Identity Development Model. Reprinted from* The Journal for Nurse Practitioners, *14(8), R. A. Owens, Transition experiences of new rural nurse practitioners, 605–611, Copyright 2018 with permission from Elsevier.*

through their experiences. The result of going through this learning process was their role transitions and change in their professional identities. Healthcare facility leaders could use this model as a guide and framework to develop supportive rural nurse practitioner transitioning and orientation programs during their first year of practice. Furthermore, nurse practitioner education program faculty can use this model as a guide for preparing nurse practitioners to enter rural practice (Owens, 2018). The following elements are included in this model and added to Illeris' (2014) theory.

Learning New Knowledge, Skills, and Roles

This learning was critical, began for nurse practitioners in their nurse practitioner programs, and continued throughout their first year of practice (see Figure 1.1). Similar to other adult learning theories, all participants expressed an attitude of self-directed learning. The nurse practitioner's scope of practice is much different from a registered nurse's scope of practice. The nurse practitioners soon learned that new knowledge and skills would be learned, and they became providers of care rather than an assistant to the provider. In addition, they discovered that practicing at a rural facility was different from practicing at an urban facility. These nurse practitioners felt it was important that they experience rural clinical practice and learned about rural nursing theory during their formal education programs. This part of the model builds on Illeris' (2014) *content* dimension.

Incentive to Learn

The nurse practitioners expressed a responsibility and motivation to learn because they desired to provide quality, patient-centered care and increased access to care (see Figure 1.1). They realized when compared to the rural registered nurse, the scope of practice for a rural nurse practitioner is different and requires acquiring new knowledge, skills, and abilities to work in a different role. This part of the model is comparable to Illeris' (2014) *incentive* dimension.

Ongoing Professional Development

Ongoing learning of new medications, treatments, procedures, protocols, evidence-based practice, and research will always occur by the nurse practitioners and is necessary for their new professional identity (see Figure 1.1). They believed in lifelong learning and sought out these learning opportunities through professional development opportunities that include conferences, internet resources, webinars, journals, electronic software, and their peers. This adds to Illeris' (2014) theory because the nurse practitioners expressed that learning never stops for maintaining their changed professional identities.

Previous Clinical Practice Experiences

The nurse practitioners credited their strong registered nurse skills, clinical expertise, knowledge, and experiences as providing a base to add new knowledge and skills (see Figure 1.1). They expressed similar and different learning needs. Individualized learning must occur for the nurse practitioners. This is similar to Illeris' (2014) beliefs as he also feels new knowledge builds on experience and is unique to the individual.

Interactions with Patients, Nursing Staff, and Other Providers

Nurse practitioners experienced close relationships and interactions with their patients and families, nurses, other providers, and interprofessional team members (see Figure 1.1). In these relationships, they felt that rural residents perceived them as nurse practitioners and providers and different from registered nurses. The interactions occurred both in the community and healthcare facilities since they knew and interacted with many of these individuals in the community. Nurse practitioners expressed a lack of anonymity, experienced role diffusion and overlap as a community members and providers of healthcare. Many discussed how they interacted with patients and families in other community settings such as schools, stores, church, and other community events. They believed that all individuals perceived them as nurse practitioners and a provider of care rather than a registered nurse. These interactions contained important socialization and learning experiences. These interactions are similar to the interaction element included in Illeris' (2014) theory.

Registered Nurse Professional Identity and Nurse Practitioner Professional Identity

Through their role transitions, learning experiences, incentive to learn, and interactions the nurse practitioners formed their new nurse practitioner professional identities (see Figure 1.1). They were able to perceive themselves as a rural nurse practitioner and no longer working in the role of a registered nurse and described the differences between the two identities. This section of the model is similar to Illeris' (2014) concept of *identity*. Through a process of transformative learning, these nurse practitioners changed their professional identities.

Work Satisfaction, Competence, and Comfort

The nurse practitioners' experience of successful transitioning to their new professional identities resulted in feelings of work satisfaction, competence, and comfort which occurred over a one-year period of time (see Figure 1.1). This element adds to Illeris' (2014) theory for this specific population.

Rural Community and Health Care Facility Environments

The social environment consisting of the rural community and healthcare facility is where the nurse practitioners' learning experiences, relationships, and interactions took place with patients, families, and other providers and interprofessional team members (see Figure 1.1). This is also similar to Illeris' (2014) theory because he views learning as *superior situatedness*, meaning it occurs in a specific situation and social setting as experienced and interpreted by the individual.

Findings of this study add to previous research and have important implications for rural nurse practitioners. Similar to rural nurses in other practice areas, rural nurse practitioners must understand rural nursing theory because it provides a foundation to add clinical knowledge and practice skills essential for providing rural residents with safe, quality, patient-centered care. Leaders at rural healthcare facilities and nursing education programs can use this model to support and prepare nurse practitioners to enter rural health care practice. Nursing education program faculty could use the model to guide curriculum and clinical experiences. With this knowledge and skill development, nurse practitioners can better understand the rural lifestyle, barriers to rural health care, and unique rural nurse characteristics, and form close interpersonal working relationships resulting in their work satisfaction.

OPPORTUNITIES TO WORK IN RURAL SETTINGS

The demand for nurses and primary care providers in both rural and urban United States communities is increasing because of several factors. These factors include changes in government health care policies and regulations, insurance, and reimbursement that focus more on providing primary care and cost effective quality care (Graves, Mishra, P., Dittus, Parikh, Perloff, and Buerhaus, 2016). In addition, there is a need to provide prevention and management for complex chronic diseases in a growing aging population (Graves *et al.*, 2016). Lastly, there is a shortage of nurses and primary care providers especially in rural areas. In 2018 the federal government reported 6,890 Health Professional Shortage Areas in the U.S. and approximately 75 million people with inadequate primary care, with 59% of primary care access problems in rural areas, and a need of 14,136 practitioners to remove the designations (US Department of Health and Human Services, 2018). Nurses and advanced practice nurses can both meet the need for improved access to healthcare in rural communities by practicing in rural health professional shortage areas.

Advanced practice nurses have an increased opportunity to work in rural health and provide access to primary care that helps meet the rural population's healthcare needs. In fact unlike other types of providers, advanced practice nurses tend to care for diverse populations such as those located in rural and underserved areas (Kippenbrock, Wen-Juo, Odell, and Buron, 2015; Rutledge, Haney, Bordelon, Renaud, and Fowler, 2014). Advanced practice nurses, such as family nurse practitioners can be valuable in filling the generalist role in rural healthcare settings since they are trained to care for patients throughout the lifespan with a wide variety of acute and chronic health conditions. As a result, nurse practitioners are being recruited to fill rural primary care provider positions (Altman, Butler, and Shern, 2015; Kippenbrock *et al.*, 2014; Rutledge *et al.*, 2014).

In order to meet the primary care needs of rural communities, advanced practice nurses must be allowed to practice in their full scope of practice so they can practice within the full extent of their education and training. As of 2018, 22 states plus the District of Columbia allowed full practice for nurse practitioners, 16 states have reduced practice for nurse practitioners, and 12 states are classified as having restricted nurse practitioner practice. During the publication of this book, several states are in the process of discussing and passing policy that allows full practice for nurse practitioners (American Association of Nurse Practitioners, 2019). All advanced practice nurses must become involved in developing and implementing policy at the local, state, and national levels that allows them to practice in the full extent of their education and training so that they can lead the efforts to provide improved rural population access to safe, quality, healthcare.

REFERENCES

Altman, S. H., A. S. Butler, and L. Shern. (Eds.). (2015). *Assessing Progress on the Institute of Medicine Report the Future of Nursing*. Washington, D.C.: The National Academies Press. doi: 10.17226/21838.

American Association of Nurse Practitioners (2019). State Practice Environment. Retrieved from: https://www.aanp.org/advocacy/state/state-practice-environment.

Bae, S. (2016). Nurse practitioners' job satisfaction in rural versus nonrural areas. *Journal for the American Association of Nurse Practitioners*, 28, 471–478. doi: 10.1002/2327- 6924.12362.

Barnes, H. (2015). Exploring the factors that influence nurse practitioner role transition. *The Journal for Nurse Practitioners, 11*(2), 178–183. doi:10.1016/j.nurpra.2014.11.004.

Bushy, A. (2012). The rural context and nursing practice. *The rural nurse: Transition to Practice*. In D. Molinari, and A. Bushy (Eds.), (pp. 3–21). New York, NY: Springer Publishing.

Chipp, C., *et al.* (2010). If only someone had told me…": Lessons from rural providers, *The Journal of Rural Health, 27*, 122–130. doi: 10.1111/j.1748-0361.2010.00314.x.

Conger, M. M., and K. A. Plager. (2008). Advanced nursing practice in rural areas: Connectedness versus disconnectedness. *Online Journal of Rural Nursing and Health Care, 8*(1), 24–38. Retrieved from: https://rnojournal.binghamton.edu/index.php/RNO/article/download/127/104.

de la Rue, M., and I. Coulson. (2003). The meaning of health and well-being: Voices from older rural women. *Rural and Remote Health, 3*(192), 1–10. Retrieved from http: //www.rrh.org.au/journal/article/192.

Graves, J. A., *et al.* (2016). Role of geography and nurse practitioner scope-of-practice in efforts to expand primary care system capacity: Health reform and the primary care workforce. *Medical Care, 54*(1), 81–89. https://doi.org/10.1097/MLR.0000000000000045.

Hauenstein, E. J., *et al.* (2014). A model to develop nurse leaders for rural practice. *Journal of Professional Nursing, 30*(6). 463–473. doi: 10.1016/j.profnurs.2014.04.001.

Heitz, L. J., S. H. Steiner, and M. E. Burman. (2004). RN to FNP: A qualitative study of role transition. *Journal of Nursing Education, 43*(9), 416–420. doi:0.3928/01484834-20040901-08.

Illeris, K. (2014). *Transformative learning and identity*. New York, NY: Routledge.

Johnson, M., *et al.* (2012). Professional identity and nursing: Contemporary theoretical developments and future research challenges. *International Nursing Review, 59*, 562–569. doi: 10.1111/j.1466-7657.2012.01013.x.

Kippenbrock, T., *et al.* (2015). The southern states: NPs made an impact in rural and healthcare shortage areas. *Journal of the American Association of Nurse Practitioners, 27*, 707–713. doi: 10.1002/2327-6924-12245.

Lee, H. J., and M. K. McDonagh. (2018). Updating the rural nursing theory base. *Rural nursing: Concepts, theory, and practice.* In C. A. Winters, and H. L. Lee (Eds.), (pp. 45–62). New York, NY: Springer Publishing.

Lee, H. J., and C. A, Winters. (2004). Testing rural nursing theory: Perceptions and needs of service providers. *Online Journal of Rural Nursing and Health Care, 4*(1), 51–63. Retrieved from http://www.rno.org/journal/issues/vol-4/issue.1/Lee_article.htm.

Long, K.A., and C. Weinert. (1989). Rural nursing: Developing the theory base. *Scholarly Inquiry for Nursing Practice, 3*(2), 113–127.

Meleis, A. I. (1975). Role insufficiency and role supplementation: A conceptual framework. *Nursing Research, 24*(4), 264–271.

Molinari, D. L., A. Jaiswal, and Hollinger-Forrest. (2011). Rural nurses: Lifestyle preferences and education perceptions. *Online Journal of Rural Nursing and Health Care, 11*(2), 16–26. doi.org/10.14574/ojrnhc.v11i2.27.

Molinari, D. L., and M. Monserud. (2008). Rural nurse job satisfaction. *Rural and Remote Health, 8*, 1–12. Retrieved from http://www.rrh.org.au.

Molinari, D. L., and M. Monserud. (2009). Rural nurse cultural self-efficacy and job satisfaction. *Journal of Transcultural Nursing, 20*(2), 211–218. doi: 10.1177/1043659608330350.

Owens, R. A. (2018). Transition experiences of new rural nurse practitioners. *The Journal for Nurse Practitioners, 14*(8), 605–611. doi: doi.org/10.1016/j.nurpra.2018.05.009.

Poronsky, C. B. (2012). A literature review of Mentoring for RN-to-DNP transition. *Journal of Nursing Education, 51*(11), 623–631. doi: 10.3928/01484834-20120914-03.

Rutledge, C. M., *et al.* (2014). Telehealth: Preparing advanced practice nurses to address healthcare needs in rural and under-served populations. *International Journal of Nursing Education Scholarship, 11*(1), 1–9. doi: 10.1515/ijnes-2013-0061.

Sabanciogullari, S., and S. Dogan. (2015). Effects of a professional identity development program on the professional identity, job satisfaction, and burnout level of nurses: A pilot study. *International Journal of Nursing Practice, 21*, 847–857. doi:10.1111.ijn.12330.

Scharff, J. E. (2018). The distinctive nature and scope of rural nursing practice: Philosophical Bases. In C. A. Winters, and H.L. Lee (Eds.), *Rural nursing: Concepts, theory, and practice.* (pp. 107–123). New York, NY: Springer Publishing.

Steiner, S. H., *et al.* (2008). Role transition during RN-to-FNP education. *Journal of Nursing Education, 47*(10), 441–447. doi: 10.3928/01484834-20081001-07.

Trede, F., R. Macklin, and D. Bridges. (2012). Professional identity development: A review of the higher education literature. *Studies in Higher Education, 37*(3), 365–384. doi:10.1080/03075079.2010.521237.

US Department of Health and Human Services, Health Resources and Services Administration, Bureau of Health Workforce. (September, 2018). *Designated health professional shortage areas statistics: Fourth quarter of fiscal year 2018 designated HPSA quarterly summary*. Retrieved from: https://ersrs.hrsa.gov/ReportServer?/HGDW_Reports/BCD_HPSA/BCD_HPSA_SCR50_Qtr_Smry_HTML&rc:Toolbar=false.

Winters, C. A., and H. J. Lee. (2018). Rural nursing: Concepts, theory, and practice. (5th ed.). New York, NY: Springer Publishing.

CHAPTER 2

Health Care Delivery Systems

Vicki Brooks

Objectives:

1. Define various Healthcare Delivery Systems in rural settings.
2. Explore challenges of Health Care Delivery systems in rural settings.
3. Describe the resources within rural Health Care Delivery systems.

Discussion Questions:

1. What is the most common healthcare delivery system in rural America?
2. What are the biggest challenges to rural healthcare delivery?
3. What collaborative measures can be done to strengthen the delivery of rural healthcare?

INTRODUCTION

This chapter will begin to explain the various healthcare delivery systems that may be present in rural healthcare environments. The National Academy of Medicine uses the term "health safety net" when describing the complicated net of public, private, professionals, and intuitions that provide care to rural and underserved, uninsured, underinsured, low-income, or Medicare/Medicaid recipients (HRSA, 2019). Rural health safety net providers can deliver healthcare in a brick and mortar building, a mobile unit, or telemedicine. Rural healthcare is a safety net providing primary care, secondary care, or tertiary care in a variety of settings, each having different levels of resources available. The rural setting may have only a hospital and/or a free-standing clinic that is delivering minimal to multilevel healthcare services. This chapter will explain the many possibilities of how healthcare safety nets can be achieved in a rural setting.

Many rural communities may have a hospital setting. This can be described as a rural hospital or a critical access hospital. The Health Resource Services Administration (HRSA) Federal Office of Rural Health Policy defines a rural hospital as one located in a non-metropolitan county or as a hospital within a metropolitan county that is a considerable distance from the urban area (HRSA, 2018). A rural hospital may be designated as a critical access (CAH) hospital. Critical access hospitals receive a special payment designation from Centers for Medicare and Medicaid Services Medicare (CMS) because they have fewer than 25 beds for patient care and very limited services (AHA, 2019). The CAH designation is designed to reduce the financial vulnerability of rural hospitals and improve access to healthcare by keeping essential services in rural communities (RHIhub, 2019). CAH hospitals are usually the only hospital provider in the community but there may be a rare instance when more than one CAH is in the same vicinity (MedPAC, 2017). In 2015, 41 percent of U.S. hospitals were located in rural areas and half of rural hospitals were designated as critical access hospitals (MedPac, 2018). As of January 2018, there were 1,353 certified CAHs in 45 states. Connecticut, Delaware, Maryland, New Jersey, and Rhode Island do not have any CAHs (RHIhub, 2019).

Many rural hospital systems rely on reimbursement from Medicare and Medicaid populations. In 2017, Medicare and Medicaid made up 56 percent of rural hospitals' net revenue (AHA, 2019). A determining factor for identifying the type of rural hospitals is the Prospective Payment System (PPS). The PPS was established by the Centers for Medicare and Medicaid services (CMS) for hospital care and payment (CMS, 2019). A PPS is a method of reimbursement in which Medicare payment is made based on a predetermined, fixed amount. These programs reimburse less than the cost of providing the proper care (AHA, 2018). The payment amount for a particular service is based on the classification system of that service (for example, diagnosis-related groups [DRG] for inpatient hospital services) (CMS, 2019). CMS uses separate PPSs for reimbursement to acute inpatient hospitals, home health agencies, hospice, hospital outpatient, inpatient psychiatric facilities, inpatient rehabilitation facilities, long-term care hospitals, and skilled nursing facilities (CMS, 2019).

HEALTHCARE DELIVERY SYSTEMS

Rural Hospitals

Rural hospitals may be structured in several ways:

1. County Hospital Districts will have a publicly elected Board of Directors,

are usually a political subdivision of the state, and have a tax levying system to support charity care (HHS, 2016).

2. County Hospitals have a governing board appointed by elected County Commissioners and are supported by a county tax budget. Some rural cities have a similar structure for their hospitals to include a city hospital, not county hospital (HHS, 2016).
3. Private 501c3 are Acute Care Hospitals and are locally governed by a board of directors and often supported by a local philanthropy or a foundation (HHS, 2016).

Depending on the community needs, there are various healthcare delivery models formed through relationships between the rural hospital and rural health clinics. Rural clinics can be a Federally Qualified Health Center (FQHC), Rural Health Clinic, Community Health Clinic, or Urgent Care Clinic. Community health system relationship integration can occur from contractual agreements and collaborations, including referrals and co-location arrangements (AHA, 2018). Agreements can provide for the purchase of clinical and/or administrative services between the rural hospital and the clinics. Collaborations can allow for sharing of clinical and administrative personnel, as well as facilitating the continuum of patient care (AHA, 2018).

Rural Health Clinics

The Rural Health Clinic Services Act of 1977 (Public Law 95-210) was passed to address an inadequate supply of physicians serving Medicare patients in rural areas and to increase the use of non-physician practitioners, such as nurse practitioners (NPs) and physician assistants (PAs) in rural areas (Medicare Learning Network (MLN), 2018). Rural Health Clinics (RHC) may be designated as a provider-based clinic; meaning they are part of the local rural hospital or rural health system. A freestanding RHC will be independent but maintain a collaborative agreement with a nearby hospital or health system. It is most common to have a provider-based RHCs to provide primary care to outlying/rural areas and rely on the resources of the hospital or health system. Any designated Rural Health Clinics are paid an all-inclusive rate (AIR) from Medicare and Medicaid for medically needed primary health services and qualified preventive health services that are provided by a Rural Health Clinic (RHC) practitioner (MLN, 2018). In 2018, the Medicare Learning Network (MLN) reported 4,700 RHCs nationwide that are providing primary care and preventive health services in rural and underserved areas. To qualify for an RHC, CMS and HRSA guidelines must be met, including the location of the clinic must be:

1. A non-urbanized area, as defined by the U.S. Census Bureau.

2. An area currently designated within the previous 4 years by the Health Resources and Services Administration as one of these types of federally designated or certified shortage areas:
   a. Primary Care Geographic Health Professional Shortage Area (HPSA) under Section 332(a)(1)(A) of the Public Health Service (PHS) Act
   b. Primary Care Population-Group HPSA under Section 332(a)(1)(B) of the PHS Act Medically Underserved Area under Section 330(b)(3) of the PHS Act or
   c. Governor-designated and Secretary-certified shortage area under Section 6213(c) of the Omnibus Budget Reconciliation Act of 1989

RHCs must:

1. Employ or contract with a Nurse Practitioner, Physician Assistant, or Certified Nurse Midwife.
2. Have an NP, PA, or CNM working at the clinic at least 50 percent of the time the RHC is open.
3. Directly furnish routine diagnostic and laboratory services.
4. Have arrangements with one or more hospitals to provide medically needed services that are not available at the RHC.
5. Have available drugs and biologicals necessary for treating emergencies.
6. Provide point-of-care specific laboratory tests on site.
7. Have a quality assessment and performance improvement program.
8. Post their days and hours of operation.

Another option for a rural health clinic is a Federally Qualified Health Centers (FQHC). The FQHC can be urban or rural but designed for an underserved population. Federally Qualified Health Centers are usually located within a community and receive funds from the HRSA Health Center Program to provide primary care services to underserved areas (HRSA, 2018). The defining legislation for Federally Qualified Health Centers is from the Consolidated Health Center Program in Section 1905(l)(2)(B) of the Social Security Act (HRSA, 2018).

FQHC must meet certain requirements, including providing care on a sliding fee scale based on ability to pay and operating under a governing board that includes patients that represent the population served (HRSA, 2018). FQHC may be a Community Health Centers, Migrant Health Centers, Health Care for the Homeless, and a Health Centers for Residents of Public Housing (HRSA, 2018). In 2017, HRSA funded 1,400 health centers that were operating in 12,000 service delivery sites. More than 27 million people in every U.S. state, the District of Columbia, Puerto Rico, the U.S. Virgin Islands, and the Pacific Basin receive care from FQHC (HRSA, 2018).

Mobile Health Clinics

Mobile health clinics (MHCs) are another way of delivering rural healthcare. MHCs can be located inside a large van, bus, or recreational vehicle. These vehicle-based clinics may be part of a rural health system, a rural health clinic, or FQHC. They travel to rural areas and/or medically underserved areas. MHCs physically drive into the designated areas of need. MHCs can be a successful and cost-effective model of healthcare delivery uniquely to assess and fulfill the needs of rural populations (Bennet *et al.*, 2017). MHCs are able to address both medical and social determinants of health which can decrease healthcare barriers and improve individual health outcomes (Bennet *et al.*, 2017). When the MHC remains financially sustainable, improving the population health, and reducing healthcare costs become viable. MHCs can serve as a bridge between the clinic and the community members, thus resolving a gap in the rural healthcare system (Bennet *et al.*, 2017).

Urgent Care Clinics

Urgent Care Clinics (UCCs) are another form of healthcare delivery in the rural setting. UCCs provide medically necessary services which are required for an illness or injury that would not result in further disability or death if not treated immediately but require prompt care (American Academy of Urgent Care Medicine (AAUCM, ND). Urgent Care Clinics provide immediate medical services, offering outpatient care for the treatment of acute and chronic illness and injury. Out of convenience, this service is becoming more common in recent years for the rural population to use UCCs as their primary care provider. UCCs can serve as primary care or medical home centers for patients living in rural or medically underserved areas. The UCCs can be sustainable in underserved areas because they are less expensive than a hospital emergency department (AAUCM). Many urgent care settings can be defined further as same-day care or walk-in care. This type of healthcare is used by patients who may lack a primary care provider or are unable to obtain an appointment with their primary care provider in a timely manner. Urgent care clinics can be part of a larger rural healthcare system or independently owned. The UC clinic may be staffed with a nurse practitioner, physician assistant, or physician (AAUCM, ND).

Nursing Home and Long-Term Care Facilities

Nursing Homes (NH), Skilled Nursing facilities (SNF), or Long-Term Care facilities (LTC) can be found in the rural health setting. NHs can be part of a hospital system or independent. Nursing Homes have also evolved over time with the length of stay (LOS) requirements from insurance coverages and the needs of the patient (CMS). Once a patient has been discharged from an acute care stay, the patient may still require some level of medical care. This can leave few options for patients. Returning home may be an option if they have family to help them further recover.

Once a patient no longer qualifies for acute care, but still requires skilled nursing care, they may be admitted to a Swing Bed. Similar to NH, Swing Bed provides post-hospital SNF care with existing hospital beds. Medicare requires a three-day qualifying inpatient hospital stay prior to admitting a patient to a swing bed in any hospital or admission to an SNF. Approved swing bed hospitals or CAHs may use any acute care inpatient bed within the hospital to provide swing bed services, with the exception to newborn nursery, intensive care unit, or psychiatric designated beds. To qualify for post-acute SNF-level care, swing bed, hospitals must meet certain criteria: examples are rural area, fewer than 100 beds, or CAH (CMS, 2019).

Medicare will pay (non-CAH) hospitals offering swing bed SNF-level services under the PPS Medicare Part A. Medicare will pay CAH swing bed services based on 101 percent of the reasonable costs of the provided services (CMS 2019). The usual deductible and copayment/coinsurance will apply to the patient if leaving a tertiary facility and returning to a CAH Swing Bed. There is no additional cost to the patient if discharged from a rural hospital visit directly into a swing bed program within the same facility (CMS, 2019).

Nursing homes, skilled nursing facilities (SNF), or long-term care facilities are usually staffed by Medical Assistants, Licensed Vocational Nurses, and a Registered Nurse Charge Nurse with a Medical Director (physician) who is required to see the patients weekly and be available for critical changes in a patient (CMS, 2019).

Hospice Care

Hospice provides end-of-life care and can be found in the rural setting. Hospice focuses on care, not curing, and is usually provided in the patient's home. Hospice is a team-oriented approach of physician, nurse, social worker, chaplain, counselor, and home health aides who work together to meet physical, spiritual, and emotional needs in or out of the hospital setting (NHPCO). Hospice services are available to patients of any age, religion, race, or illness. Hospice care is covered under Medicare, Medicaid, most private insurance plans, HMOs, and other managed care organizations (NHPCO). In 2017, there were 878 rural hospices; this is 20% of all hospices in the United States (MedPac, 2019). The number of rural hospices does not capture the size of providers, their capacity to serve rural patients, or the size of their service area (Medpac, 2019). An additional consideration is urban hospices may provide services in rural areas (Medpac, 2019). Hospice care can also be provided in hospice centers, hospitals, nursing homes, and other long-term care facilities. It would be rare to see a freestanding hospice center in a rural setting. Hospice can be within the health system or independently owned.

Palliative Care

Palliative Care is a compassionate comfort care that provides symptom relief from physical and mental stress of a serious or life-limiting illness through a coordinated interdisciplinary healthcare team (NHPCO). Palliative Care can begin at diagnosis, during curative treatment and follow-up, and at the end of life. Palliative Care services are available with curative or life-prolonging care (NHPCO). This can be delivered in or out of the hospital setting. Palliative Care can be owned by a hospital system, comingled with a hospice company, home health company, or independently owned (NHPCO). Palliative Care is seldom seen in the rural setting which is especially problematic since rural residents can be older, sicker, and have lower incomes when compared to urban residents (RHIhub, 2019).

Occupational Health

Occupational Health is a multidisciplinary team approach to facilitate the well-being and safety of employees across the lifespan by providing use of therapeutic daily activity (AOTA, 2019). Larger rural businesses may employee a nurse or nurse practitioner to provide care for the safety of their employees. In rural environments, local business may contract with the rural hospital or physical therapy, rehabilitation department to provide services from pre-employment screening to return-to-work after an injury for their employees (AOTA, 2019).

Telehealth

The Center for Connected Health Policy has defined Telehealth as the wide range of diagnosis and management, education, and other related fields of health care (NIH). These fields can include, but are not at all limited to: Dentistry, Counseling, Physical and occupational therapy, Home health, Chronic disease monitoring and management, Disaster management, Consumer and professional education.

Telehealth has slowly earned a place in the rural healthcare setting. With the advancement of technology, access to Telehealth has increased. Many people living in rural communities have internet access, Wi-Fi capability, and smart phones. This does allow for greater access to healthcare. Telehealth access may also be provided in a health clinic or hospital setting.

There are many challenges with cellular service and internet access in the rural environment. These can include frequent power outages, disruption of internet services, diminished internet speed and bandwidth. Telemedicine limitations for professionals within the hospital setting can occur with equipment deficit, connectivity and compatibility (NIH).

CHALLENGES OF RURAL HEALTHCARE SYSTEMS

There are many challenges in rural healthcare. These challenges can be further defined by the number of limited resources and availability of funds. This can mean lack of qualified healthcare providers and needed equipment. Many rural areas have a deficit in healthcare providers and lack funding for special equipment needed to meet the demands of the rural communities (HHS, 2016). Many rural communities have limited availability of medical facilities, tools, and supplies that impact the quality and quantity of services provided. Challenges within the hospital can include limited number of hospital beds, operating rooms, and laboratories equipment. Certain diagnostic imaging equipment, including X-ray machines, computerized axial tomography (CAT) scans, and magnetic resonance imaging (MRIs) may only be available during limited time frames. Essential equipment for monitoring vital signs, ventilators, defibrillators, and autoclaves may be in short supply or need of upgrading (HHS, 2016). One example of limited resources related to funds is expensive emergency medications including antivenom (Profab) for snakebites. This medication may be unavailable or may have a very limited supply in stock (Weant *et al.*, 2012). The snakebite victim will need to be transferred to a higher level of care immediately. This can create fragmented healthcare and disruptive delivery process especially in life-threatening situations.

In addition to the limited resources, rural residents often lack other means to use medical resources that are offered. Many rural residents are uninsured or underinsured which results in decreased access to specialty referrals in urban settings. Rural areas have fewer doctors, primary healthcare providers, and other healthcare workers when compared to urban areas (HHS, 2011). Whether lack of financial means, insurance reasons, or transportation issues, many rural residents are more likely to go without higher levels of care that is needed. The improvements in health status in rural areas have not kept pace with those in urban areas (White House, 2010). This can affect life expectancy and key health outcomes will vary based on race, sex, socioeconomic status, and geographic location (Centers for Disease Control and Prevention, CDC, 2013).

Many rural hospitals become overburdened as challenges intensify, accumulate, and compound each other (AHA, 2019). American Hospital Association reported in 2019, a list of rural health challenges faced by hospital. These are: the high cost of drugs, low patient volume, patient and payer mix, geographic isolation, medical surge capacity, cyber threats, regulatory burden, Medicaid expansion, health plan design, workforce shortage, aging infrastructure, and limited access to healthcare.

Maintaining a rural healthcare system that is accessible and responsive to the needs of the rural communities requires change that can be influenced by the community. It requires networks of providers and community leaders collaborating to identify needs, barriers, and the resources to create a coordinated and sustainable healthcare system (AHA, 2019). The healthcare professionals involved in the delivery of health care need to be sensitive and aware of a community's needs and culture (HHS, 2016). Many healthcare providers who were raised in the rural community continue to work in the rural area and can support a collaborative effort (MLN, 2018).

Rural hospitals and clinics serve as economic stabilizers in their communities. They can provide both direct employment opportunities and indirect reinforcement of the local economy through the purchase of goods and services (AHA, 2019). The availability of local access to healthcare is an important factor for businesses considering whether to invest or locate in a particular area. The employment generated by rural hospitals can provide support to a tax base, which helps fund services such as local education and Emergency Medical Services (AHA, 2019). Many rural hospitals are the first or second largest employer of the community (HHS, 2011).

Rural health care systems must be adaptive and responsive to short and long-term changes. Rural healthcare is complex and can differ vastly by population, geography, and state (HHS, 2011). Achieving health equity requires the hard work of many people and organizations. This includes but is not limited to federal agencies, state agencies, and private organizations working with rural communities to eliminate health disparities among the populations that experience a disproportionate burden of disease, disability, injury, and death (CDC, 2013).

BENEFITS OF A RURAL SETTING

There are many positive aspects to a rural setting. Many rural communities move at a slower pace, with less commuting, fewer traffic issues, and improved air quality. The cost of living can be much lower in rural areas, including housing and food. The size of rural communities can provide a strong social bond within the community. Community members hold healthcare providers in high regard and interact on a regular basis with them. This can be during community events, the grocery store, or school/church activities. Rural community members are more likely to take an active role in the community politics knowing their voice may have a greater impact.

Rural settings remain uniquely interesting. Rural areas account for 97% of U.S. land but house just 19.3% of the population (Census, 2018). This provides a large amount of land to spread out for those who appreciate the quiet, privacy, and open sky of the rural setting. The quietness of the rural environment and the star-lit sky can offer a deeper personal satisfaction. Being in a rural setting can provide a much-needed source of outdoor life and an opportunity to reconnect with nature. Fields, forests, and streams offer a great outdoor living view and can potentially encourage a healthier lifestyle. This exposure to nature can help reduce anger, fear, and stress while increasing feelings of contentment. Rural area settings can contribute to an increase in well-being, reducing blood pressure, heart rate, and muscle tension (Gaston *et al.*, 2013).

REFERENCES

American Academy of Urgent Care Medicine (AAUCM). (N.D.) *Understanding the scope of urgent care*. Retrieved from https://aaucm.org/what-is-urgent-care-medicine/.

American Hospital Association (AHA). (2018). *Corporate integration; merging the rural hospital into the health clinic*. Retrieved from https://www.aha.org/system/files/2018-08/2018-rural-clinical-integration.pdf.

American Hospital Association (AHA). (2019). *Rural report*. Retrieved from https://www.aha.org/system/files/2019-02/rural-report-2019.pdf.

The American Occupational Therapy Association (AOTA). (2019). *Occupational therapy*. Retrieved from https://www.aota.org/Conference-Events/OTMonth/what-is-OT.aspx.

Bennet, J., *et al.* (2017). The scope and impact of mobile health clinics in the United States. *International Journal for Equity in Health. 16*:178 doi:10.1186/s12939-017-0671-2.

Centers for Disease Control and Prevention. CDC Health Disparities and Inequalities Report. In: Morbidity and mortality weekly report. U.S. Department of Health and Human Services. 2013. https://www.cdc.gov/mmwr/pdf/other/su6203.pdf.

Centers for Medicaid and Medicate Services (CMS). (2019). *Prospective payment system*. Retrieved from https://www.cms.gov/medicare/medicare-fee-for-service-payment/prospmedicarefeesvcpmtgen/index.html.

Centers for Medicaid and Medicate Services (CMS). (2019). *Swing bed fact sheet*. Retrieved from https://www.cms.gov/Outreach-and-Education/Medicare-Learning-Network-MLN/MLNProducts/downloads/SwingBedFactsheet.pdf.

Gaston, K., *et al.* (2013). *What are the benefits of interacting with nature*? Int J Environ Res Public Health. 2013 Mar; 10(3): 913–935.

Health Resources and Services Administration (HRSA), U.S. Department of Health and Human Services. (2018). Defining rural population. Retrieved https://www.hrsa.gov/rural-health/about-us/definition/index.html.

Health Resources and Services Administration (HRSA). (2018). Federally Qualified Healthcare Centers. Retrieved from https://www.hrsa.gov/opa/eligibility-and-registration/health-centers/fqhc/index.html.

Health Resources and Services Administration (HRSA). (2018). *Health center program*. Retrieved from https://bphc.hrsa.gov/sites/default/files/bphc/about/healthcenterfactsheet.pdf.

Health and Resources and Service Administration (HRSA). (2019). *A guide for rural health care collaboration and coordination.* Retrieved from https://www.hrsa.gov/sites/default/files/hrsa/ruralhealth/reports/HRSA-Rural-Collaboration-Guide.pdf.

Medicaid and CHIP Payment and Access Commission (MacPAC). (2018). *Rural hospitals and Medicaid payment.* Retrieved from https://www.macpac.gov/wp-content/uploads/2018/08/Rural-Hospitals-and-Medicaid-Payment-Policy.pdf.

Medicare Learning Network (MLN). (2018). *Rural health clinic.* Retrieved from https://www.cms.gov/Outreach-and-Education/Medicare-Learning-Network-MLN/MLNProducts/downloads/RuralHlthClinfctsht.pdf.

Medicare Payment Advisory Commission (MedPAC). (2017). Acute inpatient services. In Health care spending and the Medicare program. Washington, DC. Retrieved from http://www.medpac.gov/docs/default-source/data-book/ jun17_databooksec6_sec.pdf?sfvrsn=0.

Medicare Payment Advisory Committee (MedPAC). (2016). *Critical access hospitals payment system.* Washington, DC. Retrieved from http://medpac.gov/docs/default-source/payment_basics/medpac_payment_basics_16_cah_final.pdf?sfvrsn=0.

Medicare Payment Advisory Committee (MedPAC). (2019). *Hospice services.* Ch.12. Washington, DC. Retrieved from http://www.medpac.gov/docs/default-source/reports/mar19_medpac_ch12_sec.pdf.

National Health Institute (NHI), *Center for Connected Health Policy.* Retrieved from https://www.cchpca.org/about/about-telehealth.

National Hospice and Palliative Care Organization. (NHPCO). (N.D.) *Hospice care.* Retrieved from https://www.nhpco.org/about/hospice-care.

Rural Health Information Hub (RHIhub). (2019). *Rural hospice and palliative care.* Retrieved from https://www.ruralhealthinfo.org/topics/hospice-and-palliative-care.

Rural Health Information Hub (RHIhub). (2019). *Critical access hospitals.* Retrieved from https://www.ruralhealthinfo.org/topics/critical-access-hospitals.

U.S. Census Bureau. (2018). *American community survey.* Retrieved from https://www.census.gov/programs-surveys/acs/.

U.S. Department of Health and Human Services (HHS). (2011). Action plan to reduce racial and ethnic health disparities. Retrieved from http://minorityhealth.hhs.gov/npa/files/plans/hhs/hhs_plan_complete.pdf.

U.S. Department of Health and Human Services (HHS). (2016). ASPE issue brief. Retrieved from https://aspe.hhs.gov/system/files/pdf/211061/RuralHospitalsDSR.pdf.

Weant, K., R. Bowers, J. Reed, K. Braun, D. Dodd, and S. Baker. (2012). Safety and cost-effectiveness of a clinical protocol implemented to standardize the use of crotalidae polyvalent immune fab antivenom at an academic medical center pharmacotherapy 2012; 32(5):433–440.

The White House Council of Economic Advisors. (2010). *Strengthening the rural economy—The current state of rural America.* Retrieved from https://obamawhitehouse.archives.gov/administration/eop/cea/factsheets-reports/strengthening-the-rural-economy/the-current-state-of-rural-america.

CHAPTER 3

Area Health Education Centers Past and Present Role in Improving Access to Care in Rural Communities

Audrey Snyder, Steven Zucker, Monica Daniels-Mika, and Dwain Harris

Objectives:

1. Analyze the role of the National Area Health Education Center (AHEC) Program in improving access to healthcare in underserved and rural communities.
2. Articulate the importance of training the rural healthcare workforce for a value-based, patient-centered, team practice environment for innovative models of care.
3. Evaluate the impact of AHEC in improving the supply and distribution of healthcare professionals in rural communities via strategic partnerships with academic programs, communities, and professional organizations.

Discussion Questions:

1. Discuss the social, political, and economic context in which AHECs evolved.
2. How did The Carnegie Commission Report on Higher Education, *Higher Education and the Nation's Health* impact rural healthcare?
3. What two education training topics have been integrated in the interprofessional education objectives in Florida AHEC example? How do they address rural health disparities?

INTRODUCTION

Since its inception and modest beginnings in the early 1970s, the National Area Health Education Center (AHEC) Program has provided our nation with a solid foundation for the decentralization of health professions education and training in underserved rural communities and inner-city urban areas. It has also played an important role in enhancing access to healthcare through (along with other federal programs such as the National Health Service Corps [CHSC)] and the Federally Qualified Health Center Programs [FQHC]) in addressing the maldistribution of health professionals in these communities. As AHEC nears the completion of its fifth decade of operations and continues to be an important part of health workforce training in these communities throughout our nation, it is important to reflect on the origins and history of this longstanding and still extremely effective program.

NATIONAL AREA HEALTH EDUCATION CENTER BEGINNINGS

The initiation of a national Area Health Education Centers (AHEC) Program was first stimulated by a 1970 Report of the Carnegie Commission on Higher Education that recommended changes in the education of health providers (Gessert and Smith, 1981). This Commission, predecessor of the Carnegie Council of Policy Studies in Higher Education, devoted a Special Report to concerns in medical and dental education as a means of addressing geographic and specialty distribution of health personnel. In this 1970 Report, the Commission also noted that America's healthcare delivery system was not keeping pace with the nation's growing population (Watts and Jones, 1990). This Landmark Report, *Higher Education and the Nation's Health*, addressed serious concerns at the time regarding an overall shortage of health workforce and the geographic maldistribution of the health workforce, and the overspecialization of the workforce as well (Daniels, 1971).

Many factors had led to these concerns. The Flexner Report of 1910 to the Carnegie Foundation for the Advancement of Teaching recommended increasing the quality of medical care by physicians by increasing admittance and graduation standards, extending training periods, and eliminating medical schools that did not meet standards, leading to a decline in the number of medical schools and medical school graduates in the country (Reynolds, 2008). As a result, the great prosperity and population growth in the nation in the decades following World War II had health planners, governmental officials, and legislators concerned with assuring an adequate supply and geographic distribution of physicians, dentists, and other personnel. This created great interest and political pressure on starting new medical schools and academic health centers in communities across the nation and in expanding enrollments in existing ones, each of which would prove extremely costly. Furthermore, there was also an acknowledgment that rural and urban inner-city communities across the nation were already suffering from serious shortages of health providers, and that this geographic maldistribution would be exacerbated by the overall shortage and would also need to be addressed. In addition, it was evident that most academic health centers were increasingly specialized, and that beyond the acutely ill patient normally seen in their teaching hospitals, they were not ideal locations for providing appropriate training in community-oriented primary care (Swanson, 1972). There was also a clear understanding that medical residents tended to remain in practice in communities near where they took their residency training, and not necessarily where they received their medical training (Pellegrino, 1973).

Medical educators grappling with these concerns had begun planning and developing local and regional approaches to address them. At the medical school of the University of North Carolina at Chapel Hill, Dr. W. Reese Berryhill, the Founding Dean of the medical school created to serve as the "medical school of the people," upon his stepping down as Dean, recognized that their mission of extending medical care throughout the state remained incomplete, and led an effort to develop and direct a new Division of Research and Education in Community Medical Care, a forerunner to AHEC (Bacon, 2013). A 1965 Position Paper by Dr. William J. Cromartie, a Division Staff Member, states "cooperating in the establishment of regional medical education centers in the larger community hospitals was one clear way of extending the service and influence of the University over the State. Regional teaching centers would greatly enlarge the opportunities for postgraduate education for the state's physicians and would bring the faculty into contact with the realities of the practice of medicine and the health needs of the community. The Center would also provide the resources for teaching larger number of students, not only in medicine but in other health professions" (Uhl, 1993). The President of the University of North Carolina System (i.e., William Friday), where this approach was being explored and developed, was an esteemed member of the Carnegie Commission (Douglas, 2005); he was a strong proponent of their proposal to establish AHECs.

The Carnegie Commission Report, which became one of the most important Special Reports, proposed several federal initiatives to address these concerns, many of which became part of Congress's Comprehensive Health Manpower Training Act of 1971. Among these, along with the creation of a National Health Service Corps (NHSC), were federal funds for construction and start-up grants for new medical and dental schools (along with a warning that too many new schools should be avoided) and federal funding support for curriculum reform and innovation. In addition to these proposed initiatives and several others, the Commission also proposed that federal funding be available to support the development of Area Health Education Centers (AHECs) in 126 targeted communities it identified across the nation (Odegaard, 1979).

The Carnegie Commission intended that the AHECs would serve as regionally based alternatives to university health sciences centers (Zwick, Wilkington, Smith, and Stiles, 1977). These AHECs would be designed to improve the quality of health training in their areas, would help to overcome problems of geographic maldistribution of health manpower, would encourage training for primary care, and would remove the pressure in many communities for the establishment of new medical schools. They would also provide educational programs and clinical training education for medical and other health professions students from the health science centers, continuing education programs for the health workforce in their respective regions and be involved in community planning for effective regional health care delivery systems (Odegaard, 1979). As described by Dr. Eugene Mayer, the Commission reasoned that these health profession education centers would result in regional manpower development programs for physicians and other health professionals (Mayer, 1989), and that their community outreach would focus on "exposing students and residents to practice in underserved communities to help improve their awareness of and interest in practice in such communities; and would also help to reduce the professional isolation of the practitioner in these practice sites, helping to recruit and retain providers and keep them up-to-date (Mayer, 1990)". The Commission Report stated "physicians, dentists, and allied health workers are likely to be attracted to areas where there are well developed AHECs" and that this should "go far in achieving more equitable geographic distribution of health manpower" (Daniels, 1971).

This Carnegie Commission proposal to develop AHECs across the nation to decentralize medical education and address the geographic maldistribution of health professionals rapidly received broad-based support from multiple directions, as it provided something for all parties concerned. As described by Mike and Ross (1975), "Medical educators and professional societies saw AHECs as a way of expanding medical education training capacities and training large numbers of health professionals in appropriate settings without enormous financial investments in additional bricks and mortar. Health planners from regional medical programs saw AHECs embodying their cooperative community approach to healthcare. And governmental and political leaders recognized AHECs value in addressing the special needs of scarcity areas" (Mike and Ross, 1975).

In a presentation read before the American Medical Association Council on Medical Education's Annual Congress on Medical Education in February, 1971 and then published in the Journal of the American Medical Association in November, 1971, Dr. Margaret S. Gordon, Vice Chair of the Carnegie Commission, described the uneven distribution of physicians and other health personnel across the nation as a grave concern to all those interested in overcoming shortages of health professions and the several reasons for believing that the development of AHECs would be a significant factor in addressing this maldistribution (Gordon, 1971). Dr. Edmond Pellegrino, an esteemed medical education leader, also presented strong arguments for the AHECs as proposed by the Carnegie Commission in an address he delivered at the Plenary Session of the American Association of Medical Colleges' 83rd Annual Meeting in Miami Beach, Florida (Pellegrino, 1973). Dr. August Swanson, Director of Academic Affairs of the American Association of Medical Colleges, clearly presented the merits of the AHEC concept. As stated by Dr. Swanson, "basic to the concept is the fact that all health professionals cannot be educated and trained in our existing, urban-located, major academic medical centers. Among the professionals who fall into this category are physicians, nurses, and physician assistants. For a variety of reasons, ranging from building space to the nature of the metropolitan environment, it is desirable to locate our health professional education enterprise over a larger part of our cultural and geographic landscape." Dr. Swanson also pointed out that "physicians who are introduced to a smaller city or rural area during their training may find it an attractive place for a life career; and that if they are not introduced to these areas, the chances are not great for their voluntarily seeking out such an environment;" and that "educating physicians in smaller and more comprehensive units, dealing principally with primary and secondary clinical care provides an essential facet of their educational experience which is hard to manufacture in a complex environment of a university center with a major tertiary care mission." Dr. Swanson also described the many ways in which an actual high-quality education program enriches the quality of life in any community (Swanson, 1972). AHEC's time had clearly come, and it was now time for the federal government to make this happen!

FROM CONCEPT TO REALITY: AHEC'S EARLY HISTORY

In President Nixon's 1971 Health Message to Congress, he talked of ways of addressing the special needs of scarcity areas and called for the development of AHECs in communities that were underserved, as the Carnegie Commission had recommended (Zwick *et al.*, 1977). U.S. Department of Health, Education and Welfare (DHEW) Secretary Richardson then enthusiastically spoke of AHECs in his testimonies to both the U.S. Senate and U.S. House of Representatives, as a particularly promising means of addressing a need to effect a geographic and specialty distribution of health professionals and of responding to health workforce needs in the service areas in which they would be located (Odegaard, 1979). In a floor debate on a proposed Health Manpower Bill, Representative Paul Rogers (D-Fla.), Chairman of the House Subcommittee on Health and the Environment, and widely known by his fellow congressmen as "Mister Health" for his leading role in passing dozens of measures promoting healthcare, including community health centers, the NHSC, and the AHECs, described the rationale and needs for AHECs and enthusiastically supported their development (Mike and Ross, 1975).

With its widespread acceptability, AHECs were embraced by Congress and soon enacted into law as Section 774(a) of the Comprehensive Health Manpower Training Act of 1971 (PL 92-157). In June 1972, a letter of announcement of an RFP for developing AHECs was distributed nationally to 85 institutions who indicated an intention to apply; 27 were selected to receive the RFP; and 11 were finally selected to receive initial federal AHEC Awards in September, 1972. These awards from the then U.S. Department of Health, Education, and Welfare (DHEW) went to AHEC Programs affiliated with medical schools in the states of California, Illinois, Minnesota, Missouri, New Mexico, North Carolina, South Carolina, North Dakota, Texas, Maine, and West Virginia (Odegaard, 1979); and are frequently referred to as the "1st Generation AHECs". In addition, eight AHECs were also started through the Veterans Administration (VA). Several others were also started through Regional Medical Programs (RMPs), under the titles of Health Services/Educational Activities (HS/Eas).

The success of the early AHECs based at the academic health centers was noted by the Carnegie Council on Policy Studies in Higher Education in its 1976 Report, *Progress and Problems in Medical and Dental Education*, which reaffirmed faith in its AHEC concept as "one of the most encouraging and impressive developments under the 1971 Legislation". The Council supported the continued growth, development, and expansion of AHECs (Zwick *et al.*, 1977). The Health Professions Educational Assistance Act of 1976 (P.L. 94-184) reauthorized the AHEC Program with new guidelines and a range of required activities (Watts and Jones, 1981) and expanded AHEC by supporting the development of 12 new academic health center based AHEC Programs, frequently referred to as the "2nd Generation AHECs". It also reasserted a preference for the "Carnegie Medical Practice Consortium" with linkages to a central medical or university health sciences center (Jossey-Bass, 1976); and also provided for support of AHECs beyond rural communities to also include the government's interest in establishing urban AHECs to meet the special needs of our nation's inner-city areas (Odegaard, 1979) as well as the development of statewide AHEC Programs (Watts and Jones, 1990). The Health Professions Training Assistance Act of 1985 (P.L. 99-129) and the Health Professions Reauthorization Act of 1988 further expanded university-based AHECs; and ongoing development and expansion of AHECs in both rural and urban communities throughout the nation have continued to date. HRSA's Division of Diversity and Interdisciplinary Education within the Bureau of Health Professions administer the National AHEC Program. Most of the other AHECs started through the VA and RMP Systems in the 1970s are no longer in existence.

EVALUATION OF AHEC'S THROUGHOUT THEIR HISTORY

AHECs have been carefully studied and evaluated throughout their 50-year history. In 1977, Dr. Charles Odegaard, President Emeritus of the University of Washington and a nationally acclaimed administrator and medical education expert, was appointed by the Carnegie Council to undertake an evaluation of the 11 initial AHEC Programs funded in 1972. In 1979, after his comprehensive and rigorous review including site visits to each of the programs as well as meetings with federal officials from DHEW, he published *Area Health Education Centers: The Pioneering Years, 1972–1978*. In the foreword to Dr. Odegaard's review, Dr. Clark Kerr, Chairman of the Carnegie Council, stated "Odegaard's evaluation is objective and at the same time very encouraging as to the accomplishments of most of the projects. The Carnegie Commission's views that AHECs would improve the quality of health care and contribute to overcoming problems of geographic maldistribution and overspecialization have been largely justified" (Odegaard, 1979). Other major early studies included the 1978 Report of the U.S. Government Accounting Office; the 1978 Report of the U.S. House of Representatives, Appropriations Subcommittee on Health; a 1980 Report to the Congress by the Secretary of the Department of Health, Education, and Welfare; and the 1980 Report of the Graduate Medical Education National Advisory Committee (GMENAC). These reports documented a significant impact on the distribution of physicians and health manpower in the areas served by AHECs (Hansen, 1983). In 1990, in his foreword to the publication *The Story of the California AHEC System: California Area Health Education Centers, 1972–1989*, Dr. Kerr stated, "there has been a lasting change in access to health care and the quality of care available to the medically underserved" (Watts and Jones, 1981). In 2010, a national review of AHECs by Bacon *et al.* stated, "the primary mission of AHEC as a workforce development program through community-based educational initiatives has remained constant" and that "within the broad goals of the Health Resources and Services Administration (HRSA) to improve access to care for the most vulnerable and underserved populations, the AHEC role may be characterized as focusing on improvements in the distribution, diversity, and quality of the health care workforce of the country. AHEC Programs are designed to prepare a workforce that is more reflective of the population and better trained to address the primary care, preventive, and other health needs of underserved communities" (Bacon, 2000). In the following decades, AHECs have continued to be developed and evolve into a truly national program with services in all 50 states, as well as in the District of Columbia and five U.S. territories, including Guam, American Samoa, the Northern Mariana Islands, Micronesia, and Palau.

AHEC PIONEERS

Throughout its continual 50-year growth from inception in 11 states in the early 1970s to the nationwide program it is today, AHEC has been blessed with many early pioneers and inspirational leaders who will forever remain part of its legacy. The National AHEC Organization continues to perpetuate the memory of three outstanding early AHEC leaders by creating honorary awards for distinguished AHEC service in their names (i.e., Dr. Eugene S. Mayer, Dr. Andy Nicholas, and Henry "Red" Koelling, MBA), which are presented at ongoing National AHEC Conferences. Dr. Mayer, Dr. Nichols, and Mr. Koelling guided the development and evolution of AHECs in North Carolina, Arizona, and South Carolina, respectively into comprehensive and long-standing statewide initiatives still vibrant and highly effective today. Other AHEC pioneers were the early federal leaders of the National AHEC Program Office (Dan Smith and Cherry Tsutsumida) and the Grants Manager Officer (John Wescott), who each provided enormous assistance for well over a decade to the initial AHEC awardees and to institutions and schools across the nation interested in joining the AHEC movement, and in assuring for Congress and the nation that accountability, both financial and programmatic, was maintained, and that policy issues continued to evolve and expand. Another distinguished pioneer in the AHEC story was Dr. Charles Odegaard, the President Emeritus of the University of Washington and a nationally acclaimed administrator and medical education expert who was recruited by the Carnegie Council in 1975 to undertake a comprehensive evaluation of the initial 11 federal "first generation" AHEC awardees. After detailed visits to each of those programs, Dr. Odegaard published in 1979 his landmark Text *Area Health Education Centers: The Pioneering Years, 1972–1978* which still serves as an invaluable resource to institutions and individuals interested in the development of AHEC, including a penetrating analysis of the strengths and weaknesses of each of the programs. His positive findings played a major role in the continued interest in and support of AHEC by the Carnegie Council and by Congress, playing a significant role in the rapid growth and expansion of AHECs into a truly national initiative.

When recognizing these many great early AHEC pioneers that were all integral to its overall success, one truly stands out. Dr. Eugene S. Mayer, longtime Director of the North Carolina AHEC Program, provided dedicated leadership to the national AHEC movement from 1972 until his death in 1994. Dr. Mayer developed his North Carolina AHEC Program into the most successful and comprehensive AHEC Program ever developed in this nation, and one which remains so today, nearly 50 years later. He also worked tirelessly on behalf of all AHECs, testifying frequently before Congress, representing AHEC at numerous high-level national medical education and health policy meetings and conferences, founding and chairing the Legislative Committee of the National Organization of AHEC Program Directors for well over a decade, and providing assistance to states across the nation in developing their AHEC Programs. In this regard, he always made himself available to discuss AHEC with university and legislative leaders from other states whenever called upon for assistance. Powered by his own great sense of social responsibility, and a person of towering wisdom, possessing clearly admirable eloquence, vision, values, and a unique style that inspired trust that was unmatched made him a valued advisor to scores of medical education faculty and administrators as well as governmental and political leaders throughout the country. His integrity and commitment were strongly respected by legions of devoted AHEC colleagues and friends throughout North Carolina and the nation. In its storied AHEC history, Dr. Mayer without question was and will always remain its true icon and the AHEC pioneer of all time.

AHEC'S AND THE TRIPARTITE PARADIGM

As AHEC nears its 50-year anniversary, it continues to be an integral component of a national tripartite paradigm to address the geographic maldistribution of health professionals. This tripartite approach includes: (1) the community and migrant health centers, also known as Federally Qualified Health Centers (FQHCs); (2) the NHSC; and (3) the National AHEC Program.

Community and migrant health centers were first proposed and funded in 1965 as part of President Lyndon Johnson's "War on Poverty" based on a unique community-based healthcare model developed in South Africa that had brought on astonishing health improvement for the poorest citizens of that country. They were developed to assure that the neglected segments of our society would have access to health services by providing funding to build and maintain facilities that would deliver care to the high number of uninsured and indigent patients residing in the economically depressed underserved areas in which high unemployment or underemployment, and high poverty rates are common; and with the lower income and fewer insured patients making the operation of a traditional private medical practice financially unfeasible. The NHSC was established in the Emergency Health Personnel Act of 1970 to provide financial incentives in the form of educational scholarships (and eventually also loan repayment) for primary care providers in return for a service commitment to practice in medically underserved communities. AHECs, as noted earlier, were first proposed by the Carnegie Commission in 1970 and funded through the comprehensive Health Manpower Training Act of 1971 as a strategy for increasing the presence of the academic health sciences centers in needy communities through a wide range of training programs aimed at exposing health professions students to their needs, challenges, and opportunities for practice in these communities.

In essence, the federally qualified health centers provide the facilities and infrastructure to deliver care in shortage areas, the NHSC provides financial incentives to recruit physicians and other primary care providers to practice in these shortage areas, and the AHECs the commitment and involvement of the academic health science centers to decentralize health professions training programs to prepare and expose future health providers for practice in these communities. Throughout the past half-century, each of these outstanding major federal initiatives have continued to evolve and remain critical components of our nation's primary care safety net system that assures an adequate supply of practitioners for the millions of Americans who live in medically underserved communities and inner-city areas throughout the nation.

AHEC PROGRAM GOALS AND VALUES

Through advocacy, academic partnerships, education, and research, the AHEC mission is to enhance access to quality health care, particularly primary and preventive care, by improving the supply and distribution of healthcare professionals via strategic partnerships with academic programs, communities, and professional organizations. While not all states participate in the AHEC system the principles of Diversity, Distribution and Practice Transformation are inherent goals in many programs and have been tailor-made to meet unique local and state challenges (California Public Health Training Center [CPHTC], 2019).

California's AHEC program (CPHTC, 2019) is an example of a large state outreach program with 13 regional centers whose core values are representative of national directives to build a healthcare community:

- *Health*: A skilled, well-distributed health workforce will improve the health of Californians.
- *Education*: Education improves individuals and communities.
- *Community*: Underserved communities have strengths and needs.
- *Diversity*: California's diversity should be reflected in its health workforce.
- *Collaboration*: Collaboration of communities and academic institutions is essential to workforce improvement and distribution.

  Innovation: New ideas contribute to success.

Colorado's six regional AHEC sites and one program office carry out its mission with an emphasis on three defined goals to increase overall workforce capacity:

- *Diversity*: Increase the potential for secondary, college, and health profession students from underrepresented populations, educationally disadvantaged, and rural backgrounds to successfully pursue a health profession career;
- *Distribution*: Increase the potential for health profession students in medicine, dentistry, nursing, pharmacy, public health, and allied health to practice in a rural or urban underserved community by immersing them in un-

derserved community experiences through Community Based Education Training Programs, Field Placements, and Interprofessional Education and Training; provide access to evidenced-based health information, accredited high-quality continuing education programs and support for health practitioners serving in rural and medically underserved areas in Colorado; and,
- *Practice Transformation*: Facilitate and support practice transformation of Colorado's healthcare system by promoting a patient-centered approach, addressing social determinants of health through a team-based, data-centered method with a focus on improving quality and community health outcomes in rural and medically underserved areas (University of Colorado Denver, 2019).

COMMON OBJECTIVES

Regardless of the location AHECs are the linkage between academic health facilities to those geographically removed. While the internet and online education provide great advances community based, outreach continues the most effective way to ensure healthcare providers are distributed throughout the U.S. The common threads include: continuing education programs for health professionals practicing in underserved areas, teaching health professions students and residents to present health information to community members and clinic patients, providing community-based clinical training, developing programs to expose high school students to college and career opportunities in the health professions, and recording, studying, and documenting outcomes for continual improvement and advances (University of Colorado Denver, 2019).

Florida's AHEC Programs: Utilizing Academic and Community Linkages to Address Pressing Community and Public Health Needs

There are AHEC Programs at five medical schools in Florida, four of which receive both federal and state funding (Nova Southeastern University, the University of Florida, the University of South Florida, and the University of Miami) and one which is funded entirely through state support (Florida State University). These five AHEC Programs, all started at different times during the 1980s and 1990s, have banded together to form a Florida Statewide Network, also known as the Florida Alliance for Healthy Communities, a partnership between these AHEC Programs and their 10 affiliated regional, community-based AHEC Centers. This Network is a unique model partnership of five academic health sciences centers, public and private universities, osteopathic and allopathic medical schools, and rural and urban inner-city AHEC Centers. These AHECs have collaborated for well over two decades to build a strong statewide approach to health workforce development to enhance access to healthcare throughout Florida, one of the largest states in the nation, through strategies aimed at recruiting, training, and retaining primary care practitioners for practice in the state's many underserved and rural areas. For example, through the Nova Southeastern University (NSU) AHEC Program (started in 1985 as Florida's first AHEC Program), an intensive tracking study of its impact in preparing health professionals for practice in underserved areas found that over 2,000 medical, dental, nursing, pharmacy, physician assistant, and other health professions students from over 20 NSU AHEC-affiliated training programs had gone into practice delivering care in underserved communities and populations in 65 of the state's 67 counties; including over 300 graduates who had practiced in critical needs sites (e.g., FQHCs, county health departments, rural clinics, rural hospitals, and other indigent care sites).

In addition to their primary focus on health workforce development, Florida's AHECs have also long recognized the enormous potential of utilizing their well-established linkages with both academic and community partners to address a myriad of other pressing community and public health needs in the state. In this regard, Florida's AHECs have been able to utilize their long-standing relationships with medical, dental, nursing, pharmacy, allied health, public health, and numerous other health professions training programs as well as with numerous statewide and local professional organizations to implement a wide range of training initiatives for students, residents, and community providers in important topics such as HIV/AIDS, immigrant and minority health, tobacco cessation, and, most recently, opioid abuse disorder. In addition, the regional AHEC's extensive local broad-based partnerships with Florida's FQHCs and other community health services providers (such as health departments, behavioral health sites, community hospitals, etc.) has enabled AHEC to implement critical community-based initiatives in their respective service areas focusing on these same and other health issues.

This AHEC ability to play a key role in developing statewide academic and community approaches to address critical areas of need is particularly well illustrated by the great success of Florida's AHECs in addressing tobacco use as the leading preventable cause of death, disease, and healthcare costs in our society. Recognizing the great potential of AHEC's vast statewide infrastructure, in 2007 the Florida Legislature incorporated the AHEC Network in its newly funded Comprehensive Statewide Tobacco Education and Use Prevention Program (381.84 F.S.), supported entirely through the Tobacco Lawsuit Settlement revenues received by the state. As a result, in just over a decade, and through collaboration with hundreds of AHEC academic and community partners throughout the state, Florida's AHEC Tobacco Use Cessation Program has become one of the largest, if not the largest, program of its type in the nation and perhaps the world. Utilizing its academic linkages, Florida's AHECs have trained over 150,000 current and future medical, dental, nursing and other health professionals to effectively address tobacco use in the clinical setting, potentially benefitting millions of tobacco dependent patients that these professionals will collectively see over their practice lifetime. Utilizing its community linkages, AHEC has provided tobacco cessation services to nearly 200,000 smokers in nearly every community located in all 67 Florida counties. Florida's AHECs have also been instrumental in bringing tobacco prevention education to over a half million children in elementary, middle, and high schools throughout the state, thereby also contributing to the significant decrease in youth tobacco use rates in the state.

As a result of their long-standing success in maximizing the use of their extensive academic and community resources and partnerships throughout the state, in 2018, Florida's AHECs were also contracted by the state to address the opioid crisis in Florida. Though just completing its initial planning and development year, these broad-based collaborative partnerships have led to the rapid development of eight distinct training curricula (including three CME accredited online training modules) for current and future health providers; and the conducting of over 130 training programs utilizing these curricula, which were attended by over 4,200 current and future physicians, dentists, pharmacists, nurse practitioners, and physicians assistants, behavioral health specialists, and other health providers throughout the state. AHECs have also developed a Physician's Pocket Guide and a Patient Education Rack Card on opioid use disorder, distributed these materials statewide; provided technical assistance integrating behavioral health treatment in over 20 primary care sites (including FQHCs) across Florida; and developed and placed social media ads focusing on the projects training programs and available resources which have been seen by over 2.1 million people across the state.

AHEC'S FOCUS IN RURAL COMMUNITIES

Since the inception of AHECs nearly five decades ago, its primary focus has always been on addressing the geographic maldistribution of health providers through the recruiting, training, and retaining of health providers in underserved rural communities. In 1999 Ricketts reported that "AHEC Programs have supported the training of 1.5 million health professions, students, and primary care residents in underserved areas, with and explicit focus in rural areas in most state programs" (Ricketts, 1999). Now, some 20 years later, these numbers would be significantly higher.

AHEC'S NURSING FOCUS

The development of the first nurse practitioner program at the University of Colorado in 1965 by Loretta Ford and Henry Silver opened the door for advanced practice nursing in many fields. This pediatric nurse practitioner program expanded the role of nursing to meet the challenge of providing primary care to all children, especially in underserved areas (Silver *et al.*, 1998). This role developed out of Dr. Ford's experience as a nurse in rural areas in Colorado.

AHECs have had a major role in decentralizing nursing education. A model program for nursing education began in North Carolina in 1974 to provide continuing education. By 1976 North Carolina had nine AHECs with nurses in eight of the nine recruited to plan and supervise nursing activities. Continuing education, new nurse preceptorships, nursing education outreach programs with nurse practitioner and nurse midwifery courses taught away from campus (McGarth, 1976) were part of their mission. Shortly thereafter they provided clinical experiences for undergraduate and graduate nursing students in the rural counties. The third focus of the nursing education program was to provide an off-campus baccalaureate program for nurses living in a nine-county area around Fayetteville. In the 10-year period 1974–1985, 10,160 participants completed a total of 379 nursing programs (Princeton and McGarth, 1989).

NATIONAL HEALTH SERVICE CORPS TODAY

As part of the tripartite paradigm the NHSC provided workforce in the rural areas. According to Elayne J. Heisler's 2018 report for the Congressional Research Service, from FY2011 through FY2017, the most recent year of final data available, the National Health Service Corps (NHSC) offered more than 39,000 loan repayment agreements and scholarship awards to individuals who have agreed to serve for a minimum of two years in a Health Professions Shortage Area (HPSA). That same year, 10,179 NHSC providers were fulfilling a service obligation in a HPSA.

Most HPSAs are located in rural areas. In fact, according to the National Association of State Offices of Rural Health, there are 4,118 primary care HPSAs in rural and frontier areas of the U.S. compared to 1,960 in metropolitan areas.

The majority of NHSC providers serve in outpatient settings, most commonly at FQHCs. Providers also serve in rural health clinics and critical access hospitals. In FY2017, the following three professional groups made up 73% of the NHSC: mental and behavioral health providers (30%), nurse practitioners, including nurse midwives (23%), and allopathic and osteopathic physicians (20%) (Heisler, 2018).

Strength of the AHEC Network in Creatively Adapting National Initiatives to Help Address Local and Regional Health Needs

The earlier mentioned programs addressing opioid abuse and practice transformation are examples of AHECs adapting national initiatives to address the local and regional needs. The AHEC Scholars program is another example. AHECs across the nation launched the AHEC Scholars program in 2018 to address healthcare quality in rural and underserved areas by using interdisciplinary curricula to implement a defined set of clinical, didactic, and community-based activities.

Spanning two years, AHEC provides its Scholars with 160 hours of experiential and didactic education to supplement their program's curricula. The education takes place in rural and/or underserved settings and focuses on six vitally important core topic areas: interprofessional education, behavioral health integration, social determinants of health, cultural competency, practice transformation, and current/emerging health issues.

The AHEC Scholars program targets 15–25 students per AHEC center who are already enrolled in either a health professions degree program or an allied health workforce degree/certificate program. One of the hallmarks of the AHEC Scholars program is its interdisciplinary approach. Scholars come from a range of educational disciplines including nursing, medicine, pharmacy, therapies, and many others. By the definition of the program, they learn alongside students from disciplines other than their own.

AHECS TODAY

The primary mission of AHECs as a workforce development program for underserved communities through community-based educational initiatives has continued for five decades. In addition, AHECs now also play a role in the transformation of the health system by training the workforce for a value-based, patient-centered, team practice environment for innovative models of care and by providing and by promoting training for the integration of oral health and behavioral health in primary care (Bateman, 2019).

Today, 56 AHEC programs with more than 223 centers operate in almost every state and the District of Columbia. The national AHEC network consists of roughly 300 AHEC program offices and centers with, currently, approximately 120 medical and 600 nursing and other health professions schools working collaboratively with AHECs to improve health care access for underserved and underrepresented populations serving over 85% of all U.S. counties (User, 2017, Bateman, 2000). In 2018 alone, well over 11,000 medical students and nearly 4,000 nursing students were among the approximately 20,000 trainees placed by AHECs at over approximately 4,000 training sites in underserved areas, of which over 2,500 were in rural areas. In 2018 as well, AHECs provided continuing education programming to over 144,000 health providers, with a strong focus on those from rural and other medically underserved communities and primary care sites, to improve the quality of care for these communities and health disparities populations. Through AHEC health career recruitment programs for underserved and underrepresented populations, over 180,000 students throughout the nation were exposed to careers in the health professions (National AHEC, 2019, Harris, 2019).

Of special note is that based on a comprehensive nationwide assessment of AHEC Programs and Centers conducted in the spring of 2019, all of the 126 original communities first identified by the Carnegie Commission have been served by AHECs; and over 90% of these communities are continuing to be served. Well over half have been serving as the headquarters of their regional AHECs service areas. The AHECs have also proved valuable in addressing state health workforce distribution and related needs that state funding has been successfully secured to supplement and enhance AHEC activities in 70% (35) of the states across the nation; and continues to be secured in over 30 states at this time. In fact, cumulative state funding totals now far exceed the annual federal support for the National AHEC Program.

For the past 50 years, through robust community-academic partnerships, focusing on outreach, exposure, education, and training of the current and future health care workforce the National AHEC organization purpose has been to create healthcare human capital to work in rural and underserved communities. AHECs have a continual focus on improving the healthcare system by working with academic institutions, healthcare settings, behavioral health practices, and community-based organizations. Through these long-standing partnerships, the AHECs employ traditional and innovative approaches to develop and train a diverse healthcare workforce prepared to deliver culturally appropriate, high-quality, team-based care, with an emphasis on primary care for rural and underserved communities (Daniels, 1979).

REFERENCES

Bacon, T. J. (2013, January 31). AHEC's success reflects enduring power of partnerships: Newsroom. Retrieved from http://news.unchealthcare.org/som-vital-signs/2013/Jan31/baconahec.

Bacon, T. J., D. J. Baden, and L. D. Coccodrilli. (2000). The National Area Health Education Center Program and primary care residency training. *The Journal of Rural Health, 16*(3), 288–294. doi: 10.1111/j.1748-0361.2000.tb00475.x.

Bateman, M. (2019). National AHEC organization letter to Congress.

California Public Health Training Center. Retrieved July 7, 2019, from http://www.cal-ahec.org/california-public-health-training-center/.

Daniels, R. S. (1971). Higher education and the nation's health policies for medical and dental education: A special report and recommendations by the Carnegie Commission on Higher Education (Clark Kerr, Chairman). New York, McGraw-Hill Book Co. Inc., October 1970. *Archives of General Psychiatry, 24*(6), 579. doi: 10.1001/archpsyc.1971.01750120095016.

Douglass, J. A. (2005). The Carnegie Commission and Council on Higher Education: A retrospective. *Research and Occupational Paper Series, Center for Studies in Higher Education, 14*(5), 1–14.

Gessert, C. E., and D. R. Smith. (1981). The National AHEC Program: Review of its progress and considerations for the 1980s. *Public Health Reports, 96*(2), 116–120.

Gordon, M. S. (1971). Health education centers: Their role in medical education. *Journal of American Medical Association, 218*(8), 1192–4. doi: 10.1001/jama.1971.03190210046009.

Harris, D. (2019). FY 2020 L-HHS Written testimony for the record on the national area health education centers program, submitted to the House Appropriations Subcommittee on Labor Health and Human Services, Education and related agencies.

Hansen, K. F. (1983). Can area health education centers promote COPC? The Colorado experience. In E. Conner and M. Fitzhugh (Eds.), *Community-Oriented Primary Care: New Directions for Health Services Delivery, Conference Proceedings* (pp. 258–63). Washington, D.C.: National Academy Press.

Heisler, Elayne J. (2018, April 26). "The National Health Service Corps," Congressional Research Service. April 26, 2018. Retrieved from https://fas.org/sgp/crs/misc/R44970.pdf.

Jossey-Bass. (1976). *Progress and problems in medical and dental education: Federal support versus federal control.* San Francisco, CA.

Mayer, E. S. (1989). The North Carolina area health education centers program. *North Carolina Medical Journal, 50*(12), 660–664.

Mayer, E. S. (1990). Academic support for rural practice: The role of area health education centers in the school of medicine. *Academic Medicine, 65*(12), 45–50. doi: 10.1097/00001888-199012000-00035.

McGarth, B. J. (1976, October). Nursing in area health education centers. *American Journal of Nursing, 76*(10), 1605–1607.

Mike, L. H., and R. J. Ross. (1975). Area health education centers: What are they and where are they going. *Medical Education, 50*(3), 242–51.

National AHEC Organization 2017–2018 Health Workforce Training Program Highlights. (2019).

Odegaard, C. E. (1979). *Area Health Education Centers: The Pioneering Years*, 1972–1978. Berkeley, CA: Carnegie Council on Policy Studies in Higher Education.

Pellegrino, E. D. (1973). The regionalization of academic medicine: The metamorphosis of a concept. *Academic Medicine, 48*(2), 119–33. doi: 10.1097/00001888-197302000-00001.

Princeton, J. C. and B. J. McGarth. (1989). Decentralized nursing education: Does it work? T*he Journal of Continuing Education in Nursing, 20*(2), 54–57.

Reynolds, P. P. (2008). A legislative history of federal assistance for health professions training in primary care medicine and dentistry in the United States, 1963–2008. *Academic Medicine, 83*(11), 1004–1014. doi: 10.1097/acm.0b013e318189278c.

Silver, H. K., et al. (1991). A program to increase health care for children: The pediatric nurse practitioner program. A*merican Academy of Pediatrics, 102*(1), S245+.

User, S. (2017, August 10). National AHEC Organization. Retrieved August 2, 2019, from https://www.nationalahec.org/.

University of Colorado Denver: Anschutz Medical Campus. n.d. Retrieved July 7, 2019, from http://www.ucdenver.edu/Pages/UCDWelcomePage.aspx.

CHAPTER 4

Health Literacy Impact on Rural Health

Laurie Anne Ferguson

Objectives:

1. Define health literacy and its impact on health outcomes.
2. Apply health literacy concepts to rural practice populations.
3. Identify resources and strategies to improve health literacy in practice.

Discussion Questions:

1. How can you improve health literacy for patients in your practice?
2. Review some patient education materials used in your practice setting. How do they rate using PEMAT? https://www.ahrq.gov/ncepcr/tools/self-mgmt/pemat.html
3. What specific patient education project do you want to implement.

INTRODUCTION

Health literacy is defined as "the degree to which individuals have the capacity to obtain, process, and understand basic health information and services needed to make appropriate health decisions" (Ratzan and Parker, 2000). All segments of the population may experience some health literacy challenges when trying to negotiate the ever-increasing complex healthcare system. Even healthcare providers can experience limited health literacy after receiving a stressful diagnosis or overwhelming health information, making it difficult to navigate the system or make decisions. However, some populations are at increased risk of limited health literacy. *Rural location*, low formal education levels, older age, ethnic and racial minorities, and poverty are some factors associated with increased rates of limited health literacy (Paasch-Orlow *et al.*, 2005a). Health literacy has been identified by the Institute of Medicine (IOM), now called the National Academies of Science, Engineering and Medicine, as well as the World Health Organization (WHO), the Joint Commission and the Agency for Healthcare Research and Quality (AHRQ), as a significant problem impacting health behaviors, decisions, and, ultimately, health outcomes. *Healthy People 2030* provides a road map for the nation to achieve the goals of health promotion and disease prevention. The overarching goals include to attain healthy, thriving lives and well-being, be free of preventable disease, disability, injury, premature death, and eliminate health disparities, achieve health equity, and attain *health literacy* to improve the health and well-being of all (Healthypeople.gov. https://www.healthypeople.gov/2020/About-Healthy-People/Development-Healthy-People-2030/Framework). To achieve the goals of reducing health disparities and extending the quality and quantity of life, changes in health behavior are often necessary. Health behavior theories regard *knowledge and motivation* as prerequisite for behavior change (Bunda and Busseri, 2019; Klonoff, 2019). Health literacy has been described as the "currency" for improving the quality of health and healthcare and improved health outcomes in the United States (Paasche-Orlow *et al.*, 2005a). The Institute of Medicine (IOM) has made one of its priorities to promote the use of understandable health information (Nielsen-Bohlman *et al.*, 2004).

Today's healthcare environment is complex and requires increased patient responsibility to negotiate various systems, make decisions about health, and follow therapeutic plans. While the traditional definition of health literacy describes individual characteristics, it is more and more apparent that the challenges of limited health literacy require system and organizational changes for a positive impact (Brach *et al.*, 2012). Even people who have above average literacy may find navigation overwhelming. In addition, most health materials are written at higher levels than most adults can understand. Everyone is at risk of difficulty navigating the healthcare system in situations of extreme stress such as receiving news of a life-threatening diagnosis.

EPIDEMIOLOGY

Illiteracy, or the inability to read, contributes to limited health literacy. However, health literacy includes the broader definition of one being able to *manage* one's own health. Koh *et al.* (2012) summarize the breadth of health literacy as encompassing print literacy (writing and reading), oral literacy (listening and speaking), and numeracy (using and understanding numbers, such as medication doses). It is estimated only 12 percent of the 228 million adults in the United States have the skills to manage their own healthcare adequately (AHRQ, 2008). Limited health literacy is associated with lower use of preventative services, increased hospitalizations, and poorer health outcomes (Berkman *et al.*, 2011). Health disparities are exacerbated by a complex healthcare system, aging populations, low health literacy rates, and increasing rates of chronic diseases (Osborn *et al.*, 2011; Rikard *et al.*, 2016).

Several system level factors contribute to the problem of limited literacy. Contributory factors include medication complexity, short office visits, increased self-care demands, care fragmentation, and insurance paperwork (Weiss *et al.*, 2005). Today's healthcare system requires patients to take increasingly more responsibility for managing their health. The challenges increase as treatment decisions are more and more complex. Within the framework of complexity, limited health literacy has been found to relate to delayed diagnoses, poor adherence to treatment regimens, and increased morbidity and mortality (Koh *et al.*, 2012; Paasche-Orlow and Wolf, 2007a; Wolf *et al.*, 2007). Treatment regimens require more time and explanation which is often difficult in busy primary care practices. Discharge instructions and patient education materials may be difficult for patients to understand. Treatment adherence and patient follow-up, which are often inadequate, are impacted by limited health literacy.

Primary providers are often charged with the role of "gatekeeper" to direct and coordinate an individual's care. However, patients may see numerous specialists. Plans of care may not be effectively communicated between specialists and generalists, thus contributing to duplication of services and medication errors. Patient/provider communication breakdown is compounded when the patient has limited health literacy skills, as the patient often relays information between providers, and the lack of electronic health records (EHRs) compatibility has not decreased this challenge. The patient may not understand the reason or necessity for referral and therefore a comprehensive evaluation does not occur or worse, a misinterpretation and errors ensue. Patient access to care may also be hampered by complicated insurance application, referral, and reimbursement forms. Consent forms developed for provider legal protection may not readable and understandable by the patient. Therefore, consent forms may not truly provide informed consent.

Providers frequently make broad assumptions about their patient's ability to comprehend information. Graduating from high school, for example, does not guarantee a patient can read at a twelfth-grade level. A fifth to sixth grade reading level is recommended for most patient education materials (National Work Group on Literacy and Health, 1998). Ryan and colleagues (2014) found 50 percent of health education materials reviewed were written above the eighth grade level. Healthcare providers often use medical jargon which is a foreign language to people outside of health services. Limited health literacy is confounded by cultural and language differences in the U.S. In addition, the fast pace of busy primary care practices does not allow for adequate time to assess and improve patients' understanding. Furthermore, many providers have not been educated in ways to enhance patients' understanding. However health literacy is not just about written materials; health literacy is also about accessing healthcare, preventative services, understanding diagnoses and treatment regimens, and the ability to act on health information to improve overall health.

IMPACT OF LIMITED HEALTH LITERACY

The consequences of limited health literacy result in declines in our nation's health status. Limited health literacy is associated with increased rates of hospitalization and poorer health outcomes (Berkman *et al.*, 2011). According to the IOM's report, *Health Literacy a Prescription to End Confusion* (Neilson-Bohlman *et al.*, 2004), consequences of limited health literacy include increased economic costs in health services, higher societal costs, and increased burden of human suffering and disease (p. 81). In addition, limited health literacy may increase stress as the shame and stigma of illiteracy which results in decreased self-efficacy and increases the psychological burden.

Limited health literacy is associated with limited health knowledge, higher rates of chronic disease, and decreased utilization of preventative services (Berkman *et al.*, 2011). A higher risk of death is related to limited health literacy (Sudore *et al.*, 2006). From an epidemiological perspective, the risk of having limited literacy and subsequent increased mortality is the same as having a chronic disease (Volandes and Paasche-Orlow, 2007). The risk is further compounded when individuals have chronic health problems and the subsequent burden of illness on individuals and their families.

Health literacy has both individual and population determinants. Contributing determinants include age, genetics, ethnicity and race, language, educational status, socioeconomic status, and environment which includes rural location and underserved areas (Neilson-Bohman *et al.*, 2004). However, health literacy can also be considered as a determinant of health as it influences patient access, communication, decisions, and treatment adherence (Pawlak, 2005). Not surprisingly, health disparity patterns tend to parallel limited health literacy (Bodie and Dutta, 2008). Many experts suggest improvement in individual health literacy decreases health disparities which in turn improves the health of the population. In order to decrease health disparities, causes need to be identified and subsequent remedies applied. To do less supports the persistence of the inequities. The problem of limited health literacy is not only immoral, but also costly for society (Volandes and Paasche-Orlow, 2007).

IMPACTING OUTCOMES

All patients should be presumed to have limited health literacy and a "universal precautions" approach should be employed, as suggested by Paasche-Orlow and Wolf (2007b). Applying "universal precautions" for limited health literacy places the burden on the clinician to routinely assume there is limited health literacy. Patient education needs to be a central priority in every patient encounter. Sadly the healthcare provider has few incentives to spend time educating patients; insurance plans reimburse based upon procedures and diagnoses. The "medicalization" of health status problems assumes the solutions are increased "medical care" when the solution may be in improving patient education and health literacy. Healthcare needs to shift from an exclusively "medicalized" focus on health status problems to include social and economic causes of poor health status and health disparities (Lantz *et al.*, 2007; Raphael, 2008). To monitor patient outcomes based exclusively on outcome markers such as obtaining laboratory tests and filling prescriptions misses the critical impact of limited health literacy on patient comprehension and treatment adherence. Over the last decade, there has been an increased recognition of the importance of health literacy as linked to health outcomes. Improvements in health literacy can positively impact access to healthcare, quality, and cost (Koh *et al.*, 2012). Several recent federal policy initiatives increased the collective attention to addressing limited health literacy including the Affordable Care Act (ACA), the Department of Health and Human Services' (HHS) National Action Plan to Improve Health Literacy, and the Plain Writing Act. The Plain Writing Act of 2012 requires all federal government published documents to be written in a clear manner that is understandable (Koh *et al.*, 2012).

To improve health literacy, efforts should be focused around three core interventions. First, simplifying written material to make it easier to understand which includes medication information. Language should be written to clearly convey information, rather than for legal protection. Second, efforts should be targeted to improve provider communication, placing the burden on the provider not the patient. Third, a focus on improving patient's ability to self-manage their care (Koh *et al.*, 2012).

In 2012, participants a IOM Roundtable on Health Literacy identified ten attributes of health literate health care organizations (Brach *et al.*, 2012). The attributes that define organizations that make it easier for patients to understand, navigate, and make informed decisions regarding their health include:

1. Has leadership that makes health literacy integral to its mission, structure, and operations.
2. Integrates health literacy into planning, evaluation measures, patient safety, and quality improvement.
3. Prepares the workforce to be health literate and monitors progress.
4. Includes population served in the design, implementation, and evaluation of health information and services.

5. Meets the needs of populations with a range of health literacy skills while avoiding stigmatization.
6. Uses health literacy strategies in interpersonal communications and confirms understanding at all points of contact.
7. Provides easy access to health information and services and navigation assistance.
8. Designs and distributes print, audiovisual, and social media content that is easy to understand and act on.
9. Addresses health literacy in high-risk situations, including care transitions and communications about medicines.
10. Communicates clearly what health plans cover and what individuals will have to pay for services. https://nam.edu/perspectives-2012-ten-attributes-of-health-literate-health-care-organizations/

Improving numeracy is an important component in improving health literacy and health outcomes (Koh *et al.*, 2012; Waldrop-Valverde *et al.*, 2009). "Computational health numeracy involves the ability to count, quantify, compute, and otherwise use simple manipulation of numbers, quantities, items, or visual elements in a health context so as to function in everyday health situations" (Golbeck *et al.*, 2005, p. 375). Health numeracy refers to using numbers in a health-related activity such as reading nutrition labels, counting calories, and understanding medicine instructions. However, health literacy is not just about arithmetic, but also about understanding how to apply numeracy skills appropriately to the situation. For example, in order to achieve better diabetic illness control, a patient needs to recognize the need to increase an insulin dose when blood sugar is high. A fairly complicated task requires recognition of normal or target blood sugar goals and appropriate insulin remediation.

Critical to improving patient knowledge is improving health literacy and a great deal of research has focused on better ways to educate patients. Printed material should be written in a clear, culturally sensitive manner at the fifth grade level or lower (National Work Group on Literacy and Health, 1998). However, beyond the printed media, utilization of communication technology provides opportunities to bridge the divide of limited health literacy. The use of technology can convey complicated ideas via pictures, video, and multimedia which transcend the spoken and written word (Barry, 2002; Woolf *et al.*, 2005).

COMMUNICATION STRATEGIES

Two interventions for promoting better understanding in patients with low literacy are *Ask Me 3*™ (Partnership for Clear Health Communication, 2008) and the *Teach Back Method* (Wilson *et al.*, 2008). *Ask Me 3*™ which is endorsed by the American Medical Association Foundation, is a tool designed to promote better communication. The *Ask Me 3*™ tool encourages asking patients the following three questions to assess: (1) What is my main problem?; (2) What do I need to do?; and (3) Why is it important for me to do this? (Cassey, 2007).

Teach Back, also called *closing the loop or show me*, is a method to assess patient's understanding about their illness and its treatment. Patients who are illiterate may rely heavily on spoken instructions, demonstration, and pictures. Using everyday language, the healthcare provider provides information and has the patient repeat back or demonstrate what has been taught (Wilson *et al.*, 2008). It is interesting to note that nurses have long used a "teach back approach" called "return demonstration." Sadly only more recently has there been nursing contribution to the health literacy literature even though the focus is the core of nursing practice. Strategies for improving communication with patients with low health literacy include asking open-ended questions, and using pictures and demonstrations. Culturally sensitive and easy to understand language is critical to enhancing patient understanding. Educational materials need to be evaluated for their clarity and understandability not simply legal compliance. Ironically medications are approved by the Food and Drug Administration (FDA) only after extensive research yet written materials have no threshold for approval and use (Rudd, 2006).

Since patients rarely admit low reading or comprehension skills, care must be taken to protect the patient from embarrassment in evaluating literacy status. Recommendations for specific strategies employed by healthcare providers to improve health literacy of patients should include the use of pictures, symbols, and media to convey information regarding health topics. Avoidance of unnecessary overload by limiting the number of items or topics discussed at one encounter is helpful to improve comprehension (Hironaka and Paasche-Orlow, 2008). The use of one to two syllable words to communicate information, along with avoiding the use of medical jargon are necessary to improve understanding and subsequently adherence. Multiple forms of communication can facilitate understanding. For instance, the use of pictures, a bulleted list of important points along with a short video/DVD can improve comprehension of complicated topics (See Table 4.1). A simple strategy of casually handing printed materials upside down can reveal patients who cannot read without causing embarrassment. Instructions on prescriptions should include the reason for taking the medication and how often to take it in specific terms. Experts suggest avoiding usage of terms like BID or TID or even two or three times per day. Written specific times medication should be taken, 8:00 a.m. and 8:00 p.m. or 8:00 a.m., 2:00 p.m., and 10:00 p.m. make directions less ambiguous. Use clear pictures in handouts as people remember what is seen longer than what is verbally spoken. However one size may not fit all. Effective education materials should be given in a cultural appropriate and sensitive manner. Clear patient education materials in one set-

TABLE 4.1. How to Plan and Develop a Health Educational Video/DVD to Enhance Health Literacy.

1. Choose relevant topic
   a. Large topics should be divided into smaller topical segments
2. Develop story board and script
   a. Content should focus on behaviors
3. Use plain language (one to two syllables words)
   a. Language should be targeted to 5th grade level
      i. Assess reading level and language: Doak, C. C., Doak, L. G. and Root, J. H. (1996). Teaching patients with low literacy skills. 2nd edition. Philadelphia: J.B. Lippincott Co. is an excellent reference.
   b. Culturally sensitive
      i. Consider food or customs common to target population
   c. Socioeconomically neutral
   d. Avoid distracting backgrounds
4. Plan video/DVD length to not exceed 8 minutes
   a. Ideal length for populations at risk for limited health literacy is 3–5 minutes
5. Recruit actor
6. Determine filming location. Choose a quiet place!
7. Consider use of green screen to allow for varied appropriate backgrounds
8. Assemble appropriate props
9. Determine appropriate and effective dress. Bold solid colored (non-print) clothes with lab coat. No distracting jewelry.
10. Consider the following: Use of B-roll
    - Filming angles
    - Focal lengths
    - Scene matching
11. Consult experts for guidance concerning filming: Top Ten Video Editing Hints can be accessed from: http://desktopvideo.about.com/od/desktopediting/tp/editrules.htm
12. Film video—record in editable segments to allow for editing and smooth transitions.
13. SPEAK SLOWLY!
14. Choose film editing software program. There are free programs and editing software for purchase.
15. Import video into video editing program
16. Edit video for clear logical sequence.
17. Insert close up demonstration shots as appropriate
18. Transition smoothly
19. Insert title and topical slides
20. Final edit and export to DVD
21. Develop accompanying brochure to reinforce key points. Terminology and pictures should duplicate video/DVD pictures and points.
22. Copyright material (Certified mail to oneself in a sealed envelope is an inexpensive way to copyright[This is not an official or enforceable way to procure copyright.])

Randall and Muneta (2000).

TABLE 4.2. Features of a Good Handout.

• Use pictures • Focus on a central message • Emphasize key points by highlighting, use of color or underlying • Utilize lots of white space • Utilize Font 12 point or greater

Adapted from Doak, Doak and Root (1996).

ting may not be understood in another. For guidance developing and assessing educational handouts see Tables 4.2 and 4.3.

At the population level, effective approaches for improving health literacy need to be interprofessional and occur in many settings including venues outside healthcare. School health programs need to incorporate instruction both on health promotion, disease prevention along with teaching skills on how to navigate the healthcare system and improve decisions about personal health.

Population level disparities in social structures are linked to limited health literacy, information technology, motivation, and ability (Berkman *et al.*, 2011). The digital divide further limits access for vulnerable populations. Bodie and Dutta (2008) posit the root causes of healthcare disparities need to be addressed to improve the issues of the digital divide, health marketing, and health communication. A healthier population is better for all.

OTHER STRATEGIES TO IMPROVE HEALTH LITERACY

The distinction between health education and health promotion, the latter having to do with a focus on behavior change, is often elusive in the literature (Whitehead, 2001). To improve health outcomes, improved knowledge as well as behavior change is needed. Kinzie (2004) provides guidance for interventions in her article titled "Instructional design strategies are needed for health behavior change." The five strategies grounded in health promotion theory include: (a) gains attention; (b) presents stimulus material; (c) provides learning guidance; (d) elicits performance and provides feedback; and (e) enhances retention and transfer. Brach and colleagues (2012) discuss best practices to improve health literacy that include clear communication and therefore written materials should incorporate the concepts of language, sentence length, tone, as well as layout and design. The tone of voice, body language, and loudness as well as the pace of communication are important to consider in both personal and video-based communication. Combining appropriate written information with audio-visual educational materials can improve patient understanding.

TABLE 4.3. How to Plan and Develop a Health Educational Pamphlet to Enhance Health Literacy.

1. Tips to remember when developing an health information pamphlet
   a. Who is your audience?
   b. What do you want them to learn?
   c. Key points should follow key points emphasized in the video/DVD
   d. Edit, edit again. Have others review your text
   e. KEEP IT SIMPLE
   f. Include meaningful information
   g. Focus on behaviors
   h. Describe the benefits of the behavior
2. Use plain language (one to two syllables words)
   a. Language should be targeted to 5th grade level
      i. Assess reading level and language, Patient Education Material Assessment Tool (PEMAT), https://www.ahrq.gov/ncepcr/tools/self-mgmt/pemat.html
   b. Culturally sensitive
      i. Consider food or customs common to target population
      ii. Socioeconomically neutral
3. Use pictures from video/DVD or pictures that help convey the message simply
4. Culturally sensitive
   a. Consider food or customs common to target population
5. Socioeconomically neutral
6. Consider using desktop publisher or other software program to assist with layout and design.
7. Leave lots of white space
8. Choose large bold, readable fonts
9. Double check your facts
10. Bullets can highlight your message
11. Best messages can be summarized in a short list
12. Provide a spot for additional or personalize information, e.g., medication name, use, and directions
13. Clearly state the benefits of adopting new behavior
14. Consider printing your brochure on high quality brochure thick paper
15. A simple brochure in black and white will cost less than $200 for 1,000. Color will add about 20%. Home printing can provide additional savings for smaller jobs.

Additional resources

- PEMAT—Patient Education Assessment Tool http://www.healthliteracyoutloud.com/2014/01/28/pemat-patient-education-materials-assessment-tool-hlol-109/
- Online course in Health Literacy: https://www.hrsa.gov/cultural-competence/index.html
- Guide for developing print materials: www.nci.nih.gov/aboutnci/oc/clear-and-simple/page1
- Online readability calculator: www.wordscount.info
- Health Literacy Translations Toolkit: www.hablamosjuntos.org/mtw/defautl.toolkit.asp
- Agency for Healthcare Research and Quality (AHRQ) https://www.ahrq.gov/topics/health-literacy.html

Schillinger, D., Machtinger, E. L., Wang, F., Palacios, J., Rodriguez, M., and Bindman, A. (2006). Language, literacy, and communication regarding medication in an anticoagulation clinic: A comparison of verbal vs. visual assessment. *Journal of Health Communication: International Perspectives, 11*(7), 651–664.

PROVIDER COMMUNICATION

Communication in patient encounters is also a provider responsibility. Patient health literacy capabilities are linked to health outcomes. Interventions must also address provider communication styles and abilities. The literature reveals that the use of medical jargon results in poor patient understanding as to treatment options and clinical outcomes. Castro, Wilson, Wang, and Schillinger (2007) found 81% of clinical encounters reviewed contained at least one unclarified jargon term resulting in decreased patient understanding. Unfortunately providers often overlook communication needs and rarely assess patient recall or comprehension (Schillinger *et al.*, 2003). Even small interventions, such as the addition of visual aids, were found to increase patient comprehension of anticoagulant treatment and medication adherence (Schillinger *et al.*, 2006).

POLICY IMPLICATIONS

Improving access is one of the most critical components of improving health in rural America and specifically in rural populations. Comprehensive health insurance coverage and promoting physical access are necessary in order to improve health for the population. However the issues of history, culture, and education are just as critical to consider in increasing access to healthcare. Know your community and the culture. What is acceptable in one community may not be okay in another. Fear and suspicion may prevent early access to care. Low levels of educational attainment, rural location, and an elderly population are risk factors for poor health literacy. The problems are multi-factorial and the challenges are great. However knowledge is power and increasing knowledge increases health of individuals and the population. Efforts to improve health literacy influences behavior and may positively impact population health outcomes.

SUMMARY

Health literacy research has explored the impact of limited health literacy on specific chronic illnesses, parenting, and medication adherence as well as provider communication. Uniform interventions between health literacy and health outcomes are challenging due to the complexity of the problem and both individual and system factors. However several causal links are associated with health literacy including access and utilization of care, patient-provider relationship, and the ability for self-care (Paasche-Orlow and Wolf, 2007a).

CONCLUSION

Although millions of Americans are able to navigate city streets, bus routes, and malls, many do not have the skills to understand and utilize our healthcare system. Nearly one half of all American adults or 90 million people are unable to comprehend health information and make informed health decisions. Limited literacy impacts health behaviors, health decisions, and ultimately health outcomes. The consequences of limited health literacy result in a decline in our nation's health status. Limited health literacy is associated with increased rates of hospitalization and poorer health outcomes (Berkman *et al.*, 2011). All patients should be presumed to have limited health literacy and universal precautions should be assumed. Patient education needs to be a central priority in every patient encounter. The concept of health literacy is central in achieving the six components of high-quality healthcare as outlined in the IOM's *Crossing the Quality Chasm*: safety, effectiveness, efficiency, timeliness, patient centeredness, and equitable treatment (Abrams *et al.*, 2009; Becker, 2009).

REFERENCES

Abrams, M. A., P. Klass, and B. P. Dreyer. (2009). Health literacy and children: Recommendations for action. Pediatrics, 124, S327–S331.

Agency for Healthcare Research and Quality [AHRQ]. (2008). 2007 National Healthcare Disparities Report. Retrieved from http://www.ahrq.gov/qual/nhdr07/nhdr07.pdf.

Barry, M. J. (2002). Health decision aids to facilitate shared decision making in office practice. Annals of Internal Medicine, 136, 127–135.

Becker, B. N. (2009). Focusing on health literacy might help us cross the quality chasm. American Journal of Kidney Diseases, 53, 730–732.

Berkman, N. D., *et al.* (2011). Low health literacy and health outcomes: An updated systematic review. Annals of Internal Medicine, 155(2), 97–107. DOI: 10.7326/0003-4819-155-2-201107190-00005.

Bodie, G. D. and M. J. Dutta. (2008). Understanding health literacy for strategic health marketing: eHealth literacy, health disparities, and the digital divide. Health Marketing Quarterly, 25, 175–203.

Brach, C., *et al.* (2012). Ten attributes of health literate health care organizations. Retrieved from https://nam.edu/perspectives-2012-ten-attributes-of-health-literate-health-care-organizations/.

Bunda, K. and M. A. Busseri. (2019). Lay theories of health, self-rated health, and health behavior intentions. Journal of Health Psychology, 24(7), 979–988. DOI: 10.1177/1359105316689143.

Cassey, M. Z. (2007). Building a case for using technology: Health literacy and patient education. Nursing Economics, 25, 186–188.

Doak, C. C., L. G. Doak, and J. H. Root. (1996). Teaching patients with low literacy skills. 2nd edition. Philadelphia: J.B. Lippincott Co.

Golbeck, A. L., *et al.* (2005). A definition and operational framework for health numeracy. American Journal of Preventative Medicine, 29, 375–376.

Healthypeople.gov. (2017). Healthy people 2030 framework. https://www.healthypeople.gov/2020/About-Healthy-People/Development- Healthy-People-2030/Framework.

Hironaka, L. K. and M. K. Paasche-Orlow. (2008). The implications of health literacy on patient provider communication. Archives of Disease in Childhood, 93, 428–432.

The Joint Committee on Standards for Education Evaluation. 1994. The program evaluation standards: How to assess evaluations of educational programs. Thousand Oaks, CA: Sage.

Kinzie, M. B. (2004). Instructional design strategies for health behavior change. Patient Education and Counseling,56, 3–15.

Klonoff, D. C. (2019). Behavioral theory: The missing ingredient for digital health tools to change behavior and increase adherence. Journal of Diabetes, Science and Technology, 13(2), 276–281. DOI: 10.1177/1932296818820303.

Koh, H. K., *et al.* (2012). New federal policy initiatives to boost health literacy can help the nation move beyond the the cycle of costly "crisis care." Health Affairs, 31(2), 434–443. DOI:10.1377/hithaff.2011.1169.

Lantz, P. M., R. L. Lichtenstein, and H. A. Pollack. (2007). Health policy approaches to population health: The limits of medicalization. Health Affairs, 26, 1253–1257.

National Work Group on Literacy and Health. 1998. Communicating with patients who have limited literacy skills. Report of the National Work Group on Literacy and Health. Journal of Family Practice, 46, 168–176.

Nielsen-Bohlman, L., A. M. Panzer, and D. A. Kindig. (Eds.). (2004). Health literacy: A prescription to end confusion. Washington, DC: National Academies Press.

Osborn, C. Y., *et al.* (2011). Health literacy explains racial disparities in diabetes medication adherence. Journal of Health Communication, 16:268–278. DOI: 10.1080/10810730.2011.604388.

Paasche-Orlow, M. K., *et al.* (2005a). The prevalence of limited health literacy. Journal of General Internal Medicine, 20, 175–184.

Paasche-Orlow, M. K., *et al.* (2005b). Tailored education may reduce health literacy disparities in asthma self-management. American Journal of Respiratory Critical Care Medicine, 172, 980–986.

Paasche-Orlow, M. K. and M. S. Wolf. (2007a). The causal pathways linking health literacy to health outcomes. American Journal of Health Behavior, 31, S19–S26.

Paasche-Orlow, M. K., and M. S. Wolf. (2007b). Evidence does not support clinical screening of literacy. Journal of General Internal Medicine, 23, 100–102.

Partnership for Clear Health Communication at the National Patient Safety Foundation. 2008. Retrieved from :http://www.npsf.org/askme3/PCHC/.

Pawlak, R. (2005). Economic considerations of health literacy. Nursing Economics, 23,173–180.

Rapheal, D. (2008). Shaping public policy and population health in the United States:

Why is the public health community missing in action? International Journal of Health Services, 38, 63–94.

Ratzan, S. C. and R. M. Parker. (2000). Introduction. In Selden C. R., Zorn, M., Ratzan, S. C. and Parker, R. M. (Eds.). National Library of Medicine Current Bibliographies in medicine: Health literacy. NLM Pub. No. CBM 2000-1. Bethesda, MD: National Institutes of Health, U.S. Department of Health and Human Services.

Rikard, R.V., *et al.* (2016). Examining health literacy disparities in the United States: A third look at the National Assessment of Adult Literacy (NAAL). BMC Public Health,16 (975). DOI 10.1186/s12889-016-3621-9.

Rudd, R. (2006). Panel 1: Health literacy, literacy, and health outcomes. In Surgeon General's workshop on improving health literacy. Retrieved from http://www.surgeongeneral.gov/topics/healthliteracy/toc.htm.

Ryan, L., *et al.* (2014). Evaluation of printed health education materials for use by low-education families. Journal of Nursing Education and Scholarship 46(4), 218–228.

Schillinger, D., *et al.* (2006). Language, literacy, and communication regarding medication in an anticoagulation clinic: A comparison of verbal vs. visual assessment. Journal of Health Communication, 11, 651–664.

Schillinger, D., *et al.* (2003). Closing the loop: Physician communication with diabetic patients who have low health literacy. Archives of Internal Medicine, 163, 83–90.

Sheridan, S. L., *et al.* (2011). Interventions for individuals with low health literacy: A systematic review. Journal of Health Communication 16, 30–54. DOI:10.1080/10810730.2011.604391.

Sudore, R. L., *et al.* (2006). Limited literacy and mortality in the elderly: The health, aging and body composition study. Journal of General Internal Medicine, 21, 806–812.

Volandes, A. E., and M. K. Paasche-Orlow. (2007). Health literacy, health inequality and a just healthcare system. The American Journal of Bioethics, 7, 5–10.

Waldrop-Valverde, D., *et al.* (2009). Gender differences in medication management capacity in HIV infection: The role of health literacy and numeracy. Aids Behavior, 13, 46–52.

Weiss, B. D., *et al.* (2005). Quick assessment of literacy in primary care: The newest vital sign. Annals of Family Medicine, 3, 514–522.

Whitehead, D. (2001). Health education, behavioural change and social psychology: Nursing's contribution to health promotion? Journal of Advanced Nursing, 34, 822–832.

Wilson, F. L., *et al.* (2008). Using the teach-back and Orem's self-care deficit nursing theory to increase childhood immunization communication among low income mothers. Issues in Comprehensive Pediatric Nursing, 31, 7–22.

Wolf, M. S., *et al.* (2006). A critical review of FDA-approved medication guides. Patient Education and Counseling, 62, 316–322.

Woolf, S. H., *et al.* (2005). Promoting informed choice: Transforming health care to dispense knowledge for decision making. Annals of Internal Medicine, 143, 293–300.

CHAPTER 5

Emergency and Disaster Preparedness

Wendy Fletcher

Objectives:

1. Identify two major origins of disasters.
2. Develop a historical timeline of emergency and disaster preparedness in the United States.
3. Discuss the types of emergency alerts or warnings and recognize situations leading to their appropriate use.
4. Use the information provided to identify vulnerabilities in one's workplace disaster plan and develop an alternative action plan for any potential system failures.
5. Utilize safety tips provided to develop a patient education piece on disaster safety.
6. Consider deficits in local public policy and advocate for improvements to mitigate risks in one's community or workplace.

Discussion Questions:

1. Disaster can strike at any time. Understanding your facility's emergency and disaster plans can better prepare you for emergencies arising from a disaster.
   a. Considering your current work environment, are there areas where you believe you are vulnerable to unforeseen events?
   b. How can you better prepare to prevent liabilities, particularly the loss of life, the ability to care for your patients (or yourself), and to safeguard your practice and patient data?
2. Necessity has proven to indeed be the "mother of invention," when it comes to public policy surrounding disaster preparedness.
   a. What is your role in shaping public policy?

   b. How can you become a greater public policy influencer?
   c. Choose a topic related to emergency/disaster planning and write a letter to your State Representative or Federal Member of Congress, advocating for a change that could reduce risks for disasters in your community.
3. Communication is the key to effectively managing any disaster. Consider the following scenarios and develop a personal and professional plan for communications during these events:
   a. A mass casualty event at a local manufacturing plant has overwhelmed your community's wireless service provider, making cell phone communications impossible.
   b. An active shooter code has been called in the medical annex building where you're currently providing patient care. You're in the room with a patient and his family when you receive the "all call" alert on your cell phone.
   c. During a spring thunderstorm, your clinic loses both land line and cell phone services, disabling your electronic medical record system. What downtime procedures do you have in place to ensure patient safety during the outage?
4. The COVID-19 pandemic of 2020 was a "wicked teacher," providing numerous opportunities for improving public health in the United States and around the world.
   a. Discuss the differences between politics and policy, and how these two factors influenced the U.S. response to the pandemic.
   b. Vaccine hesitation by providers and patients occurred during the pandemic of 2020. Choose a pro-vaccine or anti-vaccine stance (related to COVID-19 vaccines) and develop an evidence-based argument for your views. Be sure to cite your sources and level of evidence for your argument.
5. Discuss and/or develop a patient education handout about mitigating risks at home during a disaster. Work in groups of 3–5 members and be sure not to duplicate topics. Combine your efforts into one easy-to-read pamphlet or 8 × 11 handout. Be sure to consider the community you are serving and the most likely disasters to impact your patients.

INTRODUCTION

Gaining a better understanding of the history, policy, and practice of emergency preparedness can help change the lens with which one defines, prepare for and respond to disasters. This chapter will help you better understand how to recognize and mitigate risks posed by both "Mother Nature" and "human nature."

Experience can be a wicked teacher during a disaster, and when unprepared, we often find out quickly what we do not know. The old adage, "Better safe than sorry," is no better applied than in emergency and disaster planning.

Disasters and emergencies come in many forms. Healthcare workers learn basic first aid and emergency life-saving skills early on in their careers. Much of the time, that education is focused on one patient or one assignment, one shift at a time. Many of us take for granted that our disaster education actually began decades prior to our first CPR certification, nursing degree, or licensure as a healthcare professional. For most of us, learning to stay calm and safe during a disaster began as early as our first few days of kindergarten.

20th-century Education in Readiness

Anyone born before the mid-1950s likely lived through a fair share of air raid drills with blaring sirens and "duck and cover" instructions during their school days. In the wake of World War II, tensions between the United States and the (then) Soviet Union set up a 44-year period now known as the "Cold War," where the threat of military attacks on U.S. soil prompted Americans to prepare their children for the possibility of air strikes by Communist invaders.

School-goers since the 1960s may have vivid recall of standing outside their school buildings, awaiting a fire chief's "ALL CLEAR!" signal. Routine fire drills were instituted within a year of the 1958 Our Lady of the Angels School fire in Chicago, IL (Cowan and Kuenster, 1998). One of the deadliest fires in American history, 92 pupils and 3 nuns died; numerous others were injured in attempts to jump from second-floor windows after a fire near the stairwell blocked their escape. Southerners and Midwesterners may recall following teachers' advice during unpredictable seasonal storms. "Open at least 2 windows before walking safely but quickly into the hallway." This would be followed by instructions to "sit closely together along the inside wall and cover your head."

The 21st-century's New Lessons

Emergency preparedness took on a new identity after the turn of the 21st century, following terrorists' attacks on the United States on September 11, 2001. A man-made disaster with catastrophic effects, over 3,000 Americans lost their lives in a single day. Thousands of first responders and others on and near the scenes continue to suffer with long-term health issues, both mental and physical, following those attacks.

Policy changes after 9/11 were far-reaching, from changes to security screenings in airports and overhauls of mass casualty plans at every level, to post-disaster physical and mental health management. Preventing the next attack, preparing for that which "could never happen here," and survival in the aftermath became the new focus of disaster management across the nation.

Another concern facing the nation during the new century's first two decades was the uptick in school-related gun violence. While school shootings date all the way back to the 1700s and the Pontiac's Rebellion school massacre of 1764 (K12 Academics, 2020), until the 1990s, deaths or injuries at school by gunshot were considered rare. "More people have died or been injured in mass school shootings in the United States in the past 18 years than in the entire 20th century" (Antonis Katsiyannis, cited in Springer, 2018, pg. 1).

During the first decade of the new century, schools began routinely adding active shooter exercises to their emergency preparedness drills. Over 147 separate events leading to injury or fatalities in American schools drove school administrators to change their approach to school violence to one of zero tolerance. "Passive reassurance" became proactive "worst case scenario" planning in light of the rising frequency of school gunman incidents.

THE EVOLUTION OF EMERGENCY PREPAREDNESS IN AMERICA

In the United States, broad scale emergency management is tasked to the Federal Emergency Management Administration (FEMA). While not officially created until 1979, the role of the federal government in disaster relief began in the early 1800s (FEMA, 2020). When a fire devastated a large seaport in New Hampshire in the winter of 1802, threatening commerce in the northeast, the newly founded U.S. Congress provided relief by suspending bond payments for the effected merchants. The Chicago Fire of 1871 and the Great Mississippi Flood of 1927 lead to even more Federal involvement. While not directly involved at that time, Congress supported the American Red Cross in its efforts to provide relief to flood victims. Soon after, Congress began funding operations to provide flood control systems to prevent future floods along the river's banks in several states along the Mississippi River.

From 1803 to 1949, Congress passed 128 separate laws relating to disaster relief, but did not pass a comprehensive federal disaster plan until 1950. This plan authorized the president to declare a major disaster and allowed state governments to request disaster relief aid from the federal government. That same year, the Federal Civil Defense Act of 1950 created a nationwide system of civil defense authorities, mobilizing efforts to manage both natural hazards and man-made incidents following World War II and the Cold War.

It wasn't until 1965, when Hurricane Betsy caused major damage across the southeastern coast of the U.S., that Congress passed the National Flood Insurance Act of 1968, allowing homeowners to apply for and be reimbursed for damages resulting from major floods. Programs providing direct financial support to individuals and federal funding mechanisms to repair public facilities after natural disasters spurred the development of risk reduction programs throughout the 1960s and 1970s.

It was a man-made disaster in 1979 that lead to the establishment of what we now know as FEMA. An "inefficient and fragmented response" (FEMA, 2019, pg. 17) by over 100 entities following the partial nuclear meltdown of the Three Mile Island Nuclear Generating Station in Harrisburg, PA, resulted in President Carter signing an Executive Order establishing this Agency, and giving it the dual mission of emergency management and civil defense.

On September 11, 2001, terrorist attacks changed America forever. Over 3,000 lives were lost and billions of dollars in property damaged or destroyed in New York, Virginia, and Pennsylvania as hijacked aircraft were crashed into New York City's World Trade Towers, the Pentagon, and a field in rural Pennsylvania. The following year, President George W. Bush signed the Homeland Security Act, forming a new organization, the Department of Homeland Security (DHS), focusing primarily on terrorism-related preparedness. FEMA was then rolled into DHS, and its focus reverted back to the management of natural disasters.

EMERGENCY ALERTS

Some disasters are neither foreseeable, nor preventable. Early detection systems and reliable emergency alert systems, however, can help to protect the public before disaster strikes. FEMA's Integrated Public Alert and Warning System, known by the acronym IPAWS, provides public safety officials with the ability to alert the public about serious emergencies from a single platform. This includes the Emergency Alert System (EAS), wireless telephone and tablet emergency alert messages, the National Oceanic and Atmospheric Weather Radio system, and other public alert systems. Federal, state, local, tribal, and territorial emergency management systems can send and receive alerts to 100% of a service area, overshooting by no more than 1/10 of a mile, to any wireless network customers' phones nationwide (FEMA, 2020). IPAWS is used for 3 distinct types of alerts or warnings, described below.

- *Presidential*: The EAS is the national alert system that requires all communication systems that broadcast within the United States to provide the president the capability to broadcast from their platforms within 10 minutes of a national emergency. The president has the sole responsibility for determining when to activate the EAS for national-level messaging.
- *AMBER*: State and local authorities, in cooperation with EAS providers, can issue alerts meeting certain criteria in cases of child abduction. AMBER is a backronym for "America's Missing: Broadcast Emergency Response" a system named for Amber Hagerman, a 10-year old child abducted and murdered 5 miles from her Arlington, Texas home in 1996.
- *Imminent Threat*: If you are within the geographic region of an imminent threat, including inclement weather, technological incidents (chemical

spills, radiation leaks, as examples), or bio-hazard exposure, you may receive an imminent threat alert by phone, radio, TV, or siren alert. These warnings signal immediate danger and are generally accompanied (when by verbal or text notification) of specific instructions to help you avoid the imminent dangers associated with the threat. Outdoor sirens generally are used as a "take cover" warning, and require the listener to follow local rules on how and where to shelter when sounded.

Understanding the emergency alert system, ensuring that you and your staff are able to access these alerts readily, and coordinating with local officials on your role in the event of an alert should be part of your facility's emergency action plan. Keep in mind that contingency plans for caring for your own family, personal property, and pets should also be considered and detailed for various types of disasters and emergencies.

Good planning and well-rehearsed drills can alleviate some of the emotional stress when disaster strikes.

MOTHER NATURE

Weather

When "Mother Nature" strikes, her fury often involves severe weather and extreme temperatures. Two of her most damaging elements are wind and water. The most commonly occurring natural disasters in the United States over the last century have been convective storms (thunderstorms with lightning) and flooding (Statista, 2016). According to the National Weather Service website (2019), one's chances of being struck by lightning are only slightly better than winning a major lottery, approximately 1 in 1,222,000. Failure to evacuate flood prone areas however, especially entering flood waters in a motor vehicle, or remaining in a flooded area after a flood is an all-too-frequent cause of injury, infection, and death.

Safety tips for avoiding injury and death due to flooding:
"Don't drown, turn around!"
"Get to higher ground."

Flooding can occur within minutes during heavy rains or in areas with rapidly shifting or melting snow. Water in areas that are normally dry can have detrimental effects days, weeks, or months later. For this reason, it is important to assure that you have adequate insurance (even if you do not operate in a known flood plain), and that you have taken precautions to assure that important equipment, documents, and the people in your home and office are safeguarded in the event of a flood.

Wind can cause structural and property damage. Regular drills with a review of safety plans can minimize physical harm to people in the event of high winds. One of the most frequent consequences of high winds is downed power lines, particularly when wind and rain are involved. Because water and electricity can cause fatal consequences, it is important for you and your staff to know how to safely disconnect electrical service, or who to call to do so, in the event of a downed power line or other problem with your electrical service.

Earthquake

Earthquakes are a natural disaster that can happen without warning. While they can happen anywhere, they are more likely to happen in the United States along the west coast shorelines, in areas where volcanoes are present (including volcanic islands like Hawaii and Puerto Rico), and along continental fault lines (as in the Mississippi valley). There is no way to prevent an earthquake, and besides the structural damage they cause, their after-effects can include fires, tsunamis, landslides, sink holes, and avalanches.

Standard home and business insurance policies do not contain coverage for earthquake damage; it is always advisable to seek the advice of your insurance professional to assure coverage for your particular needs. If you are in an earthquake prone area, be sure you have secured heavy items and those that hang on walls. Be sure that all staff and patients present during an earthquake know to stay inside, away from doorways, and to cover their heads if possible. If they cannot get under a desk or table, where they can hold onto something with one hand and cover their head and neck with the other, have them to cover their head with their arms, holding their neck with both hands. This will stabilize their head and neck in the event of falling debris.

Patients utilizing canes should be assisted to get to the lowest possible position, cover, and hold on. Wheelchair or walker-assisted patients should not be moved. They should, if at all possible, lock their wheels, cover, and hold on to the nearest immobile object.

Staying safe during an earthquake involves these simple steps: DROP, COVER, and HOLD ON.

PANDEMIC

History of Pandemics

Perhaps the most significant of all natural phenomena, with broad and sometimes disaster-level consequences on society as a whole, is the pandemic. Nothing in human history has killed more human beings than disease-causing pathogens. Viruses, bacteria, and parasites over the millennia have been mass killers on a nearly immeasurable scale.

Plague

One of the earliest recorded pandemics was the Plague of Justinian (circa 541–590 AD). Over the following two centuries, two additional outbreaks of the same infectious bacterial disease transmitted by flea-infested rats killed an estimated 100 million people, roughly half the world's population at that time. The Black Death of the 14th century, likely caused by the same organism, *Yersinia pestis*, may have killed up to 200 million, and 20th-century smallpox, 300 million.

Influenza

In 1918, an influenza pandemic, referred to historically as the Spanish Flu, infected over 500 million people (1/3 of the world's population), and killed an estimated 50 million worldwide (CDC, 2020). Despite advances in science since the 1918 pandemic, and the invention of vaccines for seasonal influenza, the ever-changing virus continues to pose one of the world's greatest public health challenges. The emergence of a novel influenza strain as recently as 2009, (H1N1)pdm09, was first identified in a febrile eight-year old Californian and spanned the globe within three months; the outbreak began six months ahead of the traditional North American flu season. Dubbed "The Swine Flu," because of its genetic resemblance to swine influenza A, the virus infected 60.8 million people and killed an estimated 575,400 (Bean, 2020).

Seasonal influenza vaccines are updated and available months ahead of known respiratory seasons of the autumn and winter months in the United States, but the threat of another influenza pandemic is always present. As researchers are forced to "chase the mix," adapting and adjusting to the ever-changing virus, immunity is never a guarantee.

HIV

Prior to 2020, only one other virus in the last 100 years, human immunodeficiency virus (HIV), has reached pandemic proportions. Between 1981 when the first cases were reported, and 2005, 65 million infections and 25 million deaths occurred (CDC, 2006). By 2020, despite advances in treatment and post-exposure prophylaxis measures, HIV has killed an estimated 32 million people and infected 75 million, with new cases added daily (CDC, 2020).

COVID-19

On January 8, 2020, the Centers for Disease Control Health Alert Network (accessed from https://emergency.cdc.gov/han/) issued its first emergency preparedness and response bulletin providing an official concern for a reported cluster of pneumonia of unknown etiology in Wuhan City, Hubei Province, China. Epidemiological tracing linked the virus to the wet markets of Wuhan, where live animals including bats and swine (both known to be vectors for coronavirus) were routinely slaughtered upon purchase. Nine days later, the etiology had been identified as a novel coronavirus (2019-nCoV). Within three months, 3,012,484 confirmed cases in 185 countries, with 208,131 deaths were reported (Johns Hopkins, 2020). As of the time of this writing, the virus continues to be actively spreading in the United States.

The Centers for Disease Control in their April 19, 2020 Situation Summary on Coronavirus, defined a pandemic as "a global outbreak of disease. Pandemics happen when a new virus emerges to infect people and can spread between people sustainably. Because there is little to no pre-existing immunity against the new virus, it spreads worldwide" (CDC, 2020).

Pandemic Preparedness

There is no way to predict when or from where the next novel virus or mutant pathogen will arise. Preparation requires awareness of current infectious diseases, epidemiology, and the diligence to act when alerted of changing trends. Conditions can change rapidly in the early stages of any pandemic. Despite centuries of technological advances, medication and vaccine developments, diagnostic and treatment modalities, the best defenses against pandemics continue to be basic human actions. Handwashing, personal space (in the context of "social distancing"), and environmental disinfecting are still the only research-proven strategies to prevent the spread of disease.

Pandemic preparedness should be both personal- and public-focused. Education for individuals should highlight improving and maintaining strong immune systems. Ensuring a healthy diet, regular exercise, attaining normal weight, and keeping vaccines current are non-pharmacological approaches to personal wellness. As a healthcare provider, encouraging your patients to maintain clean home and work environments, stay home when sick, cover coughs and sneezes, and perform frequent handwashing using soap and water will help reduce the risk of infection.

Community-focused strategies for the public should include limiting face-to-face contacts whenever possible, maintaining personal space (6–10 feet is generally considered adequate). Advocating for and promoting flexible sick leave policies, telecommuting, and remote meetings is also advisable. Having pandemic-event policies in place and ready to implement quickly can lessen the impact of a pandemic on the community-at-large.

Healthcare providers may not have the ability to perform social distancing or face-to-face contact. Ensuring the proper use and disposal of personal protective equipment (PPE) will help reduce the risk to themselves and others. Preparation for pandemic should include PPE stocked at levels adequate to care for the anticipated workload. A 30-day supply of PPE for your current staff level is a good starting point.

General Planning for Natural Disasters

"You can't always predict, but you can prepare." Ready.gov

Assuring that you and your staff are educated in what to do in the event of a natural disaster can greatly mitigate risks and improve outcomes. General safety tips and good preparation include:

1. Have a plan and always be alert to weather, environmental conditions, and your general surroundings, as well as staying alert to current disease trends and CDC health alerts,
2. Prepare an emergency supply kit, including water, non-perishable foods, a whistle, flashlights, extra batteries, and first aid supplies to treat at least minor injuries, and a hand-crank weather radio,
3. Do regular risk reassessments and ensure active, engaged participation in all safety drills,
4. Coordinate efforts with local emergency response organizations,
5. Ensure your phones, internet access (and those of your staff members) have appropriate permissions set to receive EAS-broadcast messages.

Human Nature

Perhaps even more damaging than emergency situations caused by natural phenomenon and "Mother Nature," are those arising from both intentional actions and sometimes unintentional, nonetheless dangerous, human errors. As healthcare providers, our first duty is non maleficence, to do no harm. We uphold the values of benevolence and altruism. Sometimes our good natures can cloud our judgement and delay our preparedness, making us vulnerable to attacks by those who do not share our values or worldviews, or cherish human lives in the same ways we do.

Being aware and being prepared for human nature related events should be no less important than preparing for a natural disaster. In many ways, the plans are the same: assess the threat, plan for the unexpected, educate, communicate, and practice, in effort to mitigate (risk) as much as possible.

CYBER THREATS

Modern America is heavily dependent on computer-based technology. The cars we drive, the phones we carry, the charts we use to care for our patients, are predominantly computerized and electronic. Our dependence upon internet-based communication, computer interoperability, and cloud-based storage has become a matter of convenience that has made us vulnerable to a new kind of man-made disaster, once reserved for "hackers" looking to breech government files, can now stop your clinical workflow in its tracks and hold your entire healthcare system hostage for ransom: the cyberattack.

Cyberattacks are malicious attempts to access or damage a computer system and often lead to the loss of money, personal information, and can damage your reputation and safety, or the safety of others (FEMA, 2020). In healthcare, the most common cyberattacks occur through the use of ransomware, a type of malicious software designed to disable a computer system until a ransom is paid. Ransomware can spread quickly through an office or network system through email phishing schemes or unknowingly visiting an "infected" website.

The U.S. Department of Homeland Security is home to the Cybersecurity and Infrastructure Security Agency (CISA). As the nation's cyber-risk advisor, CISA publishes recommendations on preventing and defending against cyberattacks on its www.us-cert.gov website. This agency also coordinates with the Federal Bureau of Investigations and the Central Intelligence Agency to respond to reports of ransomware and to aid in recovery efforts (CISA, 2020).

To protect against the threat of ransomware, good planning, and common sense "Cyber-Safety" should be employed. This includes locking down or restricting permissions on work-related computers from unnecessary internet connections, installation privileges, disabling social media websites, regular software and operating system updates, frequent backups of data to a separate server or data drives that are then stored offline and off-site (CISA, 2020).

When it comes to cyber-security, just as it is with medical records and personal health information, the principle of "least privilege" should be consistently applied. System users should have the least amount of access as is necessary to perform their specified duties. Strong spam filters and configuring firewalls to block access to potential or known harmful IP addresses can also protect your clinic from a ransom situation. Recovery can be costly, both fiscally and mentally. This is why a well-trained computer specialist on your staff and emergency planning team can be a worthwhile investment.

CHEMICAL EMERGENCIES

Chemical emergencies involve agents in any form (solid, liquid, aerosol, or vapor) that are poisonous and have known toxic effects on living organisms or the environment. Currently the U.S. Centers for Disease Control lists 65 chemicals as potential poisons that may necessitate emergency intervention due to exposure. The list includes commonly known household cleaners and disinfectants such as ammonia and chlorine, chemicals used in medications such as digitalis and opioids, nicotine, as well as those agents associated with chemical warfare, such as mustard gas, ricin, cyanide, and sarin (CDC, 2020).

As a rural healthcare provider, emergencies involving chemicals are more likely to be minor and happen in your home or office due to everyday spills, splashes, or accidental inhalation, rather than from highly concentrated chemicals in your immediate environment. Chemical exposure can happen in three ways: inhalation, ingestion, or contact (American Red Cross, 2020). Exposure is not always known, as in the case of carbon monoxide. Maintaining up-to-date Safety Data Sheets, assuring safe storage and proper use of all on-site chemicals, managing spills, and disposing properly of chemical containers can reduce risks of harm.

While there are occasional reports of chemical leak incidents in hospitals, factories, and refineries, or spills from overturned transport containers on roads, rail- or water-ways, in the U.S., strict regulation and enforcement policies have limited the public's exposure to harmful chemicals. Numerous governmental agencies including the Environmental Protection Agency, the Food and Drug Administration, the Occupational Safety and Health Agency (OSHA), and the Consumer Product Safety Commission set strict standards on production, storage, disposal, safe-handling, transport, use of, and exposure to chemical products.

While chemical agents can pose significant risks to people, pets, and the environment, threats of attack or disaster by chemical agent are uncommon and unlikely. Chemical agents that pose the greatest risks are often: (1) difficult to produce in mass quantities, (2) difficult to deliver in lethal amounts, and (3) tend to dissipate readily in open air environments (FEMA, 2019). Exceptions to this "unlikely to harm" rule are opioids, including fentanyl and carfentanyl, and the chemicals mixed to produce illegal methamphetamines, including phosphine, iodine, hydrogen chloride, and various solvents.

A chemical attack could come without warning. Signs of chemical release would likely be sudden and severe, and include difficulty breathing, eye irritation, burning sensation in the airways, nausea, and problems with motor functions. Findings of dead birds, insects, or animals in the immediate area may also be indicative of a chemical agent release (FEMA, 2020).

Emergency readiness for a chemical emergency or attack focuses on adequate clean air and sheltering-in-place. If the chemical is inside a building where you are, get out as quickly as possible without going through the area of contamination. If the chemical is outside, move quickly to the closest building and close all doors and windows. If you are unable to get indoors, try to get upwind and as far away from the chemical as possible.

To prevent indoor contamination from the outside air, close all vents and turn off all fans and ventilation units. Be sure emergency supply kits include duct tape, scissors, and non-porous plastic to cover doors, windows, vents, or chimney dampers. Seal the room with plastic sheeting and duct tape until advised by authorities the threat has dissipated. Stay informed using a handheld radio, television, or cell phone if available.

RADIATION THREATS

Radiation-associated emergencies and disasters, while extremely rare, are extremely dangerous and can result in long-term health effects and death. For this reason, an understanding of the risks associated with radiation exposure and the proper emergency preparedness for a radiation event is crucial.

Nuclear Reactors

"Radiation injury in the general population due to accidents or incidents is a rare but remarkable event that merits serious study and planning in the health care system" (Cerezo, 2011). Outside of routine and diagnostic healthcare-related radiologic exposure, in the Unites States, harm to humans and the environment due to radiation is extremely rare. There are more than 90 nuclear reactors in the U.S., and the oldest in operation has been active for over 50 years. There has been one significant radiation leak from any of those reactors, in 1979, at Three Mile Island in Pennsylvania.

Nuclear Bombs

According to the Stockholm International Peace Research Institute Yearbook (SIPRI, 2019), at the start of 2019, nine independent nations possessed approximately 13,865 nuclear weapons; the U.S. and Russia account for 90% of those. Due to a lack of transparency and reliable information, the report cites the approximations as mere estimates of what likely exists, particularly in countries where policies to not comment on their nuclear arsenals have existed for decades; Israel is an example.

Strong foreign policies, tight security protocols, and swift military actions over decades have lessened the threats of long-range nuclear bomb attacks in the last half-century. Nuclear threats on a smaller scale, however, have increased, with the invention of less conventional and more mobile "mini-bombs," known as radiological dispersion devices.

Radiological Dispersion Devices (RDD)

RDDs combine the powers of a conventional explosive with radioactive materials. The technical ease of building a RDD, as compared to a nuclear bomb, makes them more appealing to terrorists. While generally less lethal, the scattered materials they deploy can result in dangerous amounts of radioactive materials and "fallout," which can take months to years to decontaminate.

Radiation Exposure Preparation

Radiation exposure requires the same air inhalation precautions as chemical emergency sheltering-in-place (see above). In addition, anyone exposed to radioactive material must undergo contact decontamination by removing clothing and shoes, showering thoroughly with soap and running water. Contaminated items should be bagged and isolated away from any living things.

Many communities have nuclear shelters. Blast shelters are designed to withstand the initial heat, fire, pressure, and radiation from a nuclear event, while fallout shelters are specifically designed to absorb the radiation given off by radioactive fallout particles (FEMA, 2020). Knowing if these shelters are available, how to access them, and how and where to shelter otherwise, should all be part of your radiation disaster plan.

BIOTERRORISM

The use of biologic warfare dates back to the 14th century BC, when the Hittites sent tularaemia-infected rams to their enemies. In the 1400s Spaniards mixed leprosy-tainted blood with wine and sold it to their French foes. In the 1700s, British soldiers passed out blankets from a smallpox ward to Native Americans, and 100 years later, Confederates sold clothing from yellow fever and smallpox patients to the Union soldiers during the American Civil War (Barras and Greub, 2014).

So while nothing new, the modern mechanisms of deployment of biologics have heightened the odds of mass casualties associated with bio-weapons. Threats and use of biological agents as weapons in the mid 1990s and early 2000s, along with the discovery of military stockpiles of bioweapons around the world, exposed civilian vulnerability to bioterrorism.

Many overt (meditated, announced, or otherwise "claimed") attacks have been carried out by those with religious, not military, motivations. Examples include the 1995 sarin gas deployment in a Tokyo subway by the religious cult known as Aum Shinrikyo, and the intentional contamination of salad bars with salmonella in various public restaurants in Oregon by the Rajneesh cult in 1984. Covert attacks using anthrax-contaminated letters in 2001 infected 22 Americans, and resulted in five deaths. The origin of the anthrax was traced to a U.S. Army laboratory at Fort Detrick, but the perpetrators were never apprehended. The anthrax letters reinvigorated the federal government's focus on preparedness for potential biological warfare.

Because attacks tend to be covert (unannounced and without known motive), healthcare providers must be able to quickly identify and report potential bioterrorism events within the populations they serve. The detection of unexplained illnesses with unusual fever, respiratory, skin, or gastrointestinal symptoms should be raise suspicion. Those which show rapid progression and dissemination, and those associated with clusters of patients in a single locale, particularly those effecting otherwise healthy populations, should raise concern and sound the alarm to public health officials. Any overt threats of attack should also be immediately reported to local and federal authorities.

There are four diseases primarily recognized with bioterrorism potential: anthrax, botulism, plague, and smallpox. Numerous others, including filoviruses (Ebola and Marburg hemorrhagic fever), arenaviruses (Lassa and Argentine fever), Q fever, brucellosis, ricin toxin, clostridium perfringens, staphylococcus enterotoxin B, and various food- and waterborne pathogens rank in the top two categories of highest priority (CDC, 2000).

Rural healthcare providers should maintain updated contact information and open lines of communication with local health departments and emergency services personnel to expedite the management of a bioterrorism or suspected bioterrorism event. Performing staff competency drills relating to site containment, proper selection and use of PPE, and assuring that all safety and personal protection equipment is in working order can mitigate the risk to clinic staff and others responding to patients in such an event.

All patients with acute illness of unknown origin should be cared for utilizing standard precautions along with the use of personal protective clothing, and equipment adequate for the mission based, upon the suspected organism. This may rapidly accelerate from gloves and gowns, up to and including self-contained air-purifying respirators. Until patients can be definitively diagnosed, extreme caution and the least possible contact with others should be exercised.

The National Institute for Occupational Safety and Health (NIOSH) regularly updates recommendations for the selection and use of respirators and protective clothing for healthcare workers and first responders. Their recommendations can be found on the CDC website and should be routinely reviewed by providers and staff.

Finally, proper decontamination of the care environment and providers, as well as the proper disposal of any contaminated (or potentially contaminated) equipment must be undertaken once the patient is removed from the clinic. Sheltering in place and protecting against exposure via thorough handwashing, wearing a facemask, and avoiding contact with others as much as possible until given further instructions by public health officials is advisable.

An adequate supply of bottled water is recommended, as many biological agents can contaminate not only air, but water and agricultural products in the immediate area.

ACTIVE SHOOTER

Active shooters can create disasters in any setting. This section will target healthcare settings. Violence against healthcare workers is a growing epidemic in the United States. Studies show that up to 75 percent of the 25,000 incidents of workplace assaults annually occur in healthcare settings (Stephens, 2019). While the majority of cases involve verbal or physical abuse, the most serious forms of workplace violence are those incidents involving an active shooter.

According to the Federal Bureau of Investigation, there were 160 healthcare-related active shooter incidents between 2000 and 2013, with 6.4 incidents per year during the first six years and 16.4 per year during the second six years, mimicking a national trend of increased gun-related violence (Stringer, 2018). In most of these cases, the shooters were not patients, but rather individuals with a previous or current relationship with an employee or provider, often of a romantic nature.

Active shooter training for yourself and all staff members should become a routine on-boarding practice, with drills updated at least annually. Being informed, having a plan of action, including coordinating efforts with security personnel and local law enforcement, is an integral part of any plan to ensure safety in the event of an active shooter emergency.

Communication skills, particularly recognizing the warning signs of potential dangers, can mitigate potential risks. Verbal threats, unusual behaviors, and weapon-carrying individuals should be immediately reported and managed per office policy. Being well-informed of any social concerns expressed by your staff members (especially where suspicion of domestic violence exists) can also help to successfully thwart an on-site incident by intervening early with notification to authorities as necessary. Gathering information and providing rapid updates to your staff can heighten their awareness, improve response times, and solidify the plan of action in a threatening situation.

Everyone on staff should be included in planning and participating in safety drills, to assure they understand what to do if confronted with an active shooter situation. These drills should include their responsibilities for the management of any patients present, particularly those with disabilities, mobility problems, or other functional needs.

In active shooter survival training, your staff will learn the three key activities to survival: RUN, HIDE, and FIGHT (Federal Emergency Management Agency, 2019):

- "RUN!" The top priority in an active shooter situation is to get away from the shooter as quickly as possible. Staff members should verbally identify at least two escape routes from their usual position within the work environment. Once out of the vicinity, they should warn and prevent anyone outside from entering the area, and notify 911 immediately, including details about the shooter, location, and weapons involved.

- "HIDE!" In the event that escape is not possible, every staff member should be able to demonstrate how and where they would hide from a shooter. Out of sight, behind locked doors (and one other barrier whenever possible), without light or noise is recommended. Staff should be instructed to remain in place until a member of law enforcement clears them to come out of hiding. It is important to remember that hiding separately, not in groups, can lessen morbidity and mortality and make it more difficult for a shooter to do harm.

Hiding in groups is NOT recommended.

While a cell phone can be used to send an alert, silent texting, not talking is recommended. Cell phone vibration and key clicks should always be turned off in active shooter situations. Most modern cell phones are equipped with shortcut keys for emergency calling, and while not recommended from a hiding place, could be used after escape or if the caller is certain they cannot be seen or heard while making the call.

- "FIGHT!" As an absolute last resort, be prepared to inflict severe or lethal injury on the shooter. If you must fight, commit fully to acting as aggressively as possible against the shooter. Improvise whatever makeshift weapons (chairs, shelving, fire extinguishers, scissors, aerosols, and books as examples) you can to distract or disarm the shooter and defend yourself. An emergency call to 911, leaving the phone on a stable surface, with the line open and the microphone function enabled would be advisable, as long as it does not delay action against the shooter or further increase the risk for harm to anyone involved.

Once the shooter has been detained by law enforcement and is no longer a threat, it is important to find a way to let the authorities know if you (or other staff members) are still present on the scene. A sign in a window, a text message or call to a team leader, or a loud, but non-threatening verbal shout for help from your position is best. If exiting the building after law enforcement has arrived, be sure to keep your hands clear and visible, and ask for help as you exit. Get to safety as quickly as possible.

A well-prepared staff with well-rehearsed, enacted response may lessen the deleterious outcomes of an active shooter situation.

MAKING PROGRESS

We've come a long way as a nation since the air raid drills of the early last century. America's disaster preparedness is now a much more coordinated effort, from the federal to the local level. While storms, floods, drought, climate change, earthquakes, and fires are still concerning and demand our attention, these threats often pale in comparison to the silent (but potentially deadly) risks of our modern world.

At the same time, modern technology and our ability to be better "connected" has proven advantageous in our plight to be better prepared for emergencies and disasters. Modern cell phones, social media, satellite and computer-based communication systems, and buried fiber-optics have improved our ability to sound the alarms of impending danger. Disaster planning resources are now readily available from any computer or cell phone from reliable resources such as FEMA, the CDC, and state Departments of Public Health via the internet.

Every community should have an emergency planning committee, even if only an informal network of first responders or other volunteers, which is often the case in rural areas. Use a collaborative approach in your participation with these groups. Teamwork and cooperation among its emergency management members will benefit the entire community in the event of a disaster.

Today's disasters and emergencies require sophisticated, coordinated efforts at multiple levels. Whether the threat is silent—as in a cybersecurity breach that disables your charting, finance, or communications systems—or as loud as tornado or industrial explosion that rocks your community, planning, practice, and good communication will help improve your responses and mitigate your risk. As a rural healthcare provider, being prepared for a disaster and for life in the days and weeks following a disaster will serve you and your patients well. There is no need to feel as helpless a child under a desk with a textbook over his head!

CONCLUSION

Planet earth, its weather, natural phenomena, and inhabitants can at times be completely unpredictable. Disasters can challenge even the most seasoned among us. The tools needed to "weather the storm," or "win the war," are those of any good healthcare provider: sharp assessment skills, critical thinking, effective communication, and the ability (and willingness) to use those skills to the benefit of others.

Effective emergency and disaster planning requires an exploration of various "what if" scenarios, accompanied by the coordination and alignment of available resources within well-defined priorities. As a healthcare provider, you will be looked to as a leader—if not THE leader—in moments of crisis. Embracing that role now will help you better prepare for later, and hopefully long before disaster strikes.

Take the time to delineate team duties, assure adequate supplies are in stock, and that all emergency kits and equipment are ready and functional. Take the time necessary to practice (even low probability) high-risk scenarios. By doing so, you will likely mitigate future risks and potentially, save lives. You'll be "safe, not sorry!"

REFERENCES

Barras, V. and G. Greub. (2014). History of biological warfare and bioterrorism. *Clinical Microbiology and Infection, 20*(6), 497–502.

Bean, M. 2020. A look back at swine flu: 8 facts about the world's last pandemic in 2009. Becker's Hospital Review, March 12, 2020. Accessed online at https://www.beckershopsitalreview.com/public-health/swine-flu-8-facts-about-the-world-slast-pandemic-in-2009.html.

Centers for Disease Control. (2000). Biological and chemical terrorism: strategic plan for preparedness and response. Recommendations of the CDC Strategic Planning Workgroup. *Morbidity and Mortality Weekly Report, 49*(RR04); 1–14.

Centers for Disease Control. (2006). The global HIV/AIDS pandemic, 2006. *Morbidity and Mortality Weekly Review, 55*(31); 841–844.

Centers for Disease Control. 2010. The 2009 H1N1 pandemic: summary highlights, April 2009–April 2010. Accessed online at https://www.cdc.gov/h1n1flu/cdcresponse.htm.

Centers for Disease Control. 2020. Emergency preparedness and response. US Department of Health and Human Services. Accessed online March 31, 2020 at https://emergency.cdc.gov/agent/agentlistchem.asp#o.

Cerezo, L. (2011). Radiation accidents and incidents. What do we know about the medical management of acute radiation syndrome? *Reports of Practical Oncology and Radiotherapy, 16*(4); 119–122.

City of Houston. (2012). Run Hide Fight. Surviving an active shooter event. Accessed online 04/19/2020 at https://youtu.be/5VcSwejU2D0.

Cowan, D. and J. Kuenster. (1998). *To sleep with the angels: The story of a fire*. Ivan R. Dee: Chicago, IL.

Cybersecurity and Infrastructure Security Agency. 2020. Ransomware. Accessed online 04/23/2020 at https://us-cert.gov/Ransomware.

Federal Bureau of Investigations. (2018). Active shooter incidents in the United States in 2018. A report of the Advanced Law Enforcement Rapid Response Training (ALERRT) Center at Texas State University and the Federal Bureau of Investigation. U.S. Department of Justice, Washington, D.C. 2018.

Federal Emergency Management Administration. (2019). We Are FEMA: Helping people before, during and after Disasters, 3rd ed. FEMA No FP112-01, catalog number 10314-1. United Stated Department of Homeland Security.

Federal Emergency Management Administration. 2020. Integrated public alert and warning system. Accessed online 04/19/2020 at http://fema.gov/integrated-public-alert-warning-system.

Johns Hopkins. (2020). Johns Hopkins Coronavirus Resource Center, accessed 4/27/2020, online at https://coronavirus.jhu.edu/map.html.

National Weather Service. (2019). Odds of becoming a lightning victim. Accessed online 4/19/2020 at https://www.weather.gov/safety/lighning-odds/.

Springer. (2018, April 19). Rapid rise in mass school shootings in the United States, study shows: Researchers call for action to address worrying increase in the number of mass school shootings in past two decades. *Science Daily.* Retrieved April 23, 2020 from www.sciencedaily.com/releases/2018/04/180419131025.htm.

Statista. (2016). Natural disasters in the U.S. 1900–2016, by type. Accessed online 04/19/2020 at https://www.statista.com/statistics/2365004/number-of-natural-disaster-in-the-us-by-type/.

Stephens, W. (2019). Violence against healthcare workers: A rising epidemic. *American Journal of Managed Care*, In Focus Blog, May 12, 2019. Accessed online at https://www.ajmc.com/focus-of-the-week/violence-against-healthcare-workers-a-rising-epidemic.

Stringer, H. (2018). Hospital shooting rates bump up need for active shooter drills: Nurses learn how to respond to open gunfire situations. Nurse.com accessed online at http://resources.nurse.com/hospital-shooting-rates-active-shooter-drills.

The American National Red Cross. (2020). Chemical emergency preparedness. Accessed online, 4/23/2020 at https://www.redcross.org/get-help/how-to-prepare-for-emergencies/types-of-emergencies/chemical-emergency.html.

World Health Organization. (2009). Whole-of-society pandemic readiness: WHO guidelines for pandemic preparedness and response in the non-health sector. WHO Press: Geneva, Switzerland.

CHAPTER 6

Healthcare for Older Adults Living in Rural America

Ruth McCaffrey

Objectives:

1. Identify specific barriers and challenges for older adults living in rural areas.
2. List evidence-based programs that can assist in overcoming these barriers and challenges.
3. Discuss how nurses are able to provide person-centered care for older adults in rural areas.

Discussion Questions:

1. List the barriers faced by rural older adults that are not barriers in urban areas. Describe how these barriers impact the health and well-being of rural older adults.
2. Discuss the issue of care giving for older rural adults. Who is most involved in care giving, what struggles do these care givers face? Why are there fewer organizations to assist in caring for older adults in rural areas?
3. What is care coordination and why is it so important for rural older adults. Name three methods that care coordination is being accomplished. How could these methods be improved? What is the nursing role in these organizations?

INTRODUCTION

Aging throughout the United States

The population of the United States is aging and the number of older adults in our society is growing as life expectancy lengthens (US Census, 2017). The

Administration on Aging (2015) found that in 2014, 14.5% of the population, or 1 in 7 people in the United States, were older than age 65. The U.S. Census Bureau speculates that this number will continue to rise until by 2020, 17.8% of the U.S, population is older than age 65 (Ortman, Velkoff and Hogan, 2014). It is estimated that each day, 10,000 baby boomers—those people born in the years following World War II—retire and begin receiving Medicare and Social Security benefits (Insured Retirement Institute, 2016). This number represents about 33% of the U.S. workforce. A child born in 2014 will live an average of 30 years longer than a child born in 1900. In 2015, 70% of men and 45% of women older than age 65 were married; 35% of women are widowed, and 20% either single never married or are divorced. Those older adults, 85 years of age and older, in the United States population are the fastest-growing cohort in the country and this group is projected to rise from 5.8 million today to 19 million in 2050 (U.S. Census Bureau, 2017).

Not only are the numbers of older adults continuing to increase, but the cost of providing care to older adults escalates yearly, as well (Bahler *et al.*, 2015). Older adults have different and unique social, emotional, and physical needs compared to younger adults. The biggest struggles for all older adults is to remain independent as they age and live overall healthy lives. Healthy People was published in 2014, continues to be updated, and specifically addressed the most important issues in caring for older adults in the following objectives:

- Person-Centered Care planning that includes caregivers and families
- Quality measures of care and monitoring of health conditions in older adults
- Fair pay and compensation standards for formal and informal care givers
- Minimum levels of geriatric training for all health professionals
- Enhanced data on certain subpopulations of older adults including those in rural areas (HHS, 2014).

The normal aging process is accompanied by numerous physiological changes. Even in the absence of disease, these physiological changes increase the older adults' vulnerability to morbidity and mortality (Sadana and Michel, 2019). Many of these alterations involve decline in functional reserves with a reduced physiological response to stressors. For example, when older adults experience a physical stressor such as infection, their immune response is slower and less effective than that of a younger person (Sadana and Michel, 2019). Normal age-related changes can adversely impact health and functionality and require corrective strategies to adapt to the changes (Ferrante, Pisani, and Murphy, 2015). Too often the older adult or family members incorrectly accept the individual's decline in functionality as inevitable. For example, they may consider confusion and cognitive decline as normal forgetfulness in old age. Many people refer to having "senior moments" that may be just common forgetting or may signal cognitive decline which is not a normal part of aging.

The Healthcare Effectiveness Data and Information Set (HEDIS) is a tool used by more than 90% of healthcare plans in the United States to measure performance in hospital and office settings for adults over 65. Medicare and other insurers use HEDIS requirements as a basis for payment. The 2017 HEDIS measurements for older adults include the following measures as essential in providing quality healthcare:

- Annual measurement of body mass index (BMI)
- Annual review and discussion of advanced care planning
- Review of all health records, including medication reconciliation upon care transition from hospital, rehabilitation center, or nursing home to home
- Annual medication reconciliation with educational review
- Annual review of medications that cause delirium or increase dementia (Luskin *et al.*, 2017).

Older adults are more likely to develop certain types of health conditions that are related to aging rather than to any specific disease process. These have been grouped and are referred to as geriatric syndromes. Understanding how to assess older adults for these syndromes and effectively Table 6.1 provides a list and short explanation of geriatric syndromes.

Another general consideration for all older adults that should be addressed by healthcare providers is End-of-Life decision making. Older adults from different ethnic and cultural backgrounds differ in what they consider important at the end of their lives. In order to provide patient-centered care providers should explore end-of-life wishes and be sure they are discussed with family members to avoid stress and frustration at the time life is ending. Healthcare providers should know state and federal laws and institutional policies regarding living

TABLE 6.1. Geriatric Syndrome.

Syndrome	Explanation
Incontinence	Acute or reversible or chronic—may be due to infection, atrophic vaginitis, delirium, psychological disorder, reduced mobility, excessive urine output, stool impaction and medications
Falls	Disturbances in sleep can contribute to falls, injuries and other health problems—Requires fall risk assessment
Cognitive Impairment	Chronic debilitating decline, loss of personality & independence—requires neurologic & laboratory evaluation—long term care and end of life planning
Frailty	Overarching geriatric syndrome increases impact of physical stress during acute medical illness or surgery—evidenced by unintentional weight loss, self-reported exhaustion, weakness (decline in grip strength), slow walking speed, low physical activity

Carlson, Merel, and Yukawa, 2015.

wills, durable power of attorney, and procedures for refusal of extraordinary measures, such as resuscitation and initiation of life support. Effective care for dying patients usually involves a team of caregivers including professionals, family members, friends, clergy, and others (Romo *et al.*, 2016).

Many older adults and their families turn to palliative care when chronic illness becomes difficult to manage (Chilton, 2019). Palliative care provides supportive medical, social, emotional, and spiritual services to patients and their caregivers. The services are provided relying on the combined knowledge and skill of interdisciplinary teams of professionals. Palliative care provides comfort, care, and a support system to both the family and patient, integrating the psychological and spiritual aspects of patient care, throughout the trajectory of illness, from the time of diagnosis until death, and encompasses end-of-life care. This includes offering help to bereaved family members after the death of a loved one. The National Consensus Project (NCP) was created through Stanford University School of Medicine (NCP, 2009). This project created a group for quality palliative care, and outlines the main goal of palliative care as the prevention and relief of suffering and the ability to support the best possible quality of life for patients and their families, regardless of the stage of the disease or the need for other therapies (NCP, 2009). The Consensus Project outlines palliative care as being delivered concurrently with life-prolonging therapies or as the main focus of care. Leadership, collaboration, coordination, and communication are key elements for effective integration of these disciplines and services (NCP, 2009), Hospice and palliative care are similar with hospice caring only for people at the very end of life while palliative care is throughout the illness process. Both hospice and palliative care are growing in popularity in the United States, in part due to the overall aging of the population.

AGING IN RURAL AMERICA

While there are many similarities between rural and urban older adults related to health care and quality of life there are also important differences that require different types of practice and attention. Population decline and aging are challenges that often face communities across the rural United States. Over recent decades, rural areas in the U.S. have seen changes in the level of aging adults related to younger adults. This is due to the movement of young adults and their children toward urban areas and the remaining of older populations and aging in place of populations left behind. For example, about two-thirds of rural communities have experienced an overall decline in population and rise in median age since 2010 (Thiede *et al.*, 2016). In rural areas of the United States, 15% of the population (about 50 million people) is over 65, as opposed to 12% in urban centers. One quarter of older Americans live in a small town or other rural area (American Society on Aging, 2016). As the entire population of the United States ages, older adults in rural areas are generally poorer, have higher levels of chronic disease, and have a dwindling supply of healthcare providers, compared to their peers in urban communities (Jaffe, 2015). Ten percent of rural elders live in poverty, rural elders account for 25% of Medicare and 30% of these elders are duel eligible for Medicare and Medicaid (US Department of Health and Human Services, 2015). In addition their support system is shrinking because many younger family members seek schooling and improved job opportunities in urban areas. The rural elderly population often does not want to leave communities in which they have lived all of their lives where they have friends and churches that know them. In addition, living in urban areas tends to be more expensive for those living on retirement incomes.

In a new study from the CDC older rural people have a higher burden of chronic disease and a higher rate of preventable death (CDC, 2017). Preventable deaths are categorized as those deaths that may have been prevented through health promotion activities. Among older rural adults, diseases such as stroke, heart disease, diabetes, and cancer could have been prevented with nutrition programs, smoking cessation programs, and weight management. These types of programs are more readily available in urban areas due to lack of transportation barriers and costs (Rural Health Hub, 2018).

Health promotion and disease prevention are a focus of nursing practice. This is more important in rural communities with fewer resources and funding. Nurses are charged with enabling people to increase control over and improve their health through patient-centered, innovative programs. Health promotion particularly in rural settings moves beyond individual behavior towards social determinants of health and environmental factors that can put barriers in the way of health. Social determinants of health are the economic, social, cultural, and political conditions in which people are born, grow, and live that affect health status. Modifiable risk behaviors include, for example, tobacco use, poor eating habits, and lack of physical activity, which contribute to the development of chronic disease.

Demographic trends such as aging rarely reverse course quickly therefore the trend of rural communities to see increases in percentages of older adults including those older old or over 85 years of age will persist. This trend will continue to be a challenge to community development in rural America for the foreseeable future (Thiede *et al.*, 2016). Elders in rural America have difficulty with obtaining the services they need, obtaining long-term care, and home-based services. In home health, long distances between clients (windshield time) increases the amount of time the home health nurse needs to see the same number as urban nurses. Care coordination is a difficult aspect for elder health in rural areas (US Department of Health and Human Services, 2015).

Patterns of rural–urban differences in elderly patient health experiences vary by race, ethnicity, and coverage type for older adults with Medicare (Center for Medicare Services, 2018). Healthcare effectiveness data and information set

(HEDIS) collects information from medical records and other data on people in Medicare advantage plans. Consumer Assessment of Healthcare Providers and Systems (CAHPS) data for Medicare beneficiaries reenrolled in fee-for-service Medicare and managed care plans collects data to measure the quality of care that Medicare patients receive. CAHPS data measures patient experience with healthcare provided, including getting the care they needed, how quickly care was provided, and how well did healthcare providers communicate. In an overall look at care received 18 of 33 rural patients received worse care on the HEDIS and CAHPS measures than urban residents. This report by the Center for Medicare Services (CMS.gov, 2018) determined that rural residents regardless of ethnicity received worse care than those in urban areas. They suggest that research is needed to understand whether this pattern reflects poorer dissemination of clinical practice guidelines to rural areas, poorer translation of those guidelines into practice, or some other cause. The findings of this report also identify that rural blacks receiving Medicare report notably worse patient experiences, and that research is needed on how to address this situation.

Some specific topics that are at the forefront of rural health for the elderly include:

- Rural geriatric palliative/end-of-life hospice care
- Grief and bereavement in the rural geriatric population
- Healthcare access and the uses of technology in this setting
- Educational and training programs for healthcare professionals on rural health topics.
- Rural primary care, prevention and screening for the elderly
- Home health and long-term care in rural environments
- Mental health and cognition issues of the rural elderly
- Nutrition for the rural elderly (Stanford University Reference Database)
- Transportation to medical appointments and grocery shopping
- Housing quality and affordability, including how to pay for needed repairs and modifications

Each of these issues presents an opportunity for nurses to overcome barriers and initiate novel methods for providing care to older adults in rural areas (Rural Health Information Hub, 2017).

Disparities in care faced by rural older adults are greatly affected by health provider shortages. In fact two-thirds of health professional shortage areas are in rural communities. This may get worse if immigration policies make it more difficult for foreign physicians to come to the United States (American Society on Aging, 2016). Rural hospitals are closing at higher rates than those in urban areas. This causes rural older adults to have less access to emergency rooms, specialists, dialysis, and primary care. Another disparity experienced by rural older adults is the opioid crisis. Opioid addiction hits rural elders in a different manner because in addition to individual older adult addiction, the opioid epidemic ravages families and turns grandparents into emergency caregivers (Benson and Aldrich, 2018). Other disparities include decreases in government spending for rural America in food assistance, housing supports and cuts to Medicare and funding for telehealth, rural hospital outreach, mental health, emergency preparedness, and chronic disease management (American Society on Aging, 2016).

Based on this information Baernholdt, Van, Hinton, Rose, and Mattsos (2012) reviewed quality of life measures in rural community dwelling older adults. In this study they found that these elders had lower overall quality of life than urban counterparts. This reduction in quality of life (QOL) occurred in three dimensions (Health-related QOL, Social Function, and emotional well-being). The lower scores on social functioning on QOL measures in rural areas measured in this study suggest that rural older adults may suffer from social isolation.

The CDC has determined that social factors are often magnified for older adults in rural areas because of lack of transportation and fewer integrated social services. One of the social problems that occur for older rural residents results is social isolation and loneliness. While elders (especially men) living in rural areas have a reputation for being stoic and fiercely independent, they often are challenged with living a socially isolated and lonely life (Hudson, 2018). While technology can improve social isolation, a study by Kaye (2017) found that being connected to others via the internet should not take the place of other types of physical connection. In this work Kaye reviewed a student-led visitation program, a wellness program, a program setting up garden beds in a low-income rural community, and a senior companion as program successful in reducing isolation and loneliness among older adults in rural areas. Some of the solutions for loneliness and isolation include screening for isolation among seniors, having providers of all types connect seniors with local social support groups, establish volunteer programs, elevate the discussion to a public policy issues, include social isolation to the determinants of health, develop respite services for caregivers, connect seniors through the internet to support groups and local services (Henning-Smith and Lahr, 2018).

One of the cornerstones of the rural population is self-reliance. In that regard, health beliefs are often based on what a person can do for themselves, what their family believes should be done, and the folk healing practices of their ancestors. These health beliefs play a role in how rural dwellers perceive their health and what treatments are sought. Health beliefs are defined as those convictions that influence health behaviors and ideas that people have about their own health and how health affects quality of life (Mosby, 2009). An example of the importance of health beliefs related to rural health, many rural areas older adults face barriers to treatment for depression because they feel that they should not "need" help and should fix problems themselves (Brennes, Danhauer, Lyles, Hogan and Miller, 2016). If they do need help, they often turn to church, neighbors, and family who are not able to supply the assistance that would reduce their depressive symptoms. That is why suicide rates for adults are higher in rural than in urban communities regardless of the method used. Rural–urban disparities appear to be increasing over time (Kegler, Stone and Holland, 2017).

Functional disability, the number of physical illnesses, and being a burden to family members were shown to be associated with suicidal behaviors in rural older adults (Fassberg, Cheung, Canetto, Erlangsen, Lapierre and Lindner, 2015). Nestadt, Triplett, Fowler, and Mojtabai (2017) performed a retrospective analysis on over 6,000 older adult suicide victims from 2003–2015. They found that in rural areas the male use of firearms increases suicide risk in these areas. A conclusion drawn by another groups of researchers (Koo, Kolves, and Leo, 2017) was that acceptability, availability, and lethality are important factors impacting choice of means of those committing suicide and that these factors should be considered when designing suicide prevention activities in older adults.

CAREGIVERS

One of the biggest challenges in providing care for seniors in rural areas is how to obtain, retain, and care for caregivers for rural elders. Family caregiving in the United States today is emerging as a major policy issue. Over $300 billion per year is the estimated economic value placed on the care provided by family and friends for older adults with chronic health conditions and disabilities (Arno, 2006). More than one in five adults, or 44.4 million people, in the U.S. provide unpaid care to an older adult family member (National Alliance for Caregiving and AARP, 2004).

Caregiving in rural areas has an additional unique challenge. Older Americans living in rural areas have fewer financial resources, health and social services, public transportation options, and fewer younger people compared with urban counterparts. There are greater distances between older adults in rural areas and services they require. Rural caregivers and care recipients not only have limited access to primary and emergency healthcare services, but also when those services are available it is more difficult to get to them. In a pilot program in Gainesville, Florida, Uber is being contracted to transport elders for care services, doctor visits, and trips to the emergency department.

Demographic information for rural family caregivers includes:

- Just over 25% of rural caregivers live in the same household as the care recipient; 60% live within a one-hour drive; 4% live between a one- and two-hour drive away; and 11% live more than a two-hour drive away.
- Forty-one percent of rural caregivers have children or grandchildren living with them.

- Fourteen percent of rural caregivers have provided care for 10 years or more, about 45% between 1 to 9 years, 18% between 6 months to one year, and about 23% for less than 6 months.
- Rural caregivers spend an average of 21 hours per week caregiving, but 19% of them spend more than 40 hours per week caregiving.
- Fourteen percent of rural caregivers and nearly 20% of their care recipients are veterans. (From Easter Seals Disability Services, 2006).

Demographic information for those receiving care in rural areas includes:

- Seventy percent of the rural care recipients were women and 30% were men.
- Twenty percent of the rural care recipients were under 50 years of age and 80% were 50 and over, with 27% of the total between ages 75 and 84.
- Nearly 74% of the rural care recipients lived in their own homes.
- Twenty-nine percent of the rural care recipients were married, 48% widowed, 13% single, and 10% divorced or separated.
- Rural caregivers themselves report that 13% of their rural care recipients' main problems or illnesses were the "results of old age", 8% of diabetes, 7% of cancer, and 7% of Alzheimer's/dementia (Easter Seals Disability Services, 2006).

One of the positive notes for rural elders and their families is that caregivers in rural areas feel stronger and less oppressed than urban family members. In a study completed by Crouch, Probst, and Bennett (2017), 1,352 rural caregivers were examined via survey and reported lower socioeconomic status than urban caregivers (measured by income, education, and employment), suggesting greater likelihood of caregiver strain. The researchers found that rural caregivers reported fewer instances of poor health than their urban counterparts. These findings may indicate differing cultural values in rural and urban respondents, rather than better health among rural caregivers. Understanding the characteristics of rural caregivers may help policymakers target interventions.

In a survey by Kaplan (2016) rural older adults have a higher level of participation than other groups. For rural elderly the religious community was the largest source of social support outside of the family. Religion correlates with improved physical and mental health among both older adults and caregivers for these older adults. These researchers found the following psychological benefits of those who participate in religion:

- A positive and hopeful attitude about life and illness, which predicts improved health outcomes and lower mortality rates
- A sense of meaning and purpose in life, which affects health behaviors and social and family relationships
- A greater ability to cope with illness and disability/less likely to have depression.

Religious issues can also be harmful to an older adult or their caregivers. Religious devotion can promote excessive guilt, inflexibility, and anxiety. Some religious groups discourage mental and physical healthcare including blood transfusions, insulin therapy, and treatment for infections and substitute religious rituals such as praying and chanting for these problems.

When providing medical care for rural older adults, the practitioner should obtain a spiritual history that determines the person's spiritual beliefs and how these beliefs influence care and health choices. This should be done for both the caregiver and care receiver to get a deeper understanding of the role of religious devotion in their lives. If there are any of the negative aspects of religion such as guilt, the healthcare provider can work with that caregiver or receiver to resolve those feelings and move toward a healthy relationship between the caregiver and care receiver.

INTEGRATING CARE FOR OLDER ADULTS IN RURAL COMMUNITIES

Rural adults over 65 years of age account for 25 percent of the Medicare population and 30 percent of those on Medicare are dual eligible for Medicare and Medicaid (Griffin and Coburn, 2014). The barriers faced by older adults when living in rural areas includes medical issues and social, societal, and community barriers. The goal for elders in rural communities and for those in healthcare should be to provide needed services to those older adults in rural areas to allow them to remain healthy and independent as long as possible and when that is no longer possible to provide a safe and secure environment for them to meet their health needs. This means that rural elders need more than medical providers, for example care providers, and services such as meals on wheels, health aides to assist with activities of daily living, and assistance with executive activities of daily living such as banking and bill paying. Caring for rural elders at the community level requires a team approach, building relationships with and between providers, and adapting cultures and services. If services are integrated without including current delivery systems, resistance may be experienced and duplication of services could waste precious time and resources. One way to maximize the ability to provide needed social services to rural older adults and keep costs under control is through care coordination.

CARE COORDINATION

Care coordination is intended to maximize the value of care being delivered and ensure that the patient's needs and preferences are known and addressed

(AHRQ, 2017). The goal of care coordination is to provide safe and effective care by sharing pertinent information among all providers involved with the patient in order to reduce duplication and the addition of unneeded services. This is more essential in rural areas given the increased poverty, lack of sufficient providers, and transportation issues and can be difficult because current healthcare systems are often disjointed, and processes vary among primary sites and specialty sites. Older patients can be unclear about why they are being referred to a specialist. Specialists do not always receive a clear reason for the referral and what tests have been completed and primary care providers do not always receive a report from the specialist on what happened at the referral visit. Many elders have multiple chronic conditions that are physical, mental, and cognitive. Rural residents tend to have many of the social and medical vulnerabilities that make the need for integrated care management so important. Sixty-nine percent of adults turning 65 will need some form of long-term care services at some point and home and community-based services are costly and complex to manage. Working in a coordinated manner to provide services for all aspects of health problems and support for in home care providers can improve the overall health of the community, provide improved health outcomes for each elder, and reduce funding needs. Care coordination can include the following activities:

- Establishing accountability and agreeing on responsibility
- Communicating and sharing knowledge
- Helping with transitions of care (home to hospital, hospital to nursing home, home to hospice care, etc.)
- Assessing patient needs and goals
- Creating a proactive care plan
- Monitoring and follow-up, including responding to changes in patients' needs
- Supporting patients' self-management goals
- Linking to community resources
- Working to align resources with patient and population needs.

Current methods used to provide care coordination include case management, patient-centered medical homes, and accountable care organizations. While these types of care coordination are not unique to older adults nor to those in rural areas, they are very helpful to these groups because of the complexity of health and well-being in older adults.

Case management is a collaborative process of assessment, planning, facilitation, care coordination, evaluation, and advocacy to meet the needs of individuals and families (Institute for Social and Economic Development, 2017). Case management uses communication, knowledge of resources and a focus on patient-centered care to complete goals such as patient safety, quality of care, and cost-effective outcomes. Case managers can be para-professionals and work with community resources to be a primary partner in patient care that is focused on patient and family choice.

The patient-centered medical home (PCMH) can transform primary care to meet extended needs of patients and families. The medical home encompasses five functions and attributes. Comprehensive care means that the PCMH meets the majority of the patient's physical and mental healthcare needs as well as including acute care, chronic care, prevention and wellness care. The team in a PCMH may include physicians, advanced practice nurses, physicians' assistants, nurses, pharmacists, nutritionists, social workers, and educators. The PCMH is patient centered and builds a relationship and is supportive of the person. It allows the patient to make their own choices based on education and information provided by the team members. The PCMH also provides coordinated care and provides assistance with transitions between levels of care. A PCMH delivers accessible services with shorter waiting times for urgent needs which is especially important in rural areas. Accessible services may be delivered based on home medical visits when required. Finally, the PCMH demonstrates a commitment to quality care and ongoing improvement. All of these attributes of the PCMH could directly affect the barriers to health and well-being for older rural dwelling adults.

One of the aspects of the Affordable Care Act of 2010 was the development of Accountable Care Organizations. These are a group of doctors, specialists, hospitals, and other healthcare providers who come together with a common goal of delivering coordinated care to Medicare patients. Using data analytics and population health management Accountable Care Organizations aim to provide the right care and the right time and avoid duplication of services, reduce healthcare costs while reducing medical errors. The Accountable Care Organization is financially successful when it meets the needs of patients by providing patient-centered care, improves patient outcomes, and saves money by providing early intervention, health promotion and disease prevention activities, and timely intervention for acute and chronic illnesses. With these goals in mind for rural based ACOs, providing basic services such as transportation, home health services, education in areas such as medication, exercise, diet and safety, are enfolded along with medical and specialist care. Currently there are 544 rural health clinics that have joined together with ACOs around the country. While costs rose per patient visit for the first two years compared to Rural Health Clinics not participating in ACOs the overall patient satisfaction and met needs of rural elders was improved. After the first two years of ACO implementation costs per visits were lower than those for rural health clinics not enrolled in ACO programs (Hofler and Ortiz, 2016). In a later review 8 of the 11 rural ACOs participating in the Advanced Payment Program (APP) providing comprehensive care for older adults in rural areas and garnered savings for Medicare (Nattinger, Mueller, Ulrich, and Zhu, 2016).

CONCLUSION

Healthcare for older adults in rural areas poses challenges that are different from those faced by elders in urban areas. The overall goal for older adults in rural areas is to remain in their homes and continue to be independent. The support systems that allow this to happen may be missing in many rural areas and older adults struggle to get their needs met. The main barriers to adequate care for older adults in rural communities include the distances between the older persons home and care providers, home health and long-term care options, lack of care coordination, social isolation, lack of access to adequate nutrition, reliance on unpaid family care givers, and housing affordability and repair. Many of these issues require creative healthcare team programs to improve life for older adults in rural areas. Support for community health centers and programs from rural health departments could be expanded to assist in the resolution of identified health issues for older adults. Many of the issues discussed in this chapter are more social in foundation than medical. Nurses can have an important impact in the development and implementation of programs that can assist older rural adults overcome barriers to adequate health and well-being.

REFERENCES

Agency for Healthcare Research and Quality (AHRQ). (2017). Care Coordination Available at https://www.ahrq.gov/professionals/prevention-chronic-care/improve/coordination/index.html Accessed on March 20, 2019.

American Society on Aging. (2016). Aging and healthcare in rural America: Overlooked needs quiet strength. Available at https://.asaging.org/blog/aging-healthcare-rural-America-overlooked-needs-quiet-strength. Accessed on March 5, 2019.

Bahler, C., *et al.* (2015). Multimorbidity, healthcare utilization and costs in an elderly community-dwelling population; a claims data based observational study. *BMC Health Services Research, 15*(23).

Benson, W., and N. Aldrich. (2018). Raising awareness and seeking solutions to the opioid epidemic's impact on rural older adults. Grant makers in Aging. Available at https://www.giaging.org/documents/170818_Benson-Aldrich_paper_for_GIA_web_FINAL.pdf. Accessed on March 5, 2019.

Carlson, C., S. Merel, and M. Yukawa. (2015). Geriatric syndromes and geriatric assessment for the generalist medical clinics. DOI: https://doi.org/10.1016/j.mcna.2014.11.003.

Centers for Disease Control and Prevention. (2017). Rural Health. Available at https://www.cdc.gov/ruralhealth/about.html. Accessed on March 5, 2019.

Centers for Medicare and Medicaid Services, Center for Medicaid and CHIP Services. Consideration for Integrated Care Models, Washington DC; CMS: SMDL#12-00.

Center for Medicare and Medicaid Services. (2018). CMS Rural Health Strategy F.

Chilton, L. (2019). Palliative care for older adults. Medscape. Available at https://www.medscape.org/viewarticle/464726. Accessed on March 12, 2019.

Crouch, E., J. C. Probst, and K. J. Bennett. (2017). Rural-urban differences in unpaid caregivers of adults. *Rural and Remote Health, 17*, 4351. https://doi.org/10.22605/RRH4351.

Easter Seals Disability Services. (2006). Caregiving in rural America. 2018. Available at Easterseals | About Disabilities. Accessed on March 12, 2019.

Ferrante, L., M. Pisani, and T. Murphy. (2015). Functional trajectories among older persons before and after critical illness. *JAMA, 175*(4) 523–529.

Griffin, E., and A. Coburn. (2014). Integrated care for older adults in rural communities. University of Southern Maine Research Center found at https://muskie.usm.maine.edu/Publications/rural/Integrated-Care-Rural-PolicyBrief.pdf. Accessed on March 25, 2019.

Henning-Smith, C., and M. Lahr. (2018). Perspectives on rural caregiving challenges and interventions. Policy Brief, Rural Health Research Center University of Minnesota.

Hofler, R., and J. Ortiz. (2016). Costs of accountable care organization participation for primary care providers: Early stage results. *BMC Health Services Research, 16*: 315.

Hudson, R. (2018). Lack of social connectedness and its consequences. *Public Policy and Aging Report 27*(4) 121–123.

Insured Retirement Institute. 2016. Boomer expectations for retirement, 2018. Available at https://www.irionline.org/resources/resources-detail-view/boomer-expectations-for-retirement-2018. Accessed on March 27, 2019.

Institute for Social and Economic Development. 2017. Available at https://www.acf.hhs.gov/sites/default/files/orr/case_management_508.pdf. Accessed on March 20, 2019.

Kasper, J., M. O'Malley, and B. Lyons. (2010). Chronic disease and co-morbidity among dual eligible: Implications for patterns of Medicaid and Medicare service use and spending. Washington DC: Kaiser Commission on Medicaid and the Uninsured.

Kaye, L. W. (2017). Older adults, rural living, and the escalating risk of social isolation. *Public Policy and Aging Report, 27*(4), 139–144.

Luskin, A., *et al.* (2017). Patient outcomes, health care resource use, and costs associated with high versus low HEDIS Asthma Medication Ration. *Journal of Managed Care, 23*(11) 1117–1124.

National Consensus Project for Quality Palliative Care (NCP). (2009). Clinical practice guidelines for quality palliative care, ed 2. National Guideline Clearinghouse. Retrieved from www.guideline.gov. Accessed on March 19, 2019.

National Council on Aging. (2018). Falls prevention facts available at https://www.ncoa.org/news/resources-for-reporters/get-the-facts/falls-prevention-facts/. Accessed on March 2, 2019.

Nattinger, M., *et al.* (2016). Financial Performance of Rural Medicare ACOs. *The Journal of Rural Health, 34*(1) 98–102.

Ortman, J., A. Velkoff, and H. Hogan. (2014). The older population of the United States. *Journal of Gerontology, 14*(2) 230–231. www.census.gov. U.S. Department of Commerce.

Romo, R., *et al.* (2016). Decision making among older adults at the end of life: A theoretical perspective. *Advances in Nursing Science, 39*(4) 308–319.

Rural Health Information Hub. (2018). Older adults who live in rural areas face problems that impact health, accessed at https://www.ruralhealthinfo.org/topics/aging. Accessed on March 13, 2019.

Sadana R. and J. P. Michel. (2019). Healthy ageing: What is it and how to describe it? In: Michel J. P. (eds.) Prevention of Chronic Diseases and Age-Related Disability. Practical Issues in Geriatrics. Springer, Cham.

Thiede, B., *et al.* (2016). Access to services diminishes in rural America as populations age Population Trends in Post-Recession Rural America. Available at https://outlook.office.com. Accessed on March 19, 2019.

U.S. Census Bureau. (2017). The nation's older population is still growing, Census Bureau reports. Available at https://www.census.gov/newsroom/press-releases/2017/cb17-100.html. Accessed on March 1, 2019.

U.S. Department of Housing and Urban Development/Office of Policy Development and Research. (2015). Senior housing and services: Challenges and opportunities in rural America.

U.S. Department of Health and Human Services. (2014). Health People 2020. Available at https://www.healthypeople.gov/. Accessed March 7, 2019.

CHAPTER 7

Health Policy for Rural Populations

Barbara Jackson

Objectives:

1. Describe the influence of rural population community members in the health policy development process.
2. Identify the role of nursing in patient advocacy for local, regional, state, and federal health policy decisions.
3. Discuss access to care and health policy equity for rural populations and with rural hospitals.

Discussion Questions:

1. Discuss how nurses can position themselves to be change advocates to improve health, health care, initiate or guide policy changes.
2. Identify a vulnerable population that lives in your general geographic region. What community, local, regional, or state conditions and/or policies exist to improve their access to health care?
3. As the ACA has been implemented and continues to evolve, describe new and changing opportunities and roles for nurses.
4. Separate into groups. Discuss political advocacy. In general, how do nurses engage in political advocacy?

   After the group agrees on a common definition of political advocacy, explore nursing literature databases. Identify an article that illustrates the work of nurses participating in advocacy.

   a. Describe the time the article is referring to (historical or current), what healthcare issues they were facing, and what population was experiencing the issue.
   b. How do nurses demonstrate the role of advocate for the population?

INTRODUCTION

To appreciate the importance of health policy for rural populations, it is imperative to recognize the various contributors to successful health policy decisions. Obviously, the persons living in rural areas provide a wealth of information to healthcare providers, who in turn can provide valuable information to legislators for the purpose of policy making. In concert with that, nurses and other healthcare disciplines must have a general understanding of the influence of politics, the legislative process, the health of the economy impacts policy decisions, and the effect of global health initiatives to influence the policy process and to inform policy makers.

RURAL POPULATION VIEWS ON HEALTH SUPPORT NEED FOR RURAL HEALTH POLICY

One way to combat the poor health practices and outcomes of the rural population is through the tireless work of the public and rural healthcare workers and social service organizations who work to decrease the barriers to quality healthcare access and to eliminate the health disparities experienced by those living in rural settings. To tackle those challenges, improve the overall health, and to accomplish the health goals, rural-specific health policies need to be in place.

In the early 2000s, the idea of patient centeredness was a new approach to health care and approximately a decade ago it became the mainstay. Healthcare systems urge primary care providers to be actively engaged with their patients when making treatment decisions about their health conditions. Not surprisingly, patient-centered care is a challenge for healthcare providers. Likewise, it is challenging for hospital and clinic administrators as well as policy makers to appreciate the dynamics that contribute to effective collaboration between clinicians and patients.

Important to an effective partnership is understanding how the patient views his or her health and what efforts the patient has made to improve the health condition. For decades, researchers have discussed the differences in how rural and urban populations view their health. A rural patient would have to experience significant impairment to their physical health to seek healthcare and to make changes in health behavior; rural patients are often dependent on relationships with family and friends (Sriram *et al.*, 2018). Having a better understanding of the rural patient's health-seeking behaviors enables the health care provider to offer more comprehensive, individualized care.

One example of a specific health problem being viewed differently by persons living in rural environments is in the area of mental health. There is an association between socioeconomic status and mental health and knowing about the financial challenges facing many in the rural population. It is important to fully understand the correlations among certain health problems. Although there are numerous programs and policies that have been developed to improve mental health, the help may not be sought by all who have access. When compared to their urban counterparts, persons living in rural areas are less likely to seek mental health care and they discuss the stigma associated with having a mental illness (Clement *et al.*, 2015). In addition to the stigma, men who live in rural areas are less likely to see mental health care if they have less resilience and grit (Creighton *et al.*, 2017).

NURSES AS POLICY ADVOCATES

Nurses can participate in shaping public policy at the local, state, and national levels and through those efforts can advance professional practice and the health of the nation. Changes in practice, education, and regulations necessitate that the nurses advocate for themselves and the profession and become politically astute. As advocates for policy change, nurses can lend their voices and expertise to support a position on health-related issues, and while doing so can protect the public and the nursing profession. While policy changes occur, nurses must remain agile and responsive so as to safeguard those policies. U.S. health outcomes trail behind other developed countries, necessitating nurses' need to advocate for policy changes for elimination of health disparities, health promotion, and disease prevention (Sonenberg and Knepper, 2017).

As the most trusted profession for the past 17 years, according to Gallup's annual survey, society as a whole, views nurses as honest and ethical. The public can depend on nurses to fight for patients and their health (Brenan, 2018). Rooted in its history, nursing has enduring values. As health and healthcare have evolved over time, so has nursing practice. Through all of the changes in individual, family, community, and population health, nurses have also adapted to fluctuations in the economic, social, and political climate.

The *Future of Nursing* report published by the National Academies of Medicine, formerly the Institute of Medicine (IOM), and the National Academies of Sciences, Engineering, and Medicine (NASEM), provided an outline of how nurses could certify a healthy nation and advocate for improvements in healthcare delivery by increasing the educational preparation of nurses (IOM, 2011; NASEM, 2021). The report described how nurses are leaders and can be change agents in addressing strategies to eliminate health disparities. The current challenge is for nurse leaders to persuade other nurses to become involved and advocate for changes in healthcare delivery and focus on the social determinants of health including poverty, transportation, education, and housing.

RURAL HEALTH POLICY MAKERS

Ensuring adequate access to healthcare for those living in rural settings is the responsibility of the insurers, healthcare practitioners, social service organizations and local, state, and federal policy makers. Many of those delivering healthcare services are highly dependent on the health policymakers to provide the needed financial and/or policy support to meet the health needs of the rural patient populations. Policymakers at the federal level set the spending priorities, appropriate necessary funds, and allocate resources to address rural health care needs. It is vital to understand the connection between policy and public health outcomes in rural populations. Public health officials are responsible for delivering healthcare, providing health programming, collecting data for statistical trending, and advancing basic public health goals in employment, housing, food security, etc. (Centers for Disease Control and Prevention, CDC Policy Process, 2021).

Although there are 11 committees that have some level of influence and authority over health policy at the federal level, none of those have a formal, specific focuses on rural health needs (senate.gov, 2021, house.gov, 2021). Instead, there is one bipartisan informally structured caucus in both the House and the Senate that focus on rural healthcare issues. Those legislators work to ensure that rural communities have a voice in the legislative process. The Congressional Rural Caucus has the mission to educate "other Members of Congress on the constantly changing face of rural America" (Smith, 2019). U.S. Senator Tina Smith, co-chair of the Senate Rural Health Caucus, vows to "help fight to lower the cost of health care, combat the opioid crisis, and address the needs that rural communities face." All of the aforementioned health issues noted by Senator Smith are not only concerns in her home state of Minnesota, but also in every state and many, many communities around the United States (Smith, 2018).

POLITICAL INFLUENCE ON HEALTH

Although health should not be a political chess piece, it has become central to political debates and legislative maneuvering. As seen in the 2016 election cycle, the divide between the rural and urban voters widened when compared to the 2008 and 2012 elections. The political candidates took notice. The rural-urban divide saw an increase in rural constituents voting Republican by a wider margin than in the urban areas (Oberhauser, Krier and Kusow, 2019). This is important when one takes the general health of rural communities into account and the focus of both political parties on health and healthcare. According to Center for Disease Control (CDC) data, approximately 15% of the U.S. population live in rural settings and experience higher rates of unintentional injury, heart disease, stroke, cancer, and respiratory disease (CDC, 2019). With less access to primary physicians/providers, specialists, and emergency care, than their urban counterparts, the ongoing health of the rural population is at greater risk (Garcia *et al.*, 2017).

APPROACHES IN ADVOCACY

Connecting what is known about the health issues, the political candidates should focus not only their campaign promises, but also on their political platforms on the needs of the rural population. Likewise, constituents need to focus on the politicians who will plan to work on legislation for all of their needs, including healthcare. Understanding the political inclinations and what prompts a politician to act on an issue will enable informants and experts of proposed legislation to choose a more successful path toward policy change.

To build stronger connections among politicians and the constituents that would most benefit from policy development, improvements should be made in interprofessional collaboration and telehealth utilization as described by Johnson and Mahan (2020). Wamsley *et al.* (2020) further explained that a formalized, structured plan for interprofessional collaboration enables the healthcare providers to develop a comprehensive plan of care for the patients they service and empowers each member of the team the ability to advocate for the patient and support the team's mission of care. Improvements in telehealth utilization reaches the most isolated and vulnerable of the rural populations and allows for access to healthcare providers not typically accessible. However, development of policies that enable that approach needs the support of well-versed advocates who can articulate to overwhelming need and benefit (Myers, 2018).

Health policies support the health of the community with the necessary resources so that community members can improve their health and eliminate those things that are detrimental to their health. Likewise, while health policies impact the health of the community, community members can influence policy decisions through organized efforts and influential political pressure. Throughout time, community members who organized their efforts were able to stimulate changes to public policy for the environment and various groups of marginalized persons (Silliman, 1997; Martinez-Alier *et al.*, 2016).

HEALTH REFORM

National health reform has been the topic of conversation and the focus of spirited discussion among legislators and healthcare experts for decades. There have been many proposals and policies presented over the years that were meant to address the vast array of issues in the U.S. healthcare system, but health reform was difficult to achieve. After many failed attempts, the Affordable Care Act (ACA) was enacted in 2010 with three primary goals in mind: to "Make affordable health insurance available to more people, expand the Medicaid program, and Support innovative medical care delivery methods designed to lower the costs of health care" (ACA, 2010).

While the ACA was voted in by a bipartisan vote, it has not ended the partisan arguments related to health reform. The current discourse over the federal government's responsibility to ensure healthcare coverage is divided unmistakably down party lines. Although the future of the ACA remains tenuous because of the political tug-of-war taking place, this broad health reform legislation remains the answer for many of the health insurance and healthcare delivery problems facing the U.S. Theories of health political science have emerged in this tenuous time of health reform discussion (Raphael, 2014). From these theories, public policy is identified as a determinate of health and acknowledges that political power and shifting power influences how decisions are made. Power struggles are known to influence a legislator's stance on an issue, which can impact access of health services for vulnerable rural communities.

FINANCING HEALTHCARE FOR VULNERABLE POPULATIONS

Income, employment, income, disability, age, and immigration status are the traits that allow for access to healthcare in the United States. Based on these traits for the amount of benefit received, this allows for disproportionate inequities for those groups that do not fit into certain categories. Medicare provides healthcare benefits for all elderly persons and people with certain chronic disabilities. On the surface, the introduction of Medicare in 1965 would appear to be the first step to healthcare for all, but it would take 45 years for healthcare reform to provide more universal coverage.

Unlike Medicare that is federally operated and provides some level of coverage for *all* elderly persons, Medicaid does not provide the same coverage for all poor persons, as is commonly believed. Instead, Medicaid provides basically 50 different coverage plans, as each state has their own set of requirements. The services covered and income eligibility differs widely state to state, which means that there are people living in poverty that are not eligible in some states in the United States. Essentially, Medicaid provides financial support for healthcare services for some extremely low-income persons, but mostly it supports persons with disabilities and the elderly in long-term care, for whom Medicare does not financially support. As an initiative of the ACA, Medicaid expansion standardized the eligibility requirements as well as coverage. It set minimum standard benefits that all Medicaid recipients must receive. After a 2012 U.S. Supreme Court ruling, states could elect to opt in or opt out to participate in the Medicaid Expansion program and as of 2020, 30+ states are part of the Kaiser Family Foundation program (KFF, 2020). However, the expansion benefits could be in jeopardy if the growing number of states that want stricter eligibility requirements are federally approved (Garfield *et al.*, 2018).

Although there are growing concerns about the actual costs of care exceeding Medicare and Medicaid reimbursement, the added penalties from hospital readmissions and reimbursement cuts may spell the demise of more hospitals. This is especially true for the small rural hospital where 45% of the total annual revenue comes from Medicare. This coupled with increasing healthcare costs and decreasing reimbursements will most certainly lead to more rural hospital closures (Janney, 2014).

EQUITY IN HEALTH POLICY

Suitable governance is necessary for public health efforts to eliminate health disparities in rural settings (Shah and Sheahan, 2016). The process of governance can derail or enable efforts to improve the human condition. Poverty, political and social problems, and social injustices are actually supported when a lack of governmental support exists which leads to distrust, apathy, and the lack of participation of those in the vulnerable situation. To achieve sufficient decision-making and involvement by the community, it is necessary for community members and organizations to openly participate in the process with their elected officials. When those elected to office and the community members unite, the community can achieve equity and improved health outcomes from the shared process.

Often, there is a disconnect between the policy-making process and the public's understanding and needs. Health equity and health promotion become increasingly political in this time of limited resources and political maneuvering. Healthcare advocates, community organizations, and informed citizens can influence initiatives for health equity and the health policy process (Achieving Health Equity, 2018). When the research evidence confirms the inequity in rural communities specifically related to the social determinants of health, the stance of the policy makers and politicians becomes more evident. Political maneuvering remains a central indicator in dispersing resources to improve the health in rural communities. It is important for community leaders, community members and other policy makers to take note of the distributed resources and what policies were supported or ignored so as to determine the next course of action to address the communities' health concerns.

A local government can potentially decrease rural health disparities if there is any inclination that equitable disbursement of resources and health policies would be founded in equity. The personal motivations of a politician are often hidden from public view, which can make collaborations between politicians and community organizations difficult, especially when the community organization is striving for policies of health equity. Political decisions are dependent on many factors, some of which pull the legislator in different directions. The legislator may want to support policies specific to a rural region or narrow area but find themselves in a tug-of-war for allocation of resources, whether it be human capital or funding. Legislators often make policy decisions that favor their economic interests in lieu of the social problems of their community.

HEALTH POLICY IN RURAL HOSPITALS

Since 2010, there have been close to 100 rural hospitals that have closed (Germack, Kandrack and Martsolf, 2019). Changes in reimbursement and healthcare delivery are the culprits. This is forcing lawmakers in rural communities to evaluate ways to provide health services to the community members while also ensuring the success of healthcare facilities. Administrators in smaller rural hospitals struggle to stay current with ever changing and improving technology, as they don't have the financial means to equip their hospitals with the latest equipment (Huang and Gramopadhye, 2016). And as more healthcare services move to the outpatient setting, hospitals are left with excess inpatient beds and no patients to fill them. This has dampened the revenue stream and forced strict cost containment but has not resulted in financially stable hospitals.

Hospitals need to seek opportunities for reduction of costs and increases in revenue to protect themselves against the added financial pressures. Decisions by hospital administrators should be made strategically so that quality of care doesn't suffer as a result of cuts. Administrators can enlist the help of the mid-level managers and staff to initiate quality improvement projects. Rural hospitals have the unique problem of low patient volumes, which can contribute to apathy of the staff resulting in poor quality measures (Mason, 2017). Rural hospital administrators also need to look for ways to assure the local patient population of the quality of care and encourage them to seek healthcare services in their community hospital rather than bypassing it for the larger urban centers. Struggling rural hospitals should be able to protect their existence through improvement efforts.

The closure of a small rural hospital has implications for the entire community. There are many fewer hospitals serving rural areas when one compares this metric to larger urban areas. When a hospital closes its doors, patients no longer have adequate access to healthcare services and are then forced to travel to a neighboring town with a hospital or much longer distances to urban hospitals that have medical specialists available to them. It is not surprising that some patients have poor outcomes by having to travel long distances for appropriate medical care (Jia and Xierali, 2015). Along with the obvious lack of healthcare services, rural hospitals are usually a major employer for the community and they support other business in the general area. The closure of a hospital will most definitely impact the local business. If one multiplies that by the 100 closures that have occurred, the impact to the rural communities is exponential.

These issues have spurred ideas in some areas that are meeting with success. Arizona has seen success in converting their failed rural critical access hospitals into standalone emergency centers with added radiology, labs, and specialty physicians (Meyer, 2017). With the rise of standalone emergency centers in urban and suburban areas, this type of center is not unique. However, as seen in Douglas, Arizona, Jim Dickson, CEO of a neighboring town's hospital, and understanding the need for healthcare services in the rural area, appealed to Arizona's Medicaid officials to allow for this emergency center to replace the hospital without the requirement of inpatient beds. Medicaid officials agreed and the center opened in April 2017, treating over 1,000 patients a month (Meyer, 2017).

In 2017, several senators reintroduced the Rural Emergency Acute Care Hospital (REACH) Act, which was aimed to allow rural hospitals to circumvent regulations that make it impossible for Critical Access Hospitals to be viable. The REACH act would allow hospitals to decrease the number of inpatient beds and be reclassified as Rural Emergency hospitals. Ultimately, the proposed legislation was assigned to the Senate Finance committee and was last discussed in May 2017, with no further action since. With the prospect of the looming closure of 20% of the remaining rural hospitals, legislators need to pass legislation that will protect the health of those living in rural areas (Mosley, 2019).

GRANT PROGRAMS

Grant programs often support health policy initiatives that support those living and working in rural settings. In recent years, the number of grant programs specifically targeted at rural areas has increased. For example, the Administration for Community Living, National Institute on Disability, Independent Living, and Rehabilitation Research and the U.S. Department of Health and Human Services (2018) sponsor a grant offering called Rehabilitation Research and Training Center on Disability in Rural Communities to "improve outcomes among people with disabilities who live in rural areas, including those from racial and ethnic minority groups." Funding is also available from the Health Resources and Services Administration's (2019) Federal Office of Rural Health Policy, which makes funds available to eligible hospitals, health clinics, or tribal organizations in high-risk rural communities to expand access points for opioid users to receive treatment. The Rural Health Information Hub website lists other sources of funding listed by topic, sponsor, or state (2019). These funding or grant opportunities provide for expansion of services through telehealth, for example, or for a specific health problem, such as cardiac or cancer care, or by patient group.

GRANTS FOR RURAL HOSPITALS

Grant opportunities exist that support the unique health problems or resource issues that rural hospitals face. Because of that, the best asset of small, rural hospitals may be a grant writer who may already be on staff, or current staff that can be trained. Because of the financial strain that rural hospitals face, there may be little to no money to hire someone new. Partnerships with community organizations or universities with healthcare-specific grant-writing expertise could benefit the rural hospital if they do not have the expertise or personnel to write grant proposals. Students in graduate degree programs focused on healthcare typically must complete practicum requirements and, when working with experienced faculty members and hospital administrators, can be a valuable resource for writing grants. Hospital administrators, including the CEOs and the boards, can identify available resources, and their system's strengths and weaknesses to help shaping a strategy that fits their organization's goals.

WORLD HEALTH ORGANIZATION AND THE INTERNATIONAL FOCUS ON RURAL HEALTH ISSUES

All one has to do is log on to the World Health Organization (WHO) website to gain insight into the organization's focus areas related to global health issues. To better understand how the WHO arrived at those issues, it is first important to recognize the WHO definition of *health*. Defined in the WHO Constitution, adopted in 1946, *health* encompasses social, emotional, and physical foundations that is "not merely the absence of disease or infirmity but a state of complete physical, mental and social well-being" (WHO, 2021). This definition is further broadened in that it is focused not only on the welfare of the individual but also the bigger community. Of the core functions, the WHO stresses the importance of monitoring global health issues, measuring trends, all the while collaborating with healthcare partners to take action. And most importantly in this context, it is vital to construct policy options based on evidence and employing ethical principles (WHO, 2020).

As an indicator of the level of individual well-being, *health* is also a gauge of successful local, state, national, and international promotion of programs and policy decisions made by governmental bodies related to the welfare of their respective communities (Brodit and Radwan, 2019). This definition infers that there are social and cultural situations that influence personal, public health, and political agendas around the world. Likewise, it confirms that although there are differences in the issues based on location, discrimination, poverty, and lack of education, these are critical public health issues. To achieve a comprehensive plan to address health needs specific to individuals in rural areas, it is essential to assess the determinants listed above as well as the contribution of personal choices and individual innate characteristics. According to the CDC, the five leading causes of death recognized for the 46 million persons living in rural regions in the United States, include diagnoses that have been induced by genetic characteristics and life choices (CDC, 2017). Diagnoses, such as high blood pressure, obesity, and respiratory illnesses related to smoking, all rooted in personal characteristics and lifestyle choices, are a significant drain on healthcare resources globally (Vineis, 2017).

Most recently, the COVID-19 pandemic has provided a global perspective on health, health practices, the need for services, and what health policies are adequate and inadequate in the changing landscape of disease and global health. Numerous studies have been conducted to evaluate the state of healthcare and the pandemic's effect on healthcare systems, healthcare providers, individual patient health, and population health across the globe. A few such studies have explored the psychosocial impact of COVID-19 (Sun, Lin, and Operario, 2020), opportunities for improvements in population health (Goldfield *et al.*, 2020), the impact of not investing in healthcare resources prior to a crisis (Maani and Galea, 2020) and health equity and policy outcomes resulting from the pandemic (Lynch, 2020).

CONCLUSION

Access to healthcare, needed services, and the healthcare system are critical for achieving health equity, and these are the same essential factors across the globe (Brodit and Rodwan, 2018). Two major means for patients to experience access to adequate healthcare is the realization of well-informed legislators and the availability of sufficient health policies to streamline processes, provide ample services, and support the procurement of providers. Nurses and other health professionals are situated perfectly to provide the expertise and understanding of the needs of patient populations in rural settings as well as the knowledge in the process necessary to participate in policy making.

REFERENCES

Achieving Health Equity in the United States. (2018, November 13). Retrieved from https://www.apha.org/policies-and-advocacy/public-health-policy-statements/policy-database/2019/01/29/achieving-health-equity.

Affordable Care Act (ACA). (2010). Retrieved from https://www.healthcare.gov/glossary/affordable-care-act/.

Brenan, M. (2018, December 20). Nurses again outpace other professions for honesty, ethics. Gallup: Politics retrieved from https://news.gallup.com/poll/245597/nurses-again-outpace-professions-honesty-ethics.aspx.

Brodit, K., and H. Radwan, (2019). Global health equity. *Journal of Best Practices in Health Professions Diversity, 11*(2), 150–154. doi:10.2307/26894215.

Centers for Disease Control and Prevention (CDC). (2019). *Rural Health.* Retrieved from https://www.cdc.gov/ruralhealth/about.html.

Centers for Disease Control and Prevention (CDC), (2021), CDC Policy Process, Office of the Associate Director for Policy and Strategy,Centers for Disease Control. Retrieved from https://www.cdc.gov/policy/analysis/process/definition.html.

Clement, S., *et al.* (2015). What is the impact of mental health-related stigma on help-seeking? A systematic review of quantitative and qualitative studies. *Psychological Medicine, 45*(1), 11–27.

Creighton, G., *et al.* (2017). "You've gotta be that tough crust exterior man": Depression and suicide in rural-based men. *Qualitative Health Research, 27*(12). 1–10.

Garcia, M.C., *et al.* (2017). Reducing potentially excess deaths from the five leading causes of death in the rural United States. *Morbidity and Mortality Weekly Report: Surveillance Summary, 66*(2), 1–7. Doi: http://dx.doi.org/10.15585/mmwr.ss6602a1.

Garfield, R., R., *et al.* (2018). Implications of work requirements in Medicaid: What does the data say? *Issue Brief, Kaiser Family Foundation*, KFF.org. Retrieved from https://kymedicaidtracker.com/wp-content/uploads/2019/05/Issue-Brief-Implications-of-Work-Requirements-in-Medicaid-What-Does-the-Data-Say.pdf.

Germack, H., R. Kandrack, and G. Martsolf, (2019). When rural hospitals close, the physician workforce goes. *Health Affairs, 38*(12): 2086–2094.

Goldfield, N. I., *et al.* (2020). COVID-19 crisis creates opportunities for community-centered population health: Community health workers at the center. *The Journal of Ambulatory Care Management, 43*(3): 184–190.

House.gov. (2021). Committees. Retrieved from https://www.house.gov/committees.

Huang, Y. and A. Gramopadhye. (2016). Recommendations for health information technology implementation in rural hospitals. *International Journal of Health Care Quality Assurance, 29*(4): 454–474.

Institute of Medicine (IOM). (2011). *The Future of Nursing: Leading Change, Advancing Health.* Washington, DC: The National Academies Press.

Janney, C. (2014). Small rural hospitals face big changes under the Affordable Care Act. *Journal Star.* Retrieved from https://www.pjstar.com/article/20140125/News/140129435.

Jia, P. and I. Xierali. (2015). Disparities in patterns of health care travel among inpatients diagnosed with congestive heart failure. *Preventing Chronic Disease; Public Health Research, Practice, and Policy, 12*(150): 1–12.

Kaiser Family Foundation (KFF). (2020). Status of State Medicaid Expansion Decisions: Interactive Map. Retrieved from: https://www.kff.org/medicaid/issue-brief/status-of-state-medicaid-expansion-decisions-interactive-map/.

Lynch, J. (2020). Health equity, social policy, and promoting recovery from COV-ID-19. *Journal of Health Politics, Policy and Law, 45*(6): 983–995.

Maani, N., and S. Galea. (2020). COVID-19 and underinvestment in the health of the US population. *The Milbank Quarterly, 98*(2).

Martinez-Alier, J., *et al.* (2016). Is there a global environmental justice movement? *The Journal of Peasant Studies, 43*(3): 731–755.

Mason, D. (2017). Rethinking rural hospitals. *JAMA, 318*(2): 114–115.

Meyer, H. (2017). Reexamining Policy: There ought to be options, other than just close or the status quo, to help them transform to best meet community needs. *Modern Healthcare In-Depth* retrieved from https://www.modernhealthcare.com/indepth/arizona-hospital-shows-path-for-saving-rural-healthcare-policy-changes-needed/.

Mosley, D. (2019, February 21). First Opinion: 1 in 5 rural hospitals are at risk of imminent closure. Lawmakers could help some stay open. *STAT* retrieved from https://www.statnews.com/2019/02/21/lawmakers-act-prevent-rural-hospitals-closing/.

Myers, C. R. (2019). Using telehealth to remediate rural mental health and healthcare disparities, *Issues in Mental Health Nursing, 40*(3): 233–239.

National Academy of Sciences, Engineering, and Medicine (2021). *The future of nursing 2020-2030: Charting a path to achieve health equity*. Washington, DC: The National Academies Press. https://doi.org/10.17226/2582.

Oberhauser, A. D. Krier, and A. Kusow. (2019). Political moderation and polarization in the heartland: Economics, rurality, and social identity in the 2016 U.S. presidential election, *The Sociological Quarterly, 60*(2): 224–244.

Raphael, D. (2014). Beyond policy analysis: The raw politics behind opposition to healthy public policy. *Health Promotion International, 30*(2): 380–396.

Senate.gov. (2021). Senate Committee and Subcommittee Assignments. Retrieved from https://www.senate.gov/committees/committee_assignments.htm.

Shah, G. and J. Sheahan. (2016). Local health departments' activities to address health disparities and inequities: Are we moving in the right direction? *International Journal of Environmental Research and Public Health, 13*(1): 1–12.

Silliman, J. (1997). Making the connections: Women's health and environmental justice. *Race, Gender and Class, 5*(1):104–129.

Smith, A. (2019). Purpose, mission, and goals: Congressional rural caucus. Retrieved from https://ruralcaucus-adriansmith.house.gov/about-us/purpose-mission-goals.

Smith, T. (January 17, 2018). Sen. Smith "proud" to be joining leadership of bipartisan rural health caucus [press release]. Retrieved from https://www.smith.senate.gov/sen-smith-proud-be-joining-leadership-bipartisan-rural-health-caucus.

Sonenberg, A. and H. Knepper. (2017). Considering disparities: How do nurse practitioner regulatory policies, access to care, and health outcomes vary across four states? *Nursing Outlook, 65*(2), 143–153.

Sriram, U., *et al.* (2018). Support and Sabotage: A qualitative study of social influences on health behaviors among rural adults. *The Journal of Rural Health, 34*(1): 88–97.

Sun, S., D. Lin, and D. Operario. (2020). Need for a population health approach to understand and address psychosocial consequences of COVID-19. *Psychological Trauma: Theory, Research, Practice, and Policy, 12*(S1): S25.

Vineis, P. (2017). *Health without borders: Epidemics in the era of globalization.* Springer.

Walmsley, G., *et al.* (2020). Identifying practical approaches to the normalisation of interprofessional collaboration in rural hospitals: A qualitative study among health professionals. *Journal of Interprofessional Care, 1*(10): 1–10.

World Health Organization (WHO) 2020. Basic Documents (49th ed). World Health Organization. Retrieved from https://apps.who.int/gb/bd/.

World Health Organization (WHO) 2021. World Health Organization Constitution. Retrieved from https://www.who.int/about/who-we-are/constitution.

CHAPTER 8

Telehealth: An Answer or Question for Rural Health

Jill D. Cochran

Objectives:

1. Understand the history of telehealth and how telehealth is used in various healthcare setting.
2. Discuss the legal and financial challenges of providing telehealth services.
3. Describe support service and resources for telehealth adoption in rural areas.

Discussion Questions:

1. The caring aspect of nursing is fundamental to our profession and to our practice. Bedside care, touch, and therapeutic touch are incorporated into principles and practices of our discipline. How can nurses convey the essence of nursing care through telehealth?
2. What policy changes are needed to support nurse practitioner's practice in telehealth?
3. How will technological care impact medical and nursing errors and how could this be minimized?

INTRODUCTION

Being a nurse or a nurse practitioner (NP) in rural areas is especially challenging. Daily practice requires creative solutions when a patient's needs surpass available resources. Rural health disparities, socioeconomic status, and geographic isolation are just a few of the obstacles in providing health care in rural areas (Rural Health Information Hub, 2017; Center for Disease

Control and Prevention, 2018). Shortages of specialty and allied health services increase the difficulty of rural patient care. Rural patients deserve the same opportunity for positive health outcomes. However, the barriers often outnumber the opportunities. As nurses, we hold ourselves to the same standard of patient care regardless of resources. Our patients deserve the same outcome potential regardless of allied health and specialty care availability.

The level of chronic illness is higher in certain rural areas, especially diabetes, heart disease, and respiratory illnesses (James, 2017; Warshaw, 2017; National Rural Health Association, n.d.; Rural Health Information Hub, n.d.-c). Rural residents have multiple barriers to accessing health care services, including long travel distances, limited public and personal transportation, and absences from work due to travel time (Warshaw, 2017). For example, a new onset type 1 diabetic patient in a rural pediatric practice may need to be sent to a larger center with specialized care to initiate and manage care and family education and training. Many patients do not want to go back to the specialist in the larger areas as they may report a 15 minute or less visit for a four or more hour trip. Many patients feel that it is not worth the trip and that the specialist never really gets to know them. If patients miss appointments, often the specialist will not see them again. This returns management of that condition to the already overwhelmed primacy care provider.

Lack of resources for managing complex patients is only one of the issues that rural nurses face. Treating patients with chronic illness is more than keeping current with guidelines and management of conditions. It involves experience in chronic care management. The need for specialty care among the rural population has facilitated advancement for consultation via technology from providers that have that expertise. Nurses are known advocates for patients in need. Telehealth is one of the resources nurses and nurse practitioners use to improve outcomes for their patient population.

HISTORY AND BEGINNINGS

As communication has evolved, healthcare has attempted to keep up with it. In 1876, Alexander Graham Bell patented the telephone, a device for electronic speech transmission. The Lancet discussed the timely issues of unnecessary office visits and using the telephone to prevent these visits ("Notes, Short Comments," 1878).

In 1924, the concept of telemedicine was featured on the cover of Radio News as a futuristic goal (Telemedicine, Institute of Medicine [US] Committee on Evaluating Clinical Applications of, and Field, 1996). In 1948, radiologic images were transmitted between two Pennsylvania sites that were 24 miles apart (Gershon-Cohen and Cooley, 1950). From 1959 through 1964, video communications expanded from cross campus medical education (Benschoter *et al.*, 1967; Wittson and Benschoter, 1972) to supplying needed health services to Norfolk State Hospital (see, e.g., Bashshur *et al.*, 1975; Perednia and Allen, 1995). Since then, the progress of health technology has broken the technological growth curve.

In Charleston, West Virginia, Barbara McKee, Director of Care Management at Charleston Area Medical Center, initiated much of the early telehealth services in West Virginia. McKee describes the telehealth origination in West Virginia:

> "In rural West Virginia, telehealth was started by two physicians who were brothers after seeing a demonstration at the world's fair. Mountain Doctor Television (MDTV) started in 1995 and was based in a larger center in Charleston. The first outreach was in two of the state's medical schools and used more for communication and information sharing. As the technology and concept developed, eleven primary care centers were equipped with the equipment to use the services. The most requested specialty was dermatology. Psychiatry and psychology were a close second. Phone lines were used and required separate lines with varied technological requirements. Billing was not an issue since most of the patients of the primary care clinic were on reduced payment schedules which were usually not available in specialty practices. Equipment seemed compact, but required a room for storage. Specialists were recruited by the hub site and were usually intrigued by the concept and agreed to go to the studio in the educational center of the hospital. This usually took a morning or afternoon from their practice. The patient sat with the rural provider and the provider presented the patient's case and reason for specialty consult and then performed a physical exam. The user-friendly concept of the method didn't always transfer to the specialist's disposition. Many of the specialists were not accustomed to taking a history and observing an exam by a nurse practitioner. Once a specialist refused to have a nurse practitioner present a patient and another physician from the clinic was summoned to present the patient. Most of the specialists were amazing and helped bridge the gap in care for our patients" (B. McKee, Personal Communication, January 8, 2019).

WHAT IS TELEHEALTH?

The definition of telehealth has changed with the times. In the beginning, telehealth was synonymous with a video patient-and-provider interaction. Now telehealth refers to a field of technological means that provides and reports patient care. The Health Resources and Services Administration (HRSA) defines telehealth as "the use of electronic communication and information technologies to provide or support long-distance clinical health care, patient and professional health-related education, public health, and health administration" (HRSA, 2019). HRSA describes telehealth as the use of electronic information and telecommunication technologies to support and promote long-distance clinical healthcare, patient and professional health-related education, public health and health administration. Technologies include video conferencing, the Internet, store-and-forward imaging, streaming media, and terrestrial and wireless communications (American Telemedicine Association, n.d.).

Telehealth and telemedicine have often been used interchangeably. However, the American Telemedicine Association further describes the term telehealth as differing from telemedicine because it encompasses a larger assortment of services. Telehealth is provider training, continuing medical education and other services that are not patient specific. The Association describes telemedicine as the use of medical information exchanged from one site to another using electronic communications to improve patient outcomes (American Telemedicine Association, n.d.). How telemedicine or telehealth is defined is usually more dependent on the payer and the organization than the service (The Medicare Learning Network, 2018; HealthIT.gov, 2017b).

Telehealth today is at a cross-sectional point of technology and patient care. Advances in technological equipment and ease of use have progressed faster than the ability to acquire and utilize the methods. The Institute of Medicine (IOM) recognizes the significance of technology in an accelerating healthcare environment. The IOM states that use of Information Technology (IT) must be at the center of patient care and help the redesign of healthcare systems to substantially improve quality of care (IOM [US] Committee on Quality of Health Care in America, 2001). Information technology, including the Internet, holds enormous potential for transforming the healthcare delivery system, which lags significantly compared to other aspects of social Internet use (IOM, 2005). While noting the potential of IT to improve patient care, Nesbitt (2012) noted the need for additional research and incentives to support the continuing and evolving role of IT on healthcare transformation (Board on Health Care Services, IOM and Nesbitt, 2012).

TELEHEALTH APPLICATIONS

Telehealth has traveled across many areas of healthcare. Uses of telehealth seem endless in theory, but perhaps more limited in actual day-to-day application (Mid-Atlantic Telehealth Resource Center, n.d.; Health Resources and Service Administration, 2019; Olson and Thomas, 2017). Current uses of telehealth have spanned from outpatient to inpatient to patients' homes.

HEALTH CARE EDUCATION/CONTINUING EDUCATION

Training nurses and nurse practitioners in telehealth has a wide base of support though multiple specialties. Rural health nursing education has been a proponent of telehealth and telehealth education for years. Future uses, such as residencies for nurse practitioners through telehealth, are not fully explored (Nursing Education in Telehealth, 2006; Rutledge, Haney, Bordelon, Renaud, and Fowler, 2014; Rutledge *et al.*, 2017). Telehealth could be a viable option for future nursing training. In 2016, the American Medical Association adopted policy to incorporate telehealth into training medical students (American Medical Association, 2016).

PRIMARY CARE

In the early 1980s, primary care was associated with quality of care and a primary care team (*Journal of Public Health Policy*, 1983). Primary care can be described as health services that range from prevention to common illness treatment and wellness. Providers of primary care are primarily physicians, nurses, nurse practitioners, and physician assistants. Relationships in primary care are usually long term and provide coordination of care among the specialty and allied health team members (HealthCare.gov, n.d.). Telehealth is a perfect fit for patients and providers in primary care.

SYNCHRONOUS

Synchronous is a live two-way audiovisual link between a care provider and a patient (HealthIT.gov, 2017b). One of the earlier uses of telehealth was specialty consults. Many primary care facilities have the capability to connect with specialists for various conditions. This is specific to the area and the medical need. Rural areas are most deserving of this provision. The constant need for specialty care in rural areas makes telehealth a win-win situation for the patient, rural provider, and the offsite specialists. It allows the primary care provider and the specialist to see the patient at the same time and discuss the condition.

Pediatric Neurology Telehealth Clinic

The pediatric neurologist conducts monthly clinics with an associated facility. Once a month, the "home clinic" provides pediatric neurology consults with a rural clinic. Patients are checked in and recorded as if the clinic is the sole provider of the visit. The patient is presented from an exam room to the pediatric neurologist at the larger center. The presenting provider does the physical exam while the specialist observes and can request additional information during the evaluation, (see Figure 8.1). The patient is followed by both the specialist and the local provider. Specialty tests that must be approved are handled at the rural base site where the patient is usually in their medical home.

The use of telehealth for individual primary care is accelerating. Many private insurances offer the services, but state and federal programs are more limited in coverage. Individual telehealth services are for non-emergent illnesses. Most providers have specific conditions or symptoms that can be evaluated in telehealth. While telehealth may be a quick solution to a non-urgent issue, it is not recommended to replace primary care (MDLive, n.d.). Seeing a specialist or sub-specialist with telehealth is not as common as primary care visits, however, it is expected to increase.

ASYNCHRONOUS

Asynchronous is where video conferencing is a transmission of a recorded health history from one practitioner to another or to a specialist. It may be referred to as "store and forward" videoconferencing (HealthIT.gov, 2017b).

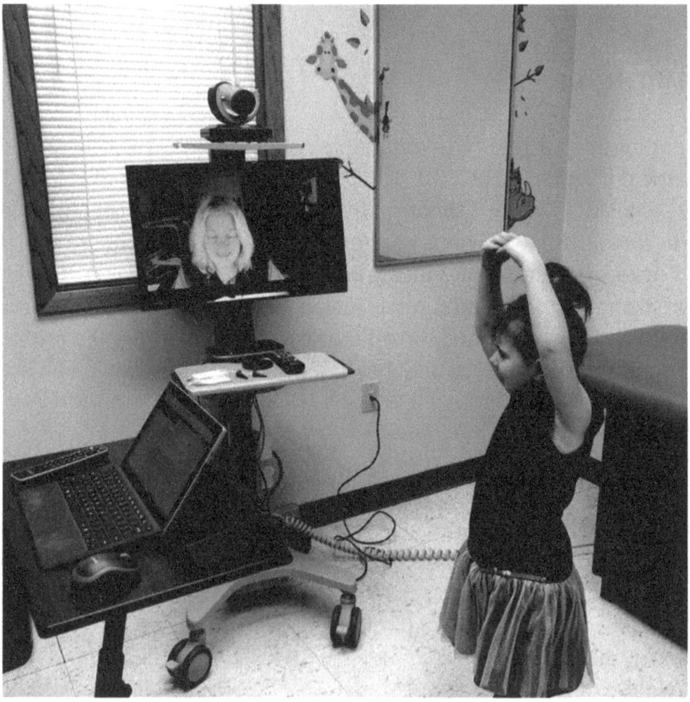

FIGURE 8.1.

FIGURE 8.2.

Example

Congestive heart failure is difficult to manage and requires multi-specialty care. With asynchronous methods, a practitioner would present the patient as a case, without the patient being present. A team of specialists would hear the case and suggest plans of care for the patient's conditions. Other consults occur as the group learns from each other's complex patients. Rural areas such as West Virginia often lack in team specialty care. Extensions for Community Healthcare Outcomes (ECHO) was created with grants and collaboration of primary care clinics and state medical schools, (see Figure 8.2). ECHO provides primary care providers with access of team specialty for several chronic disease process. ECHO provides clinical support for conditions such as Hepatitis C/HIV, chronic pain management, chronic lung disease, and endocrine disease.

REMOTE PATIENT MONITORING (RPM)

Electronic tools are used to record medical data and personal health data in one location which will be reviewed by a provider at a later time in another location.

Example

Heart monitors, glucose monitoring, oxygen saturation monitoring, EEGs, digital radiology and tele-radiology, sleep recording (HealthIT.gov, n.d.). A patient with syncopal episodes may need cardiac monitoring for several weeks. Providers can prescribe a digital heart monitor that transmits data back to them in real time or near real time.

Mobile Health (eHealth)

Example

Patients can track their health through applications that are provided by their primary care provider. This app will show the patient information about previous visits, medication, labs, and vaccinations. Patients and providers can usually send secure messages through the app.

This application involves healthcare and public health information provided through mobile devices. Models of eHealth include patient portals, texts about public health issues and reminders for preventive health care such as flu immunization, mammograms, and colonoscopies (HealthIT.gov, 2017b).

Hospitals

With one-fifth of the US population living in a rural area, rural hospitals are well utilized for emergent and necessary care (HealthIT.gov, 2017). Critical Access Hospitals (CAH) is a designation given to a rural hospital by Centers for Medicare and Medicaid Services (Balanced Budget Act of 1997). CAH are designated to improve access to healthcare and reduce the financial vulnerability of rural hospitals. Conditions that are required for CAH designation are (Rural Health Information Hub, n.d.-a):

- Have 25 or fewer acute care inpatient beds
- Be located more than 35 miles from another hospital
- Maintain an average length of stay of 96 or less hours for acute care patients
- Provide 24/7 emergency care services

Rural hospitals have an enormous responsibility to patients, providers, and communities. These hospitals must engage and collaborate with communities to facilitate network development between local and distant entities. Small rural communities often have isolated unmet needs. Rural hospitals often attempt to compensate for the unmet needs of the communities and populations. Small rural hospitals can become experts in the subject matter and coordinate the healthcare environment of all involved via telehealth services.

Specialty services are scarce, yet integral to rural health care. For example, small rural hospitals may have some specialty care physicians, but not enough to cover continual 24-hour call in a hospital. Additional services, such as occupational therapy, dieticians, and speech therapy may also not be available in small hospitals. Hospitals contract with telehealth specialists to provide coverage especially when the specialist is needed but not available (Schadelbauer, 2017). This keeps healthcare in the rural communities and generates revenue to maintain the hospital's financial status.

Synchronous

Telestroke

Strokes in any geographic location are a life-threatening condition that requires urgent and decisive care. The level of decision making may be more than a provider in a rural emergency department can provide, depending on its expertise and scope of practice. For example, tissue plasminogen activator (tPA) is the standard of care for a non-hemorrhagic strokes. However, the window for administration and accuracy of the stroke type is integral for treatment or non-treatment with tPA. Telemedicine for strokes, or telestroke allows rural hospitals the same level of expertise as larger centers (Mid-Atlantic Telehealth Resource Center, n.d.; HealthIT.gov, 2017a).

EMERGENCY MEDICINE TELEHEALTH FOR TRAUMA

Victims of trauma in rural areas are twice as likely to die from life-threatening injuries as patients in urban areas (Mid-Atlantic Telehealth Resource Center, n.d.). Telehealth in the ED can provide assistance and consultation from a large array of trauma specialists. When the consulting specialist sees the actual patient, it facilitates better and more accurate communication. Visual presentation helps the provider describe the case and assists the specialist in assessing the patient's response to the intervention in real time (Mid-Atlantic Telehealth Resource Center, n.d.).

Asynchronous

Teleradiology

Teleradiology is the ability to send radiographic images from one location to another. A radiologist receives the image and can provide immediate diagnosis or consultation to the provider. This application of radiologic technology is one of the most widely used and accepted applications of telehealth in hospital and healthcare settings. Uses include traditional x-ray images, ultrasounds, and contrast studies that may require live viewing (Mid-Atlantic Telehealth Resource Center, n.d.).

SPECIFIC CONDITIONS THAT HAVE BENEFITED FROM TELEHEALTH

Mental Telehealth

The prevalence of mental illness is similar between urban and rural residents. However, the available services show a stark difference (HRSA, n.d.). Less than 10% of all psychologists and 20% of medical social workers practice in rural areas. More than 60% of rural Americans live in a mental health professional shortage area. Sixty-five percent or more of rural Americans receive mental health care from their primary care provider. In many communities, law enforcement is the crisis responder for mental health issues (Mohatt, n.d.; Watson and Fulambarker, 2012). The mental health provider shortage is second to the stigma of mental health. The perceived stigma of mental health increases barriers beyond resource shortages. It is no surprise that primary care providers deliver more than half of rural America's mental healthcare.

The higher rate of substance abuse in rural areas challenges the mental health community for support and means of rehabilitation (Rural Health Information Hub, 2018). Telehealth is a capable tool to provide much-needed support and treatment in rural areas. The convenience and confidential nature of telehealth have been reported as advantages for patients in early studies (King *et al.*, 2009).

Telepsychology provides psychological services using telecommunication techniques. Telepsychology uses multiple means of communication. The services may be synchronous or asynchronous. The American Psychological Association developed guidelines specific to the practice of psychology (American Psychological Association, n.d.). Regional telehealth associations provide current and user-friendly tools to find telepsychology providers in specific geographic areas (Mid-Atlantic Telehealth Resource Center, n.d.-a; Mohatt, n.d.; Rural Health Information Hub, 2018a).

OTHER SPECIALTY CARE

The role of telehealth has grown exponentially in other disciplines and specialty groups. Collaboration among disciplines promotes the necessary team concept in patient care. Locations such as hospitals, primary care centers, homes, ICUs, and hospice centers are only the beginning of locations that request and provide consultations. Location is no longer a set variable in the equation (Mid-Atlantic Telehealth Resource Center, n.d.).

Use of telehealth in Medicare patients increased significantly between 2014 and 2016. Almost 90,000 Medicare Fee-For-Service beneficiaries utilized 275,199 services from telehealth. The largest growth was among the oldest (85 and older) population of beneficiaries (CMMS, 2018). During this time, 80% of the population using telehealth services was white, non-Hispanic. End stage renal disease accounted for the largest increase in users (Centers for Medicare and Medicaid Services, 2018).

Currently, there are about 200 telemedicine networks and 3,500 service sites in the U.S., with over half of the hospitals in the nation using some form of telehealth. As technology continues to advance, more hospitals will likely follow the trend and implement telemedicine in some form. Resources for the public to access further information. It is intentionally designed to be user-friendly (Dostie, 2017).

CHALLENGES: PAYMENT, SCOPE OF PRACTICE

Financial

Federal/Medicare

While the uses of telehealth are endless, policy and payment limit access for services. Home monitoring may save money, but if it is not a paid entity of the patient's insurance, it is not a service. Reimbursements for services do not correspond with technology. Regardless of the benefits of any technological advance in healthcare, sustaining the method is key to use and advancement

Payment for telehealth service has progressed in various ways. At the origination of telehealth, the face-to-face encounter was the only acceptable form of securing payment. As the technology developed and usability confirmed the need for the process, payment began to follow. Medicare is usually the standard for other payers to follow in billing practices (CMMS, 2018). However, state-to-state Medicaid or other payers may not adhere to the same standards. This provides opportunities for policy initiatives at both state and national levels.

Medicare published an informational report on Medicare and telehealth describing who is eligible for services in telehealth (CMMS, 2018):

> "(1) The populations of Medicare beneficiaries, such as those who are dually eligible for the Medicare program under title XVIII of the Social Security Act (42 U.S.C. 1395 et seq.) and the Medicaid program under title XIX of such Act (42 U.S.C. 1396 et seq.) and those with chronic conditions, whose care may be improved most in terms of quality and efficiency by the expansion, in a manner that meets or exceeds the existing in-person standard of care under the Medicare program under such title XVIII, of telehealth services under section 1834(m)(4) of such Act (42 U.S.C. 1395m(m)(4)) (Section 1)".

Medicare policies define geographic and practice settings that are billable. Under Section 1834(m), statutes prohibit Medicare payment for telehealth services if the originating sites are not in a rural HPSA for a county outside of a Metropolitan Statistical Area. Additional requirements involve supplemental federal funding. The statute generally allows payment for only live face-to-face encounters (Tuckson *et al.*, 2017; Centers for Medicare and Medicaid Services, 2018).

Two characteristics of the telehealth process involve the originating site and the distant site. The distant site refers to where the physician or licensed practitioner delivering the service is located at the time the service is provided via telecommunication system. The originating site is where the eligible Medicaid member receives the services provided via a telecommunication system (National Consortium of Telehealth Resource Centers, 2018).

State/Medicaid

The big picture of telehealth policy is in constant change. Payment policies differ by state and payer. Each state can choose how they cover telehealth services. Reimbursements are dependent on several aspects of the service and how it is provided. Six questions describe the services (National Consortium of Telehealth Resource Centers, 2018; Center for Connected Health Policy, 2018b):

- Who is paying? Third party payer Medicare, Medicaid, private payer, self-pay?
- What modality? What technology provides the service?
- What type service? Is it a service that payers allow and that has a CPT/HCPCS Code?
- Who is the direct recipient of the service? Patient or other provider? Provider to provider?
- Where is originating site? Geography, what type of facility (medical or non-medical)?
- What type healthcare provider is delivering the service? Physician, NP, PA, and psychologist, health educator, dietician?

The National Telehealth Policy Resource Center was developed to provide national resources for telehealth. To further elevate telehealth practice, the Center for Connected Health Policy (CCHP) became a national resource for research and policy to advance state and national health care policies that promote better systems of care (CCHP, n.d.). The CCHP website provides an interactive tool that describes current states laws and reimbursement through state payers such as Medicaid (CCHP, 2018a). Using the tool, each state defines the six questions that allow payment for service. The tool links the information to the individual state manuals for further information.

For example, using the CCHP web tool, the rural state of West Virginia outlines the requirements for payment (West Virginia Department of Health and Human Resources Bureau for Medical Services, 2016):

- Who is paying? West Virginia State Medicaid
- What modality? Live video/audio. Only real time communication.
- What type service? Outpatient or inpatient E&M services, behavioral health services (RHCs and FQHC are not authorized to serve as a distant site)
- Who is direct recipient of care? Patient is receiving care that is designated by E&M Services
- Where is originating site? Services are not limited to non-metro statistical professional shortage areas as defined by CMS telehealth guide. No exclusion in state geography.

Authorized originating sites for West Virginia:

- Offices of physicians or practitioners
- Private Psychological Practices
- Hospitals
- Critical Access Hospitals (CAH)
- Rural Health Clinics (RHCs)
- Federally Qualified Health Centers (FQHCs)
- Hospital-based or CAH-based Renal Dialysis Centers (including satellites)
- Skilled Nursing Facilities (SNF)
- Community Mental Health Centers (CMHC)
- What type healthcare provider is delivering the service: Physicians or licensed practitioners in West Virginia eligible to provide services

The originating site must bill with the correct Telehealth code with telehealth Modifier (GT). The originating site may bill E&M services that precede the telehealth service and other Medicaid covered services (Center for Connected Health Policy, 2018a). Distant site Appropriate CPT/HCPCS code (West Virginia Department of Health and Human Resources Bureau for Medical Services, 2016). Since Medicaid is specific to each state, any billing outside the state would be denied coverage.

SCOPE AND LAW

Reimbursement for services is a challenging job that changes frequently. A larger challenge for nurse practitioners with telehealth services is the scope of practice and state law where the NP practices. The impact of policy and regulation on rural health and rural nurse practitioners varies from state to state and payer to payer.

The nurse practitioner accessing telehealth may be in one state and the patient in another. The patient and nurse practitioner may be in one state, and the nurse practitioner has to send the medication electronically to another state. Depending on the scope and laws of both states, this could be an issue. Even with a DEA number, it is difficult to send scheduled IV-V meds. At this point in time, the nurse practitioner must be licensed and credentialed in both states and have prescribing privileges for each state (NursingLicensure.org, n.d.).

Compact licenses are emerging for Registered Nurses, but not as quickly for the Advanced Practice Registered Nurses (APRN). The APRN Compact was developed to support legislation for practice among member states while allowing states to retain autonomy and authority to enforce the State Nurse Practice Act (National Council of State Boards of Nursing, Inc., n.d.). More legislative work is needed to complete the process. Adding telehealth services to the proposed legislation further complicates the practice.

Even when the law designates that NPs have billing rights in that state, the insurance companies are national and often do not adhere to the state laws. Some private insurances will only bill under a collaborating or supervising physician. In states where practice is autonomous, insurance may not recognize that state individually, and even though the state law requires it, they pay on a case-by-case, or region-by-region basis. Some private insurance further cause issues by charging a specialty co-pay for NPs in primary care.

National organizations such as the American Association of Nurse Practitioners (AANP) work to prevent insurance denials and promote access to nurse practitioners by private insurance. AANP formed the Multistate Reimbursement Alliance (MSRA) to track issues surrounding insurance credentialing, contracting and reimbursement. Through the AANP, MSRA provides a toolkit to help NPs navigate the denial process and report reimbursement issues (AANP, n.d.-b).

In 2017, the Veterans Administration (VA) services worked with AANP to bridge the gap in providing telehealth services to veterans by qualified nurse practitioners (Hebert, 2017). Organizations like AANP discuss the barrier among states with outdated scope or practice abilities. This prevents a more unified ability to access national licensing and credentialing (AANP, n.d.-a).

Current research suggests that expanding the scope of practice for nurse practitioners may improve access, supply, and quality of care. In rural populations, outcomes suggest that the quality of patient outcomes is not reduced when the scope of practice is expanded (Ortiz *et al.*, 2018). However, national licensing for nurse practitioners has not occurred to date. This is a large barrier for nurse practitioners and restricts opportunities in telemedicine. Even more importantly, patient access to health services is negatively impacted.

LEGAL IMPLICATIONS

As corporations expand telehealth as a healthcare business, additional care must be taken to maintain integrity within the business and the process. The same laws that govern non-virtual business govern telehealth entities. Adherence to the originating site specifications and designation for that state and provider is mandatory.

The billing process must contain accurate evaluation and management (E&M) codes as well as a telehealth designation codes similar to office visit billing. The visit and the documentation should be equal to the same type of service performed in office (CCHP, 2018a). In addition, the distant site must use appropriate CPT/HCPCS codes (West Virginia Department of Health and Human Resources Bureau for Medical Services, 2016).

Concerning referrals, the Anti-kickback Law prevents referrals to another entity in which the provider has a financial interest (The Stark Law [42 USC § 1395nn]). This is still enforced in telehealth visits.

Standards of clinical practice such as malpractice insurance, peer review, and quality improvement must be part of the process. Any medical device used in patient care should have FDA approval (Dorsey and Topol, 2016).

Telehealth providers must insure quality of care. Concerns about the quality of health care providers are common (Farr, 2018). The Wall Street Journal reported misdiagnosed skin problems and links with doctors that were not in the United States and did not have licenses to practice where the patient was located (Beck, 2016).

SECURITY OF CARE

The convenience of accessing healthcare in a private home environment seems ideal, but some patients fear loss of security (Powell, Henstenburg, Cooper, Hollander, and Rising, 2017). Security is a general concern among current and prospective uses of telehealth. Online information about telehealth advises patients what to ask their telehealth provider about privacy safeguards (Telemedicine privacy and security, n.d.).

Security is a not only a concern for patients, but also a concern for providers (Hall and McGraw, 2014). Fear of violation of patient privacy and security is inhibiting physicians from using telehealth (Healthcare data security worries discourage virtual care use, 2018).

Recent data breaches increase the vulnerable aspect of telehealth and electronic medical records (Healthcare IT News, 2018). The explosion of technology and communication has exceeded the ability to protect the process. HIPAA compliant procedures may be outdated before they are published (Luxton, Kayl, and Mishkind, 2012; Baker and Bufka, 2011). Goodman (2016) notes in his book *Future Crimes*, "Will the dependence on technology open doors for medical hackers? Can we trust technology with the lives of our patients? . . . Lone individuals with ill intent can reach out and have a negative effect on tens of millions at anywhere and at any time." With innovative progress come futuristic concerns.

It would seem common knowledge that routine text messaging, email, or video chatting is not appropriate for telehealth services. HIPPA has specific requirements for privacy in telehealth methods. The system should be constantly monitored to prevent any breach of electronic protected health information (ePHI) whether accidental or malicious. Only authorized users should have access to the ePHI and the transmission (HIPAA Journal, n.d.). Secure electronic communications between patient and provider must be maintained with or without an intervening healthcare provider (Federation of State Medical Boards, 2014). Secure communication should also protect the integrity of the ePHI (Zhang, 2016).

Federal regulations provide HIPAA enforcement and data breach notifications (HITECH Act Summary, 2017). Translating these regulations into the telehealth framework is a daunting task. Organizations like the National Consortium of Telehealth Resource Centers assist telehealth providers in creating and maintaining secure and confidential means of providing care (National Consortium of Telehealth Resource Centers, 2019). Privacy and security are key in advancing telehealth services for both the provider and the patient.

MALPRACTICE AND MALPRACTICE COVERAGE

Malpractice issues are of concern in any practice. Telehealth is no exception (Schlachta-Fairchild, Varghese, Deickman, and Castelli, 2010). Location of the services can impact the cost of malpractice insurance (National Consortium of Telehealth Resource Centers, 2017).

Cyber liability from data breaches and telehealth malpractice coverage are new necessities as telehealth expands into everyday practice. Common questions for providers include: Who provides the insurance and how much is needed? Does the cost outweigh reimbursement for providing the service? (Do I need additional malpractice insurance for telemedicine? 2018). What should it cover? (A cyber insurance policy checklist, 2018). The CCHP is one of several organizations to help guide providers through the legal jungle of telehealth (CCHP, n.d.).

THERAPEUTIC RELATIONSHIPS AND PERSONAL INTERFACE

The technological benefits of access are weighted with the loss of personal touch. If a patient does not feel connected with the provider, he/she most likely will not continue seeing that provider or using the service (Rowe, 2017). It seems as if consumers want aspects of healthcare that are on opposing ends of the spectrum; personal interaction, yet the convenience of video interaction. Regardless of the venue, patients prefer personalized healthcare in a way that fits the culture and desires of each patient. Patients hold a nostalgic vision of a community provider that knows him/her and circumstances of each family (Leaf, 2018). It is a reasonable concept that telehealth with the patient's usual provider would be well accepted (Welch, Harvey, O'Connell, and McElligott, 2017).

Creating and maintain a personal connection is key for telehealth use. Medical blogs suggest methods that help the provider initiate and maintain an atmosphere of connection both personally and technologically (Becker's Health IT and CIO Report, 2014). Similar blogs advise patients about using telehealth and how to get the most out of the visit. Taking notes and having questions prepared prevents the "stage fright" of the video and helps the patients stay focused on their concerns (Team, 2018).

The personal bond between the patient and the provider is a bridge for communication and healing. New technologies may increase access, but decrease therapeutic relationships. Newer may not always be better. Mehta (1999) discusses how the physician-patient relationship may be at stake with the use of telehealth. The patient's particular issue may not fit telehealth. The impact of telehealth on relationships with patients, access to healthcare, capacity for equitable treatment, cost, and quality of life must be assessed. These concerns will determine the use of this technology as a viable means of providing quality healthcare (Fleming, Edison, and Pak, 2009). Nurses and nurse practitioners have an enormous challenge to maintain the same level of personal connection virtually as they have in person.

ADOPTION OF TELEHEALTH AMONG THE POPULATIONS

The global market for telemedicine is expected to continue to increase. More than 76% of hospitals connect with patients and practitioners, and that number is expected to rise (AHA, 2019). Kaiser Permanente estimated 210,383 telehealth visits during 2015–2017. Of the telehealth visits, 74% were on a smart phone with a median time of 8 minutes (Brohan, 2018). Ninety-three percent of 1,274 of the patients surveyed said that the digital session met their needs. Today, 52% of the more than 100 million Kaiser Permanente patient encounters each year are virtual visits (Byron, 2018).

It was theorized that millennials would choose telehealth options for care and as an alternative to face-to-face encounters, if the option were available (Farr, 2018). Young adults, age 18–34, did see telemedicine as the best option for them (Ellison, 2014). Many had concerns about insurance coverage for the service (Wicklund, 2018). However, 82% of consumers in Reston, Virginia, were not using the technology (Well, 2016). In contrast, another study noted that 56% of claims for telehealth visits were associated with individuals 31–60 years old in 2016. Other age groups were much lower at approximately 19% each for age ranges of 41–50 and 51–60 (Fair Health, Inc., 2018). Convenience and short waiting times are positive factors in consumer use of providers with telehealth. However, symptoms seem to dictate whether consumers want the quick access to telehealth versus an in-person visit. More than 90% want an in-person treatment for blurred vision and toothache, while more than 78% wanted in-person visits for muscle aches, injuries, and joint pain (Consumers like telehealth, but still prefer face-to-face healthcare, 2018). Mental healthcare is the most utilized service and accounted for nearly one-third of the telehealth visits. The next most common use of telehealth was for acute upper respiratory infections (A New View of Place of Service Trends and Medical Pricing, 2018).

The geriatric population has the greatest need for telehealth services. Issues with mobility, transportation, and medication reconciliation are only a few of the issues facing geriatric patients. As noted in Figure 8.3, obtaining an accurate medication history may involve actually seeing the medications and pill bottles that the patient has in order to obtain an accurate medication list. Telehealth and video monitoring could bridge the gaps in providing care for this vulnerable population (Merrell, 2015). Telehealth in veteran health services has shown positive outcomes in the use of video technology for geriatric patients (U.S. Department of Veterans Affairs, n.d.). Telehealth also has the potential to improve access to education about chronic disease self-management (Banbury *et al.*, 2014).

Older adults and geriatric patients may feel inadequate or have a fear of the complexity of electronic devices. Concerns about user-friendly support may prohibit use of telehealth platforms (Vaportzis, Clausen, and Gow, 2017). The ability to effectively use and understand telehealth practices is not the only concern of the aging population. Apprehensions about cost and confidentially have been identified in geriatric studies (Kayyali, Hesso, Ejiko, and Nabhani Gebara, 2017). Perceived need of the service and privacy are also two aspects of hesitancy of use in geriatric groups (Buckley, Tran, and Prandoni, 2004).

Initiation of a telehealth-based program in an emergent care environment demonstrated that older patients had similar satisfaction scores as younger patients (Greenwald, Stern, Clark, and Sharma, 2018). Older people with little computer experience can be supported to use telehealth equipment. Identifying and addressing individual barriers is helpful in this population (Cimperman, Brenčič, Trkman, and Stanonik, 2013). Various projects have facilitated easing

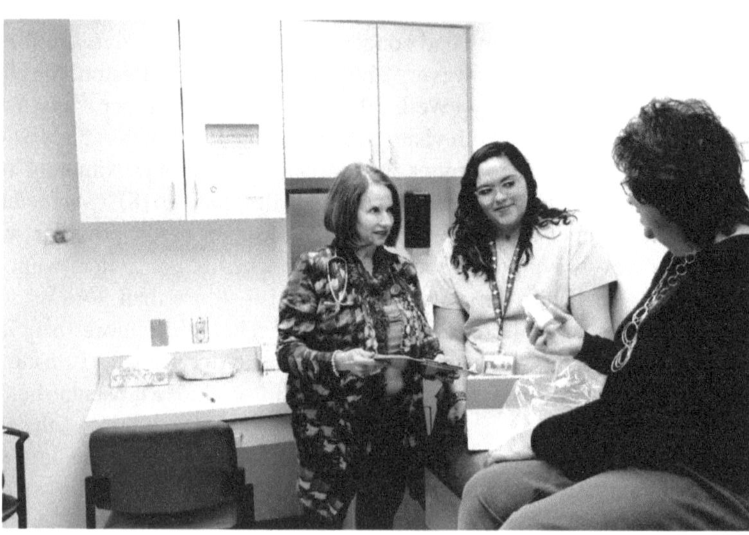

FIGURE 8.3.

TABLE 8.1. Resources for Telehealth Services.

Assistance	Agency	Methods	Web Address
Provides information on financial support for originating funds and regulations for getting started	The Office of National Coordinator for Health Information Technology (ONC) The Office of the National Coordinator for Health Information Technology (ONC) The Office of the National Coordinator for Health Information Technology (ONC)	Updated web information	https://www.healthit.gov/sites/
Provides funding resources and interactive mapping tools	Federal Office of Rural Health Policy within the Health Resources and Services Administration (HRSA)	Location services of resources and existing services	https://www.hrsa.gov/rural-health/telehealth/index.html
Policy, research, care standards, development and implementation are only a few of the areas covered in the compendium	The Office of National Coordinator for Health Information Technology (ONC) in coordination with (HRSA)	Developed Federal Telehealth Compendium Information on a rage of telehealth activities across various agencies.	https://www.healthit.gov/
Statistical support from HRSA provides needs assessment information on medically underserved areas and rural health status regions	HRSA	Updated statistics national and regional	https://data.hrsa.gov/.
Provides assistance, education, and information for organizations or individuals seeking to provide distanced health care	The National Consortium of Telehealth Resource Centers	Regionalized resources are available for the site and bring the resources close to the desired location	https://www.telehealthresource-center.org

(continued)

TABLE 8.1 (continued). Resources for Telehealth Services.

Assistance	Agency	Methods	Web Address
Technological requirements for EHR and Telehealth	ONC	Website with updated specifications for EHRs and telehealth	https://www.healthit.gov/faq/what-recommended-bandwidth-different-types-health-care-providers
Assists healthcare organizations, networks, and providers with the integration of telehealth technologies.	Center for Connected Health Policy: The National Telehealth Policy Resource Center (CCHP)	Analyzes and reports on telehealth policy issues and provides telehealth policy resources throughout the U.S.	https://www.cchpca.org/
Promotes access to medical care for consumers and health professionals through telehealth for network members	American Telemedicine Association (ATA)	Offers events, education, policy information, and advocacyy	http://www.americantelemed.org/home
Assists healthcare organizations, networks, and providers with assessing and implementing cost-effective telehealth technology to serve rural and medically underserved populations	National Telehealth Technology Assessment Resource Center (TTAC)	Serves as a telehealth resource center funded by the Office for the Advancement of Telehealth (OAT)	http://telehealthtechnology.org/

the use of telehealth in the geriatric population, and software to assess medical literacy and enhance communication is in development (HIT Leaders and News LLC, n.d.). Technological and medical literacy must be considered in all aspects of care.

SUPPORT SERVICES/RESOURCES FOR TELEHEALTH CARE IN RURAL AREAS

Multiple agencies and organizations provide support for telehealth. The resources may be regional or national. The following list is not all-inclusive, but it is representative of the type of resources available. (See Table 8.1).

Startup requirements vary with time and progress. Technological resources (such as computers) will need to be fairly new to support telecommunications (Reifsneider, 2018). Internet speed in 2018 was 10 megabits per second (mbps), and will probably become faster in the years to come. Many companies will assist with the start-up process (10 things to know about starting your telemedicine practice, 2017). Depending on the type of business arrangement chosen, financial management is similar to any medical practice, but will require some additional adjustments. Electronic medical records platforms may be standard in certain telehealth businesses. If it is a private telehealth practice, the EHR may be one of several different platforms that fit the individual's practice.

CONCLUSION

As technology advances, providers will continue to capitalize on mechanisms to improve healthcare. As in the development of any new and innovative treatments, the unintended consequences are not fully known. Nurse practitioners must embrace technology and integrate it into care while considering any adverse reactions of the intervening technology. Telehealth providers must prepare for power failure, computer glitches, and user failures. We must cautiously open the door to futuristic care in the name of meeting healthcare access and demands of the underserved (IOM, 2011). But as in the usual state of resource scarcity, we must be prepared to use personal intelligence with or without artificial intelligence. Our minds, knowledge, and experience cannot be replaced, but it can and must be augmented for the best interests of the rural population.

The transformation induced by this innovation calls on the healthcare professional to evaluate the benefits and implications of telehealth services. Botrugno (2017) challenges providers to keep high the standard of healthcare against the economic interests of private stakeholder vendors. In fact, the quality of our care depends on it.

REFERENCES

10 things to know about starting your telemedicine practice. 2017. Retrieved from https://www.mendfamily.com/part-1-10-things-know-starting-telemedicine-practice/.

A cyber insurance policy checklist. (2018). Retrieved from https://resources.infosecinstitute.com/cyber-insurance-policy-checklist/.

A New View of Place of Service Trends, and Medical Pricing. (2018). *FH healthcare indicators™ and FH medical price index™.*

American Association of Nurse Practitioners. (n.d.-a). 2019 state policy priorities. Retrieved from https://www.aanp.org/advocacy/state/2019-state-policy-priorities.

American Association of Nurse Practitioners. (n.d.-b). Multistate reimbursement alliance (MSRA): Enhancing NP support for insurance credentialing, contracting and reimbursement. Retrieved from https://www.aanp.org/practice/practice-management/business-resources-for-nurse-practitioners/multistate-reimbursement-alliance-msra?lockdown=true.

American Hospital Association. (2019). Fact sheet: Telehealth. Retrieved from http://dhhr.wv.gov/bms/Provider/Documents/Manuals/Chapter%20519%20Practitioner%20Services/Policy_519.17_Telehealth_Services.pdf.

American Medical Association. (2016). AMA encourages telemedicine training for medical students, residents [Press release]. Retrieved from https://www.ama-assn.org/press-center/press-releases/ama-encourages-telemedicine-training-medical-students-residents.

American Psychological Association. (n.d.). *Guidelines for the practice of telepsychology*. Retrieved from https://www.apa.org/practice/guidelines/telepsychology.

American Telemedicine Association.Telemedicine glossary. Retrieved from http://thesource.americantelemed.org/resources/telemedicine-glossary.

Badowski, M. E., *et al.* (2018). Providing comprehensive medication management in telehealth. Pharmacotherapy, 38(2): e16. doi:10.1002/phar.2071 [doi].

Baker, D. C., and L. F. Bufka. (2011). Preparing for the telehealth world: Navigating legal, regulatory, reimbursement, and ethical issues in an electronic age. *Professional Psychology: Research and Practice, 42*(6): 405–411. doi:10.1037/a0025037.

Balanced Budget Act of 1997, Pub. L. No. 105-33, 111 stat. 251 (1997).

Banbury, A., *et al.* (2014). Multi-site videoconferencing for home-based education of older people with chronic conditions: The telehealth literacy project. *Journal of Telemedicine and Telecare, 20*(7): 353–359. doi:10.1177/1357633X14552369.

Barbosa, I. A., and M. J. P. D. Silva. (2017). Nursing care by telehealth: What is the influence of distance on communication? *Revista Brasileira De Enfermagem, 70*(5), 928-934. doi:S0034-71672017000500928 [pii].

Bashshur, R. L., P. A. Armstrong, and Z. I. Youssef. Telemedicine: Explorations in the Use of Telecommunications in Health Care. Springfield, Ill: Charles C. Thomas; 1975.

Beck, M. (2016). Study of telemedicine finds misdiagnoses of skin problems. *The Wall Street Journal*. Retrieved from https://www.wsj.com/articles/study-of-telemedicine-finds-misdiagnoses-of-skin-problems-1463344200.

Becker's Health IT and CIO Report. (2014). The human touch of telemedicine: A primer on secure, reliable, patient-centric telemedicine solutions. *Becker's Hospital Review*. Retrieved from https://www.beckershospitalreview.com/healthcare-information-technology/the-human-touch-of-telemedicine-a-primer-on-secure-reliable-patient-centric-telemedicine-solutions.html.

Benschoter R. A., C. Garetz, and P. Smith. (1967). The use of closed circuit TV and videotape in the training of social group workers. *Social Work Education Reporter, 15*(1):18–20.

Board on Health Care Services, Institute of Medicine and Nesbitt, T. (2012). The evolution of telehealth: Where have we been and where are we going? *The Role of Telehealth in an Evolving Health Care Environment: Workshop Summary*. Washington (DC): National Academies Press. Available from: https://www.ncbi.nlm.nih.gov/books/NBK207141/.

Botrugno, C. (2017). Towards an ethics for telehealth. *Nursing Ethics*. https://doi.org/10.1177/0969733017705004.

Bradford, N. K., L. J. Caffery, and A. C. Smith. (2016). Telehealth services in rural and remote Australia: A systematic review of models of care and factors influencing success and sustainability. *Rural and Remote Health, 16*(4): 4268. doi:4268 [pii].

Brohan, M. (Oct. 2018, -10-19T14:26:40-06:00). Kaiser patients keep telehealth visits short and sweet. Retrieved from https://www.digitalcommerce360.com/2018/10/19/kaiser-patients-keep-telehealth-visits-short-and-sweet/.

Brown, J. D., A. J. Goodin, and J. C. Talbert. (2018). Rural and Appalachian disparities in neonatal abstinence syndrome incidence and access to opioid abuse treatment. *The Journal of Rural Health: Official Journal of the American Rural Health Association and the National Rural Health Care Association, 34*(1): 6–13. doi:10.1111/jrh.12251.

Buckley, K., B. Tran, and C. Prandoni. (2004). Receptiveness, Use and Acceptance of Telehealth by Caregivers of Stroke Patients in the Home. *Online Journal of Issues in Nursing*. Vol. 9 No. 3; Available: www.nursingworld.org/MainMenuCategories/ANAMarketplace/ANAPeriodicals/OJIN/TableofContents/Volume92004/No3Sept04/ArticlePreviousTopic/TelehealthforStrokePatients.aspx.

Byron, J. (2018). We do video visits—NCAL research spotlight. Retrieved from https://spotlight.kaiserpermanente.org/we-do-video-visits/.

Center for Connected Health Policy. (n.d.). About CCHP. Retrieved from https://www.cchpca.org/about/about-cchp.

Center for Connected Health Policy. (2018a). Current state laws and reimbursement policies. Retrieved from https://www.cchpca.org/telehealth-policy/current-state-laws-and-reimbursement-policies?jurisdiction=78&category=128&topic=All.

Center for Connected Health Policy. (2018b). State telehealth laws and reimbursement policies. Retrieved from https://www.cchpca.org/sites/default/files/2018-10/Fall_2018_50_State_Infographic_FINAL.pdf.

Center for Disease Control and Prevention. (2018). MMWR rural health series | MMWR. Retrieved from https://www.cdc.gov/mmwr/rural_health_series.html.

Centers for Medicare and Medicaid Services. (2018). *Information on Medicare telehealth*. Washington, D.C.: Centers for Medicare and Medicaid Services.

Chaet, D., *et al.* (2017). Ethical practice in telehealth and telemedicine. *Journal of General Internal Medicine, 32*(106*e Official Journal of the American Telemedicine Association, 15*(8): 797–803. doi:10.1089/tmj.2009.0035.

Forbes, R. C., *et al.* (2018). A cost comparison for telehealth utilization in the kidney transplant waitlist evaluation process. *Transplantation, 102*(2): 279–283. doi:10.1097/TP.0000000000001903 [doi].

García Marqués, S., *et al.* (2017). Tools assessment and diagnosis to infant colic: A systematic review. *Child: Care, Health and Development, 43*(4): 481–488. doi:10.1111/cch.12454.

Geronimo, A., *et al.* (2017). Incorporation of telehealth into a multidisciplinary ALS clinic: Feasibility and acceptability. *Amyotrophic Lateral Sclerosis and Frontotemporal Degeneration, 18*(7–8): 555–561. doi:10.1080/21678421.2017.1338298 [doi].

Gershon-Cohen J., and A. G. Cooley. (1950). *Telediagnosis. Radiology, 55*:582–587.

Goodman, M. (2016). Surviving progress. Future crimes (pp. 447–499). New York: Anchor Books.

Greenwald, P., *et al.* (2018). Older adults and technology: In telehealth, they may not be who you think they are. *International Journal of Emergency Medicine, 11*(1): 1–4. doi:10.1186/s12245-017-0162-7.

Hale, T. M., and J. C. Kvedar. (1999). Virtual mentor. Retrieved from http://www.bibliothek.uni-regensburg.de/ezeit/?2162995.

Hale, T. M., and J. C. Kvedar. (2014). Privacy and security concerns in telehealth. AMA Journal of Ethics, 16(12): 981–985. doi:10.1001/virtualmentor.2014.16.12.jdsc1-1412.

Hall, J. L., and D. McGraw. (2014). For telehealth to succeed, privacy and security risks must be identified and addressed. *Health Affairs* (*Project Hope*), *33*(2): 216–221. doi:10.1377/hlthaff.2013.0997.

Haltigan, J. D., *et al.* (2012). The infant crying questionnaire: Initial factor structure and validation. *Infant Behavior and Development, 35*(4): 876–883. doi:10.1016/j.infbeh.2012.06.001.

Health Care Fraud Prevention and Enforcement Action Team. (n.d.). Comparison of the anti-kickback statue and Stark law. Retrieved from https://oig.hhs.gov/compliance/provider-compliance-training/files/starkandakscharthandout508.pdf.

Health Resource and Services Administration. (n.d.). Quick Maps—Mental health professional shortage areas (HPSA). Retrieved from https://data.hrsa.gov/hdw/Tools/MapToolQuick.aspx?mapName=HPSAMH.

Health Resources and Service Administration. (2019). Telehealth programs. Retrieved February 2019 from https://www.hrsa.gov/rural-health/telehealth/index.html.

Health Resources and Services Administration. (2018). Telehealth programs. Retrieved January 2019 from https://www.hrsa.gov/rural-health/telehealth/index.html.

Healthcare IT News. (2018). The biggest healthcare data breaches of 2018 (so far). Retrieved from https://www.healthcareitnews.com/projects/biggest-healthcare-data-breaches-2018-so-far.

HealthCare.gov. (n.d.). Primary care. Retrieved from https://www.healthcare.gov/glossary/primary-care/.

HealthIT.gov. (2017a). Benefits for critical access hospitals and other small rural hospitals. Retrieved from https://www.healthit.gov/topic/health-it-initiatives/benefits-critical-access-hospitals-and-other-small-rural-hospitals.

HealthIT.gov. (2017b). Telemedicine and telehealth. Retrieved from www.healthit.gov/topic/health-it-initiatives/telemedicine-and-telehealth.

HealthIT.gov. (n.d.-a). Meaningful use and MACRA. Retrieved from http://healthit.gov/policy-researchers-implementers/meaningful-use-regulations.

HealthIT.gov. (n.d.-b). Meaningful use definition and meaningful use objectives of EHRs | providers and professionals. Retrieved from http://www.healthit.gov/providers-professionals/meaningful-use-definition-objectives.

Hebert, D. (2017). "RE: RIN 2900-AQ06—Authority of Health Care Providers to Practice Telehealth (82 Fed. Reg. 45756, October 2, 2017)." Received by Michael Shores, November 1, 2017.

HIPAA Journal. (n.d.). HIPAA guidelines on telemedicine. Retrieved from https://www.hipaajournal.com/hipaa-guidelines-on-telemedicine/.

HITECH act summary. (2017). Retrieved from https://www.usfhealthonline.com/resources/key-concepts/hitech-act-summary/.

HIT Leaders and News LLC. (n.d.). Health literacy principles in telehealth. Retrieved from https://us.hitleaders.news/health-literacy-principles-in-telehealth/.

Institute of Medicine (US) Committee on Quality of Health Care in America. (2001). Crossing the quality chasm: A new health system for the 21st century. Washington, DC: The National Academies Press. Retrieved from: https://www.ncbi.nlm.nih.gov/books/NBK222274/.

Institute of Medicine (US) Committee on the Robert Wood Johnson Foundation Initiative on the Future of Nursing, at the Institute of Medicine. (2011). The future of nursing: Leading change, advancing health. Washington, DC: The National Academies Press. Retrieved from http://www.ncbi.nlm.nih.gov/books/NBK209880/.

Institute of Medicine. (2004). Quality through collaboration: The future of rural health. Washington, DC: The National Academies Press. Retrieved from: http://www.nationalacademies.org/hmd/Reports/2004/Quality-Through-Collaboration-The-Future-of-Rural-Health.aspx.

Institute of Medicine. (2005). Quality through collaboration: The future of rural health. Washington, DC: The National Academies Press. doi:10.17226/11140 Retrieved from https://www.nap.edu/catalog/11140/quality-through-collaboration-the-future-of-rural-health.

James, C. V. (2017). Racial/ethnic health disparities among rural adults—United States, 2012–2015. *MMWR. Surveillance Summaries, 66* doi:10.15585/mmwr.ss6623a1.

Kaltwasser, J. (2015). Patients fear fraud, loss of privacy as health records go digital. *MD Magazine*. Retrieved from https://www.mdmag.com/physicians-money-digest/practice-management/patients-fear-fraud-loss-of-privacy-as-health-records-go-digital.

Kayyali, R., *et al.* (2017). A qualitative study of telehealth patient information leaflets (TILs): Are we giving patients enough information? *BMC Health Services Research, 17*(1), 5. doi:10.1186/s12913-017-2257-5 [doi].

King, V. L., *et al.* (2009). Assessing the effectiveness of an internet-based videoconferencing platform for delivering intensified substance abuse counseling. *Journal of Substance Abuse Treatment, 36*(3): 331–338. doi:10.1016/j.jsat.2008.06.011.

Kruse, C. S., *et al.* (2017). Telehealth and patient satisfaction: A systematic review and narrative analysis. *BMJ Open, 7*(8), 016242. doi:10.1136/bmjopen-2017-016242 [doi].

Kulkarni, R. (2018). Use of telehealth in the delivery of comprehensive care for patients with haemophilia and other inherited bleeding disorders. *Haemophilia: The Official Journal of the World Federation of Hemophilia, 24*(1): 33–42. doi:10.1111/hae.13364 [doi].

Kurth, E., *et al.* (2011). Crying babies, tired mothers: What do we know? A systematic review. *Midwifery, 27*(2), 187–194. doi:10.1016/j.midw.2009.05.012 [doi].

Langarizadeh, M., F. Moghbeli, and A. Aliabadi. (2017). Application of ethics for providing telemedicine services and information technology. Medical archives (Sarajevo, Bosnia and Herzegovina), 71(5): 351–355.

Leaf, C. (2018). Why hasn't telemedicine taken off? Hey, blame this guy. *Fortune*. Retrieved from http://fortune.com/2018/07/03/whats-holding-up-telemedicine.

Luxton, D. D., R. A. Kayl, and M. C. Mishkind, (2012). mHealth data security: The need for HIPAA-compliant standardization. *Telemedicine and E-Health, 18*(4): 284–288. doi:10.1089/tmj.2011.0180.

Mars, M., and R. E. Scott. (2017). Being spontaneous: The future of telehealth implementation? *Telemedicine Journal and E-Health: The Official Journal of the American Telemedicine Association, 23*(9): 766–772. doi:10.1089/tmj.2016.0155 [doi].

Medicare Learning Network. (2018). *Telehealth services*. Washington, D.C: U.S. Department of Health and Human Services.

Mehta, S. J. (1999). Virtual mentor. *American Medical Association Journal of Ethics*. Retrieved from http://www.bibliothek.uni-regensburg.de/ezeit/?2162995.

Merrell, R. C. (2015). Geriatric telemedicine: Background and evidence for telemedicine as a way to address the challenges of geriatrics. *Healthcare Informatics Research, 21*(4): 223–229. doi:10.4258/hir.2015.21.4.223.

Mid-Atlantic Telehealth Resource Center. (n.d.-a). Find telehealth providers. Retrieved from https://www.matrc.org/find-telehealth-providers.

Mid-Atlantic Telehealth Resource Center. (n.d.-b). How can I use it? Retrieved from https://www.matrc.org/resources/how-can-i-use-it.

Mohatt, D. (n.d.). *Rural mental health: Challenges and opportunities caring for the country* [PowerPoint slides]. Retrieved from: http://govinfo.library.unt.edu/mental-healthcommission/presentations/rural.ppt.

National center for health workforce analysis (NCHWA). (2017). Distribution of U.S. healthcare providers residing in rural and urban areas. Washington: Federal Information and News Dispatch, Inc. Retrieved from ProQuest Curriculum Essentials Retrieved from https://search.proquest.com/docview/2035229589.

National Consortium of Telehealth Resource Centers. (2017). Considerations for telehealth providers when negotiating for malpractice insurance. Retrieved from https://www.telehealthresourcecenter.org/event/considerations-for-telehealth-providers-when-negotiating-for-malpractice-insurance/.

National Consortium of Telehealth Resource Centers. (n.d.). HIPAA and Telehealth Fact Sheets. Retrieved from https://www.telehealthresourcecenter.org/fact-sheets/.

National Consortium of Telehealth Resource Centers. (2018). Telehealth Reimbursement. Retrieved from https://www.telehealthresourcecenter.org/wp-content/uploads/2019/01/Reimbursement-Jan.-2019.pdf.

National Consortium of Telehealth Resource Centers. (n.d.). Locate a telehealth resource center. Retrieved from https://www.telehealthresourcecenter.org/who-your-trc/.

National Council of State Boards of Nursing, Inc. (n.d.) About the APRN compact. Retrieved from https://www.aprncompact.com/about.htm.

National Learning Consortium. (2013). *Continuous quality improvement (CQI) strategies to optimize your practice*. (No. 2017).HealthIT.gov. Retrieved from https://www.healthit.gov/sites/default/files/tools/nlc_continuousqualityimprovementprimer.pdf. (cqi).

National Rural Health Association. (n.d.) About rural health care. Retrieved from https://www.ruralhealthweb.org/about-nrha/about-rural-health-care.

Notes, Short Comments, and Answers to Correspondents. (1878). *The Lancet.* 111(2841): 221–224.

Nursing education in telehealth. (2006). *Journal of Telemedicine and Telecare, 12*(2): 55–56. https://doi.org/10.1258/135763306776084437.

NursingLicensure.org. Nurse practitioner license requirements: Change is in the air. Retrieved 3/14/2019 from https://www.nursinglicensure.org.

Office of the National Coordinator for Health Information Technology and Federal Office of Rural Health Policy—Health Resources, and Services Administration. 2016. *Federal telehealth compendium*. Washington, D.C.: Health Resources and Services Administration.

Olson, C. A., and J. F. Thomas. (2017). Telehealth: No longer an idea for the future. *Advances in Pediatrics, 64*(1): 347–370. doi:S0065-3101(17)30009-9 [pii].

Ortiz, J., *et al.* (2018). Impact of nurse practitioner practice regulations on rural population health outcomes. *Healthcare* (Basel, Switzerland), *6*(2), 65. doi:10.3390/healthcare6020065.

Perednia, D. A., and A. Allen. (1995). Telemedicine Technology and Clinical Applications. *Journal of the American Medical Association, 273*(6):483–487. [PubMed].

Polinski, J. M., *et al.* (2016). Patients' satisfaction with and preference for telehealth visits. *Journal of General Internal Medicine, 31*(3): 269–275. doi:10.1007/s11606-015-3489-x [doi].

Powell, R. E., *et al.* (2017). Patient perceptions of telehealth primary care video visits. *Annals of Family Medicine, 15*(3): 225–229. doi:10.1370/afm.2095.

Privacy, confidentiality and security archives. Retrieved 3/14/2019 from https://www.telehealthresourcecenter.org/knowledgebase_category/privacy-confidentiality-security/.

Reifsneider, D. (2018, -05-14T11:43:34-08:00). Telehealth: What do I need to know to get started? Retrieved from https://www.simplepractice.com/blog/getting-started-telehealth/.

Rimal, D., J. H. Huang Fu, and D. Gillett. (2017). Our experience in using telehealth for paediatric plastic surgery in western Australia. *ANZ Journal of Surgery, 87*(4): 277–281. doi:10.1111/ans.13925 [doi].

Rowe, N. (2017). Telehealth connections: It's not just about the technology. *Arizona Telemedicine Program*. Retrieved from https://telemedicine.arizona.edu/blog/telehealth-connections-it-s-not-just-about-technology.

Rural Health Information Hub. (n.d.-a). Critical access hospitals (CAHs) introduction. Retrieved from https://www.ruralhealthinfo.org/topics/critical-access-hospitals.

Rural Health Information Hub. (n.d.-b). Resources from the CDC MMWR rural health series. Retrieved from https://www.ruralhealthinfo.org/resources/cdc-mmwr-rural-health.

Rural Health Information Hub. (n.d.-c). United States. Retrieved from https://www.ruralhealthinfo.org/states/united-states.

Rural Health Information Hub. (2017). Rural health disparities. Retrieved from https://www.ruralhealthinfo.org/topics/rural-health-disparities.

Rural Health Information Hub. (2018a). Rural mental health. Retrieved from https://www.ruralhealthinfo.org/topics/mental-health.

Rural Health Information Hub. (2018b). Substance abuse in rural areas. Retrieved from https://www.ruralhealthinfo.org/topics/substance-abuse.

Rutledge, C.M., *et al.* (2014). Telehealth: Preparing advanced practice nurses to address healthcare needs in rural and underserved populations. International Journal of Nursing Education Scholarship, 11(1). doi: 10.1515/ijnes-2013-0061.

Rutledge, C. M., *et al.* (2017). Telehealth and eHealth in nurse practitioner training: current perspectives. *Advances in medical education and practice, 8*, 399–409. doi:10.2147/AMEP.S116071.

Schadelbauer, R. (2017). *Anticipating economic returns of rural telehealth*. Retrieved from https://www.ntca.org/sites/default/files/documents/2017-12/SRC_whitepaper_anticipatingeconomicreturns.pdf.

Schlachta-Fairchild, L., *et al.* (2010). Telehealth and telenursing are live: APN policy and practice implications. *The Journal for Nurse Practitioners, 6*(2): 98–106. doi:10.1016/j.nurpra.2009.10.019.

Services, V. T.VA telehealth services home. Retrieved from https://www.telehealth.va.gov/.

Shen, J., and A. Naeim. (2017). Telehealth in older adults with cancer in the United States: The emerging use of wearable sensors. *Journal of Geriatric Oncology, 8*(6): 437–442. doi:S1879-4068(17)30171-6 [pii].

Simonnet, H., *et al.* (2014). Parents' behavior in response to infant crying: Abusive head trauma education. *Child Abuse and Neglect, 38*(12): 1914–1922. Retrieved from https://search.ebscohost.com/login.aspx?direct=true&db=eoah&AN=33246237&site=ehost-live.

Stabler, M. E., *et al.* (2017). Neonatal abstinence syndrome in West Virginia substate regions, 2007–2013. *The Journal of Rural Health, 33*(1): 92–101. doi:10.1111/jrh.12174.

State estimates of adolescent marijuana use and perceptions of risk of harm from mari-

juana use: 2013 and 2014. the CBHSQ report: National survey on drug use and health: The NSDUH report; 2016 ASI 4096-10.240. 2016. Retrieved from https://statistical.proquest.com/statisticalinsight/result/pqpresultpage.previewtitle?docType=PQSI&titleUri=/content/2016/4096-10.240.xml.

Talbot, J. A., *et al.* (2018). Patterns of telehealth use among rural Medicaid beneficiaries. *The Journal of Rural Health: Official Journal of the American Rural Health Association and the National Rural Health Care Association,* doi:10.1111/jrh.12324.

Team, H. (2018, -05-25T08:00:15+00:00). Building doctor-patient relationships via telehealth. Retrieved from https://www.healthsplash.com/blog/building-doctor-patient-relationships-via-telehealth/.

Telemedicine, Institute of Medicine (US) Committee on Evaluating Clinical Applications of, and Field, M. J. (1996). FIGURE 2.1, telemedicine circa 1924. Visionary cover of radio news depicting an imagined "radio doctor" who could see and be seen by his patient. Retrieved from https://www.ncbi.nlm.nih.gov/books/NBK45445/figure/a20006365mmm00001/.

Telemedicine, Institute of Medicine (US) Committee on Evaluating Clinical Applications of, and Field, M. J. (1996). *Evolution and current applications of telemedicine.* National Academies Press (US). Retrieved from https://www.ncbi.nlm.nih.gov/books/NBK45445/.

Telemedicine privacy and security. Retrieved from https://chironhealth.com/definitive-guide-to- telemedicine/telemedicine-info-patients/privacy-and-security/.

Telehealth services: What can online doctors treat? (n.d.). Retrieved from https://www.mdlive.com/patients/telehealth-services/.

Telligen and gpTRAC. (2014). Telehealth: Start-up and resource guide.

Tuckson, R. V., M. Edmunds, and M. L. Hodgkins. (2017). Telehealth. The New England Journal of Medicine, 377(16): 1585–1592. doi:10.1056/NEJMsr1503323.

Umer, A., *et al.* (2018). Capturing the statewide incidence of neonatal abstinence syndrome in real time: The West Virginia.

Vaportzis, E., M. G. Clausen, and A. J. Gow, (2017). Older adults perceptions of technology and barriers to interacting with tablet computers: A focus group study. *Frontiers in Psychology, 8,* 1687. doi:10.3389/fpsyg.2017.01687experience. *Pediatric Research,* doi:10.1038/s41390-018-0172-z.

Warshaw, R. (2017). Health disparities affect millions in rural U.S. communities. Retrieved from https://news.aamc.org/patient-care/article/health-disparities-affect-millions-rural-us-commun/.

Watson, A. C., and A. J. Fulambarker. (2012). The crisis intervention team model of police response to mental health crises: A primer for mental health practitioners. *Best Practices in Mental Health, 8*(2), 71. Retrieved from https://www.ncbi.nlm.nih.gov/pubmed/24039557.

Welch, B. M., *et al.* (2017). Patient preferences for direct-to-consumer telemedicine services: A nationwide survey. *BMC Health Services Research, 17*(1), 784. doi:10.1186/s12913-017-2744-8.

Well, A. (2016). American well: Telemedicine technology solutions. Retrieved from https://www.americanwell.com/.

West Virginia Clinical and Translational Science Institute. (n.d.). Project echo. Retrieved from wvctsi.org/programs/community-engagement-outreach/project-echo/.

West Virginia Department of Health and Human Resources Bureau for Medical Services. (2016). 519.17 telehealth services. Retrieved from http://dhhr.wv.gov/bms/Provider/Documents/Manuals/Chapter%20519%20Practitioner%20Services/Policy_519.17_Telehealth_Services.pdf.

What Is Primary Care? (1983). *Journal of Public Health Policy, 4*(2): 129–134. doi:10.2307/3342428.

Wittson, C. L., and R. A. Benschoter. (1972). Two-way television: Helping the medical center reach out. *American Journal of Psychiatry, 129*(5):136–139.

Wilson, F. A., *et al.* (2017). Reimbursements for telehealth services are likely to be lower than non-telehealth services in the United States. *Journal of Telemedicine and Telecare, 23*(4): 497–500. doi:10.1177/1357633X16652288 [doi].

Zhang, B. (2016). The benefits and risks of telemedicine. Risk Management. Retrieved from http://www.rmmagazine.com/2016/08/01/the-benefits-and-risks-of-telemedicine/.

Zundel, K. M. (1996). Telemedicine: History, applications, and impact on librarianship. *Bulletin of the Medical Library Association, 84*(1): 71–79.

CHAPTER 9

Rural Nursing: American Indians and Alaska Natives in Indian Country

Loretta J. Heuer and Misty L. Wilkie

Objectives:

1. Recognize the unique cultural beliefs, values, and traditions of rural American Indian and Alaska Native (AIAN) populations.
2. Distinguish the disparities and social determinants of health affecting the individual and community health of rural AIAN communities.
3. Describe the structure of health services available for rural AINA.

Discussion Questions:

1. Knowing the historical context and experiences of AIAN people, what are three areas you, as a nurse, could positively influence the social determinants of health for this population?
2. What are the priority issues for rural AIAN people and how can nurse practitioners and nurses address those issues?
3. Name two examples of tribal sovereignty and how it affected the tribal communities.
4. Describe three positive attributes of rural AIAN people and communities.

INTRODUCTION

Historically, the federal government used the terms Indians, or American Indians, to identify people whose ancestors were originally in the Americas before colonization. In May 2016, President Barack Obama signed Public Law No: 114-157, H.R. 4238 which amended two 1970s federal acts that defined minorities with outdated or insensitive terms. The Department of Energy Organization Act described minorities as "a Negro, Puerto Rican, American Indian, Eskimo, Oriental, or Aleut or is a Spanish speaking individual of Spanish descent." A line in Minority Business Enterprises Acts contained the words "Negroes, Spanish speaking, Orientals, Indians, Eskimos and Aleuts." The bill is amended by inserting the words "Asian American, Native Hawaiian, Pacific Islanders, African American, Hispanic, Native American or Alaskan Natives" (Congress.gov, 2016). However, the federal, state, and tribal governments continue use of differing terms to describe Native people so when interacting with individuals from Native American/American Indian and Alaskan Native population, nurses need to ask how they identify their heritage (Moss, 2016). Throughout this chapter, the authors will use the term American Indian and Alaskan Natives (herein referred to as AIAN), to align with the federal government classification on Census 2020, which refers to all individuals who identify with the original peoples of North and South America and maintain tribal affiliation or community attachment (United States Census, 2020).

NATIVE AMERICAN AND ALASKAN NATIVE TRIBES

The Bureau of Indian Affairs (BIA) recognizes 574 American Indian and Alaskan Native tribal sovereign nations located across 35 states. Federally recognized tribes have formal nation-to-nation relationships with the U.S. government and as sovereign nations, each has its own unique governance structure, culture, history, social systems, and world views (National Conference of American Indians [NCAI], 2020; Saenz, 2020). As federally recognized tribal entities, they are eligible for funding and services from BIA by virtue of their status as Indian tribes (Sweeney, 2020).

Thirteen states created a formal legislative process to recognize 66 American Indian (AI) tribes. State-only tribal recognition acknowledges their status within the state, but it does not guarantee state or federal funding. State recognized AI tribes are not federally recognized, but federally recognized tribes can be state recognized (Saenz, 2020). Additionally, some states do not have a formal recognition process; however, they acknowledge the historical and cultural contributions the tribe(s) have made to their states (Salazar, 2016).

American Indians and Alaskan Natives must be enrolled members of the tribes to receive services from either the tribe or federal government, yet there are many Indigenous people who do not belong to a tribe, either by choice or circumstances (Moss, 2016). Tribal membership criteria vary by tribe and can be based on shared customs, traditions, language, and blood quantum or lineage requirements (Thornton, 1997). In the 2000 U.S. Census, almost one million AIANs did not respond to the tribal affiliation part of the race question. Leibler and Zacher (2013) studied why AIs did not respond to the tribal affiliation section of the Census 2000 race question. The authors reported three main reasons which included some AI individuals are generally unresponsive survey participants and they chose not to complete all the questions; there was a misunderstanding of the meaning single race; and finally, tribal non-respondents identified with multiple racial or ethnic heritages. Further, AIs residing on reservations may avoid participating in the Census because they mistrust the federal government (RHO, 2010). Yet, if they do not report one or more tribal affiliations and are not enrolled in a tribe or tribes, they are unable to receive tribal, state, or federal financial or service support (Thornton, 1997). As rural nurse practitioners or nurses, knowing the distinctions between membership in federal or state tribes involves understanding the funding sources, government accountability, and access to health care for AI patients (Moss, 2016).

REGIONAL DIFFERENCES

To track diverse Indigenous groups as they migrated across the U.S., anthropologists and geographers divided AI tribes into nine geographic areas and each area shared similar culture, languages, habitats, and characteristics (Taylor and Sturtevant, 1992). Depending on the resource, there may be slight variations to names and inclusions but the main groupings are Northeastern Woodlands, Southeastern Woodlands, Southwest, Great Basin, California, Pacific Northwest, Northwest Plateau, Alaska, Northern Great Plans, and recently added, Urban (Moss, 2016). The social, cultural, language, economic, and political governance of AIAN tribes differ from geographical region to region, but it should also be noted these differences are found between tribes within each region. This chapter provides an overview of AIANs with a description of life on rural tribal lands when statistics are available.

TRIBAL LANDS

Approximately 368 treaties were negotiated and signed between the US government and AI tribes and approved by U.S. Senate between 1777 to 1868 (Taylor, 2019). Many of the AI nations relinquished millions of acres of land to the U.S. government because they were guaranteed protection from attacks on their lands, tribal sovereignty, religious freedom, self-governance, education, health care, housing, and other services. Moreover, the U.S. consented to manage and protect AI tribes' resources, including lands and timber (Grover, 2014). While these treaties remain legally binding, the U.S. government continually fails to fulfill the promised duties as noted in the high rates of poverty, crime, suicide, and poor health indicators on rural reservations (Taylor, 2019).

There are 334 federally and state recognized AIAN reservations across the U.S. These lands are known as reservations, pueblos, rancherias, missions, villages, and communities. Reservations have defined geographic areas with established boundaries lines like county or state lines. Some reservations are made up of only trust lands while others include trust lands, fee lands owned by tribal nations, individual Natives, and non-Natives. Reservations are frequently referred to as "Indian country" and federal government and tribal nations have primary jurisdiction (Luna-Firebugh, 2007; NCAI, 2020a). Most AIAN reservations are in rural, remote geographic areas with adverse weather conditions (Lindquist, 2016).

The focus is frequently on the negative aspects of the reservations with little attention and understanding of the positive features, of which there are many. First, each reservation is considered a cultural base because AIANs do not share one native language or culture. For most, their own reservation is the only place they can speak to others in their native language and share their traditional way of life. It is where their traditional arts and crafts are created, ceremonies are performed, and original stories are shared with tribal members. Second, their culture is reflective of their relationship to the land on the reservation. Third, life on the reservation includes strong family and community ties. Fourth, social services and assistance programs on reservations are administered through the tribal government or other federal agencies. When they leave the reservation, it can be overwhelming to understand and negotiate the political and social service systems off the reservation. Moreover, if AIANs move away from the reservation, they become ineligible for services such as health care unless they return to their native homelands (Gilio-Whitaker, 2019; Sandefur, 1989).

DEFINING THE AMERICAN INDIAN AND ALASKAN NATIVE RURAL POPULATION

In 2017 an estimated 5.7 million people identified as AIAN and comprised 1.7 percent of the United States population. Of the AIAN population, 2.8 million identified as one race while 2.9 million represented one or more other races (United States Census Bureau, 2018a, B02010). There are widespread misunderstandings regarding the number of AIANs who reside in rural America. For example, a commonly cited statistic is 72 percent of the AIAN people live in urban areas but in contrast the majority, 54 percent of AIAN people live in rural and small-town areas (Dewees and Marks, 2017), and 68 percent AIAN population live on or near their tribal homelands (Pettit et al., 2014). The differing statistic stems from outdated Census definitions and poor data quality so rural AIAN are "twice invisible" because of the lack of federal agencies, private foundations, and policymakers' familiarity with rural areas and their communities (Dewees and Marks, 2017). Moreover, the National Congress of American Indians created the term "Asterisk Nation" because rather than having a data point for AIANs, an asterisk is frequently used when reporting racial and ethnic data due to various data-collection and reporting issues (NCAI, 2019). Broadcasting frequently uses the term "other" but recently during the CNN's live 2020 election coverage, they posted an on-air graphic that used the phrase "something else" to refer to voters who were not white, Latinx, Black, or Asian (Zornosa, 2020).

AMERICAN INDIAN AND ALASKAN NATIVE DEMOGRAPHICS

The AIAN population living on reservations are younger; the median age is 29 as compared to 38 years old for the total U.S. population. Nearly 29 percent of the AIAN population are under the age of 18 as compared to 21.9 percent of the total U.S. population. Some states have higher proportions of young AIAN people. For example, in South Dakota, nearly 41percent of the 91,902 population is under 18 years old (NCAI, 2020).

Life Expectancy

While tribal communities have experienced an overall rise in their average life span, 73.0 years compared to 78.5 years for U.S. all races, they still lag more affluent communities by as much as 20 percent (IHS, 2019). Dwyer-Lindgren *et al.* (2017) calculated life expectancy by county from 1989 to 2014 and described the trends in geographic disparities, socioeconomic and race factors, behavioral and metabolic risk factors, and health as factors. The authors reported that geographically, the Oglala Lakota County, South Dakota, which includes the Pine Ridge American Indian reservation, had the lowest life expectancy in the country in 2014 at 66.8 years. Additionally, three other counties with tribal communities included Todd County, Rosebud Sioux Tribe (68.5 years), and Buffalo County, Crow Creek Sioux Tribe (69.0 years) located in South Dakota along with Sioux County, northern Standing Rock Sioux Tribe reservation (68.6 years), ranked in the bottom five counties for life expectancy (Mwaniki, 2018). However, one of the five counties with the highest life expectancy was Aleutian East Borough in which Alaska Natives comprise about 37 percent of the population.

Dwyer-Lindgren *et al.* (2017) also reviewed the extent to which several factors contributed to the inequality in life expectancy. They found that risk factors such as obesity, lack of exercise, smoking, hypertension, and diabetes account for 74 percent of the variation in longevity. Socioeconomic factors, a combination of poverty, income, education, unemployment, and race, were independently related to 60 percent of the inequality, and access to and quality of health care accounted for 27 percent. By only viewing the national life expectancy level, the massive differences between communities are hidden, especially in a country as diverse as the United States.

Family and Extended Family

There are approximately 574,313 AIAN families living on or near reservations (NCAI, 2020). In 2017, 37.7 percent of AIANs were married couple families. The average family size was 3.69 as compared to 3.04 for White families. The average AINA household size was 3.02, which was higher than the 2.46 for White households (United States Census Bureau, 2018b, S0201).

In the past, tribal societies valued children as they represented renewal of life. The extended family network included blood-related and non-blood related members and they were included in child raising. However, colonization disrupted the traditional structure, gender roles, and meanings of AIAN families. The removal of children and their placement in boarding schools altered child-rearing practices, and they lost their culture and identity. As the boarding school children became adults, they were confused about their cultural identity and how they fit in the world. As struggling adults, they turned to unhealthy coping mechanisms which created the cycles of broken families (Becenti and Gladue, 2018). As a result, the splitting of AIAN families continued as 25–35 percent of all children were removed from the homes and 85 percent were placed with individuals outside of their families, extended families, and communities (NICWA, 2018). To protect the interests of the AIAN children and their families, the 1978 Indian Child Welfare Act was signed into law and mandated AIAN children are to be placed with relatives, a tribal member and/or AIAN family unless there are extenuating circumstances (Dorgan, 2019). Although the Child Welfare Act was enacted, AIAN children continued to be removed from the homes at three times the rate of non-Native youth and 56 percent were adopted by non-Native families' external of Native communities (NICWA, 2018).

American Indian and Alaskan Natives continue to have strong social ties with immediate and extended family members. They believe healthy families are balanced in spiritual, emotional, physical, and social domains of life. These dimensions within the individuals and families are viewed as being inseparable from the community and the land. Rural nurse practitioners and nurses need to understand the AIAN family history and culture when providing health care services for families, and communities. The *Extended Family Tribal Best Practices, A Toolkit with Best Practices, Research and Resources* provides guidance on engaging AIAN families in the health care system (Becenti, and Gladue, 2018).

Language Fluency

In 2018, 26.9 percent of those identifying as only AIAN and 20.5 percent of AIANs identifying with more than one race spoke a language other than English in their homes (United States Census Bureau, 2018b). Of the 150 Indigenous languages, the seven most popular languages still spoken on Native lands include Navajo, Yupik, Sioux, Apache, Rio Grande Keresan, Cherokee (Tsalagi), and Choctaw. Navajo is the most used AI language and continues to be spoken by 170,000 people (Lee, 2014). Some Indigenous languages are spoken mostly by elders. Since tribal elders are the keepers of the language, cultural knowledge, and oral literature, these languages will disappear after their death (McCarty *et al.*, 2015; Wyman *et al.*, 2014). As one elder shared, "our language is dying and once our language dies, we die" (Grayshield *et al.*, 2015). The revitalization of language is central to the cultural because it provides Tribal members with a sense of awareness and a strong identity (Boyer, 2019). To preserve their languages, AIAN tribes and Tribal Colleges and Universities developed a variety of programs to generate interest in their language heritage, examples include the Diné Bí Oltá Navajo, a youth immersion language and cultural program (Notah, 2017; Slate, 2019), Montana's Blackfeet Community College developed a Native American language application for Apple iPhone and Android users (Blackfeet Community College Develops Montana's First Language App, 2013, 2019), Muscogee (Creek) Nation developed Mvskoke, a Language Mobile app which is free on Apple store or Google Play Store (Muscogee [Creek] Nation, 2016), the Nishnaabemwin Pane Immersion Program (Austin, 2019), the Native American Studies Lakota Dakota Language Program (Sitting Bull College, 2020), and the Zuni Language Materials Collections developed by the University of New Mexico (Wise and Kostelecky, 2018).

WORLDVIEWS AND VALUES ASSOCIATED WITH AIANS, INTERGENERATIONAL POVERTY, AND TRAUMA

Worldview is a set of beliefs and values that are honored and held by an individual, group, or society. The differing worldviews between groups contributes to opposing understandings of knowledge, connectedness, and science. Therefore, it is important to understand the core traditional AIAN and Western worldviews to achieve cultural harmony and develop respectful relationships. American Indian and Alaskan Natives view life as a journey along a path and the purpose is to follow the pathway as faithfully as possible without drifting from it into wrongdoing, sickness, or evil. This path is the way of wisdom, health, and beauty, and the goal is a life that culminates in the maturity and fulfillment of embodiment in old age (Gill, 2002). American Indian and Alaskan Natives focus on a holistic understanding of the whole that emerged from the time of their existence and experiences whereas, traditional western worldviews focus on science and tend to compartmentalize knowledge and place a larger emphasis on understanding the larger, related picture (Four Arrows and Navaez, 2015; Indigenous Corporate Training, Inc., 2016). American Indian and Alaskan Natives values are interwoven into their worldview, culture, lifestyle, religion, and everyday actions but there are opposing values between AIANs and non-Natives (See Table 9.1 for Contrasting Cultural Values). Besides understanding the differences between AIAN and non-Native culture and values, health care providers need to be familiar with the worldviews of intergenerational poverty and trauma that occur on rural reservations (Schultz and Kroeger, 1996).

Many AIANs live in intergenerational poverty and experience trauma on rural tribal lands which effects their worldview and values. Intergenerational poverty worldview and values are reflected in decision making, conflict resolution, financial decisions, and meeting new people. Worldview of intergenerational poverty focus encompasses local surroundings and if AIAN suffered from trauma, the world is also viewed as unpredictable and limited. Individuals from intergenerational poverty make decisions based on needs of entertainment and relationships; if they are traumatized then there are additionally safety concerns. Money is used for entertainment and based on relationships. In conflict resolution, there is the need to fight or have someone who will fight for you. There are many stereotypes associated with poverty such as the poor are lazy, they do not like to work, they abuse the social system, and they do not value education. When meeting individuals who live in poverty, these preconceived stereotypes often impact middle-class health-care providers' perceptions and communication with patient and family members. If trauma has occurred, it becomes even more difficult for the individual to "navigate the middle-class world" because they have difficultly trusting others and prefer

TABLE 9.1. Contrasting Cultural Values between American Indian and White Populations.

American Indian	White
Non-materialistic	Material comfort
Group/tribal emphasis	Individualism
Generosity	"Getting ahead in Life"
Cooperation	Competition
Respect for age	Youth
Importance of extended family	External conformity (peer pressure)
Non-verbal	Freedom
Modesty	Efficiency
Patience	Progress
Indirect criticism	Direct criticism
Spiritual/mysticism	Religion

Randall and Muneta (2000).

not to talk with new people unless something is needed (Douglas, 2011; Payne, 2019). Frequently individuals living in poverty have an overwhelming feeling of hopelessness because they do not believe their life will get better (Payne, 2019).

AMERICAN INDIAN AND ALASKAN NATIVE TRIBAL RELIGIONS AND SPIRITUALITY

Indigenous spiritualities are viewed as "lifeways" in which AI traditional beliefs, sacramental practices, and spirituality are incorporated into all aspects of daily life (Garroutte *et al.*, 2014; Jocks, 2019). These practices are passed down orally to the next generation and each tribe has a creation story that explains the beginning of the world and the origin of human beings. These stories connect the tribe's relationship to the land, other beings, and the Creator (Brown and Cousins, 2001). The ideal is to have balance and harmony with the environment, community, and spirits (Garroutte *et al.*, 2014). When the European settlers arrived, they believed Indigenous practices were irrelevant and forced conversion to Christianity with severe consequences if AIs refused (Harvard University, 2020).

The Native American Church was created in the US and members practice a combination of Christianity and traditional AI beliefs with peyote as the sacrament of choice (Garroutte *et al.*, 2014; Barry-Bratcher, 2019). In the Native American Church, peyote is considered sacred because it helps to clear the participant's mind for a closer relationship with God's spirit (Andrews, 2013). By 1882, the federal government banned AIAN religious practices, but many of the tribes living on isolated rural reservations retained their religious beliefs, customs, and traditions. It was not until the legislative passing of the 1978 American Indian Religious Freedom Act that AIANs were able to publicly practice their religions again (Jocks, 2019; Weiser, 2020).

Tribal religions and spirituality are localized according to geographic location and creation story (Schultz and Kroeger, 1996; Sullivan, 2003). American Indian and Alaskan Native ceremonies emerge from specific worldviews and tribal nations have different ceremonies for healing, offering thanks, celebrating, clearing the way, and blessing. Traditional healing ceremonies are the Sun Dance, Ghost Dance, sweat lodges, Pipe Ceremony, Smudging Ceremony, and Vision Quests. The healing ceremonies interconnect harmony and balance and many times the individual, family, and friends actively participate (Portman and Garrett, 2006).

For many tribes, the Medicine Wheel or Sacred Hoop is a powerful symbol of spirituality and represents the circle of life. The circle encases a cross signifying the four directions and each direction represents a distinctive color such as black, red, yellow, and white (Andrews, 2013; Bartlett, 2018). Depending on the Tribal beliefs, the four directions can also represent the stages of life, seasons of the year, aspects of life, elements of nature, animals, or ceremonial plants. The teachings related to the Medicine Wheel are used in everyday life, guiding how to make decisions, create change on physical or emotional levels, and create a state of balance (Bartlett, 2018).

Some AIANs safeguard their religious practices and ceremonies and are hesitant to discuss them with non-Natives; nevertheless, nurse practitioners and nurses need to understand and respect AIAN's spiritual beliefs because they influence patients' satisfaction and treatment compliance (Randall and Muneta, 2000; Tighe, 2014). Hodge and Wolosin (2015) studied the spiritual satisfaction of 1,284 hospitalized AI patients in the service areas of admissions, room quality, food service, nursing, administration of tests and treatments, treatment of visitors and families, physicians, and discharge. In order of significance, discharge process, physicians, room quality and nurses were highly associated with satisfactorily addressing AI's spiritual needs.

COMMUNICATION AND HUMOR

The AIAN worldview of illness, health, communication, and relationships with healthcare professions differs from the non-Native population. American Indian and Alaskan Natives view health holistically—physical, spiritual, mental, and emotional health are in unity. They view people, community, nature, and spirituality as being interconnected and interrelated and illness may be a result of disharmony between the sources of life. To communicate and connect with nurse practitioners and nurses, AIANs may tell stories to describe their problem or illness that is occurring in their bodies. They will also use storytelling to introduce themselves, their family, and community to new healthcare providers. In turn, it is expected that healthcare providers will listen carefully to the stories and share their own information about self, family, and friends to form a relationship. Forming a trusting relationship with the healthcare provider is needed before AIANs may be willing to accept medical knowledge, recommendations, and protocols are understood and used by members of the Native communities (Kalbfeishch, 2009).

Another way to build relationships with AIANs is to understand the importance of humor in the Native culture as laughter is considered good medicine and can help with healing. According to Lindquist (2016), Indian humor is culturally distinct and complex, and it is at the heart of Native resilience and survivability. It is embedded in life lessons and provides Native people with a healthy escape. If non-Native nurse practitioners and nurses plan to use humor when providing cultural competence care, they need to have formed a connection and trusting relationship with the Native community. Additionally, what is viewed as humor in one culture may not be viewed as humorous in other cultures (Dean, 2003).

In the Native culture, laughing and joking with one another are signs of close and trusting relationships but humor can be used in many circumstances.

For example, there are times that humor may be used to express deep pain instead of an indication of well-being. Non-Native nurse practitioners and nurses need to listen for hidden messages and think about what remains unsaid (Dean, 2003). According to Lindquist (2016), everyone enjoys laughing and it is not only good medicine, but it is good for soul as it eases the tribulations of life's journey.

COMMUNITY POPULATIONS

Lesbian, Gay, Bisexual, Transgender, Queer, and Two Spirit Community

When the Europeans arrived in America, they documented encounters with Indigenous males, females, and sometimes intersexed individuals who crossed gender lines in terms of dress, occupations, gender, and other societal roles. Gender crossing Indigenous individuals were documented in more than 130 tribes in every region of North America and were often viewed as sacred beings, whose dual genders were a gift from the Great Spirit (Hemmilä, 2016; Wigington, 2019). Most American Indian tribes acknowledged three to five gender roles which included female, male, Two Spirit female, Two Spirit male, and transgendered. Each tribe had their own specific word in their language to refer to gender crossing individuals. For example, in Navajo it is Nádleehí (one who is transformed), Lakota is Winkté (indicative of a male who has a compulsion to behave as a female), Niizh Manidoowag (two spirit) in Ojibwe, Hemaneh (half man, half woman) in Cheyenne (Brayboy, 2017).

With the conversion to Christianity, gender crossing Indigenous individuals were considered "deviant" in terms of gender and/or sexuality. Violence and ridicule were used by non-Natives to make them conform to European norms. Furthermore, many Native communities adopted negative attitudes toward homosexuality (Lang, 2016). Finally, at the 1990 Indigenous lesbian and gay international conference, the term "Two Spirit" was adopted from the Ojibwe Language so Lesbian, Gay, Bisexual, Transgender, and Queer (LGBTQ2) could be identified within their respective tribes but not grouped with other races (Jacobs *et al.*, 1997). Not all AIAN LGBTQ2s identify with the Two-Spirit movement so nurse practitioners and nurses need to be comfortable with having open dialogs about how they identify with their gender, sexuality, and heritage.

The health status of AIAN LGBTQ2 people is reflective of the general AIAN population. Health issues related to physical and mental health include a high prevalence of chronic illness, and premature mortality related to poverty, socioeconomic deprivation, racism, and discrimination (Lang, 2016). These socioeconomic issues increase the risk for HIV infection and can impact the health of AIANs who have and are at risk for HIV infection. From 2012–2016 there was a 63 percent increase in screening and 34 percent increase in HIV diagnoses among AIAN. Most of the new HIV diagnoses were among AIAN gay and bisexual men. Rural providers can utilize the Social Media Toolkit to develop and implement a social media plan to combat the HIV epidemic in Indian Country (Foley *et al.*, 2020a). Additionally, there is a need to increase the education and usage of HIV medications because AIANs have lower viral suppression rates when compared to others diagnosed with HIV (CDC, 2019a). The *Toolkit for Advancing the Uptake and Use of PrEP in Indian Country* is a useful tool to start the discussions and action steps for integrating PrEP into Tribal communities (Foley *et al.*, 2020b).

Indian Health Service is addressing the spread of HIV and sexually transmitted diseases in Indian country through the development a *Tribal HIV/STD Training Kit and Policy Guide*. This advocacy kit assists tribal health advocates and decision-makers address sexual health challenges in their communities through programmatic and policy changes (IHS, n.d.a). Moreover, existing tribal laws may discriminate against Two Spirit or LGBTQ individuals. The *Tribal Equality Toolkit* was developed for tribal leaders to use as a guide to facilitate the development or revision of tribal laws to incorporate an inclusive definition of family, address hate crimes based on sexual orientation and gender identity, and prohibit discrimination in employment, housing, and family matters (Native American Program of Legal Aid Services of Oregon *et al.*, 2013).

AMERICAN INDIAN AND ALASKAN NATIVE VETERANS

American Indian and Alaskan Natives volunteer to serve in the U.S. military at greater numbers per capita than any other racial or ethnic group. There are many reasons why AINA join the military, but one motivating factor may that they are searching for better economic opportunities (John, 2018). Heuer *et al.* (2016) surveyed 511 North Dakota AI high school students on their plans for future education and employment. Twenty-one percent planned to enlist in the military, and the main reason listed was funding for college. As of September 2012, there were 31,155 AIAN on active duty, reserve, and National Guard members (NCAI, 2020). Of AIAN service members, there is a higher concentration of female service members (20%) than all other racial groups (15%) (National Center for Veterens Analysis and Statistics [NCVAS], 2020).

Veterans are individuals who have served in the active military, naval, or air services and who were discharged or released under honorable conditions (Crotwell Pullis *et al.*, 2019). According to the United States Census Bureau's 2017 American Community Survey data, 140,000 Veterans identify as single race AIAN which comprised 0.7 percent of 19 million Veterans. The proportion of AIAN Veterans was higher at 11.3 percent as compared to 9 percent of other races. The median age of AIAN was younger at 59 compared to 64 for

Veterans of all other races. While a higher percent of AIAN Veterans completed some college credit, respectively 44.3 percent vs. 37.1 percent, 11 percent completed a bachelor's degree compared to 16.3 percent of Veterans of other races. The median personal income for AIAN veterans was the lowest at $29,847 as compared to $38,792 for Veterans of all other races. American Indian and Alaskan Natives Veteran's unemployment rate was higher at 5.5 percent as opposed to 3.5 percent for Veterans of other races. The lack of health insurance was higher in AIAN Veterans (7.4%) than all races (2.9%). Thirty percent of AIANs reported service-related disabilities in contrast to 20.6 percent of Veterans of other races (NCVAS, 2020).

Rural and AIAN Veterans are returning to their rural communities with multiple medical and combat-related issues which requires significant ongoing care. Veterans living in rural areas encounter a number of challenges such as access to healthcare and other services due to rural delivery such as hospital closings; lack of housing, education, employment, and transportation options; greater geographic and distance barriers; limited broadband internet; higher uninsured rates and difficulty of safely aging in place (U.S. Department of Veterans Affairs, 2020). Veterans Affairs (VA) and Indian Health Service (IHS) have signed a Memorandum of Understanding to improve the health status of Native Veterans and to reimburse IHS for direct healthcare services for enrolled AIAN. The VA, IHS, and tribal partnerships have made significant contributions in the areas of reimbursement dollars, VA Central Mail Out Pharmacy, outreach and training events, suicide prevention, and educational presentations on posttraumatic stress (VA-Center for Applied Systems Engineering, 2016).

GRANDPARENTS RAISING GRANDCHILDREN

American Indian and Alaskan Native grandparents, by tradition, have played a role in raising grandchildren because they were essential in passing down cultural knowledge, upholding traditional values and teachings, and facilitating development of a strong and healthy cultural identity among youth. However due to significant societal changes, grandparent roles have been expanding. Nationally, those identifying only as AIAN are disproportionately represented with 7.5 percent living with grandchildren and 50.5 percent being responsible for raising grandchildren while 2.5 percent of White grandparents live with grandchildren and 38.8 percent are raising their grandchildren (United States Census, 2018b). However, on Native lands, over 56 percent of grandparents live with their grandchildren and have sole responsibility for them (HAC, 2013).

While their lives are enriched as primary caregivers for their grandchildren, AIAN grandparents are more likely to be single, experience persistent poverty, reside in rural and reservation communities with limited access to resources, employment opportunities, and services (Bailey *et al.*, 2019; Probst *et al.*, 2004). As the grandparents take on the second round of parenting, they encounter a number of challenges and decisions because if retired, they are raising their grandchildren on fixed incomes and if employed, they may need to remain in the workforce long past retirement age. Additionally, they need to learn how to navigate the school systems, bridge the generational and technology gaps, court systems for custody and mental health services. In small towns and reservations, grandparents may not seek assistance because they are not aware of available community resources, ashamed or embarrassed of their adult child's behavior, or raising young grandchildren with behavioral and emotional problems. Grandparents raising grandchildren with mental and developmental behaviors are at greater risk themselves for depression, insomnia, hypertension, diabetes, and other chronic health problems (Bailey *et al.* 2019; Cross *et al.*, 2011).

With the national opioid epidemic, it is expected the number of grandparents raising their grandchildren will continue to rise. To support grandparents in their second round of parenting, the S.1091—Supporting Grandparents Raising Grandchildren Act was signed into law. This law established a Federal Advisory Council that is charged with identifying, promoting, coordinating and disseminating information, resources, and best practices to help grandparents and other relatives meet the health, educational, nutritional, and other needs of the children in their care as well as maintain their own physical and mental health and emotional well-being; ensure the needs of AIAN are addressed; and finally, submit a report outlining the best practices, gaps in services, and identification of additional federal legislation to congress (Congress.gov, 2018).

FEDERAL INDIAN LAW, TRIBAL GOVERNANCE AND PUBLIC SAFETY

The U.S. Code Title - 25 Indians along with several other titles, particularly Title 5 Government Organization and Employees, Title 18 Crimes and Criminal procedures, Title 28 Judiciary and Judicial Procedure, and Title 42 Public Health and Welfare include pertinent laws that frame the rights, responsibilities, and relationships between the Tribes, states and federal government (Selden and Martens, 2008). The federal Indian law addresses a variety of issues including criminal and civil jurisdiction, cultural practices, sovereignty, governance, and jurisdiction (Hoss, 2019). Many non-Native federal and state judges, law clerks, and members of Congress described their knowledge and experience with Federal Indian Law and sovereignty as none to limited. Yet these non-Native professionals make significant decisions that impact the health, welfare, and self-government of tribal nations and their citizens (Campisteguy *et al.*, 2018).

JUDICIAL SYSTEM AND LAW ENFORCEMENT

Most tribal nations have their own tribal courts and tribal law enforcement based on their unique histories and cultures. They establish and operate their own tribal justice system including the development and implementation of laws and codes. Tribal governments have jurisdiction over civil matters that occur on the reservations but have limited criminal authority. When a criminal act occurs, which government system has jurisdiction depends on the crime, identity of the accused, identity of the victim, location of the crime, and the federal statute and criminal law (Hoss, 2019). Tribal courts normally do not have criminal jurisdiction over non-Natives, but in 2013, Congress restored tribal criminal jurisdiction over non-Natives who have committed acts of domestic violence against AINAs within Indian Country (NCAI, 2020).

In Indian Country, 108 tribal nations have a form of judicial system and 175 tribal nations established formal tribal court systems (Newton *et al.*, 2019 as cited in NCAI, 2020). Some of the tribal courts resemble Western-style judiciaries which apply written laws and rules court procedures but an increasing number of tribes are returning to their traditional means of resolving disputes through the use of peacemaking, elder councils, and sentencing circles (Tribal Court Clearinghouse, n.d.). American Indians consider disputes to be a symptom of spiritual as well as physical illness and understand the connection between dispute resolution and the need for physical and spiritual healing. As a result, some tribes implemented Tribal Healing to Wellness Courts to holistically address alcohol, drug abuse, and criminal issues through ongoing judicial supervision, comprehensive drug testing, interdisciplinary team-based management, and community support (Garrow *et al.*, 2018).

On rural reservations, there are 229 tribally operated law enforcement agencies that employ nearly 3,629 full-time personnel, including approximately 2,500 sworn officers and 27 BIA police agencies (FBI.gov, 2018; United States Department of Justice, 2019). Law enforcement in Indian Country encounter many challenges, such as complicated jurisdiction boundaries, answering to multiple authorities, high crime rates, lack of resources, operating with limited resources, and patrolling some of the most isolated tribal lands frequently without backup from partner law enforcement agencies (Luna-Firebaugh, 2007).

The 80 jails in Indian country held an estimated 2,540 inmates midyear 2016. The infractions included violent offenses such as domestic violence, aggravated/simple assault, rape or sexual assault, other violent assaults, burglary, larceny-theft, public intoxication, DWI//DUI, and drugs (Minton and Cowhig, 2017). In the criminal justice system, the incarceration rate of AIANs is 38 percent higher than national rates (Greenfeld and Smith, 1999; Frosch, 2015). Additionally, AIAN youth are overrepresented in federal and state detention facilities while their White equivalents are underrepresented. Excluding youth in Indian country facilities, 3 percent of AINA girls and 1.5 percent of AIAN boys were incarcerated in juvenile facilities, yet they encompass less than 1 percent of all youth nationally (Sawyer, 2019). At every level, AIAN girls were more likely than White adolescents to be referred for juvenile court, detailed, adjudicated, and received harsher offenses for similar violations (Wiltz, 2016). According to the U.S. Commission on Civil Rights, AIANs are subjected to higher rates of differential treatment by the criminal justice system because they lack access to adequate counsel and because of racial profiling (Tighe, 2014; Bell, 2017).

DISCRIMINATION AND RACISM

The undercounted AI numbers by the U.S. Census and the geographical isolation of the tribal lands contributes to the invisibility of the population (Connolly *et al.*, 2019). The invisibility of the AIAN population was reconfirmed by the Reclaiming Native Truth project, which reported 62 percent of non-Natives believed AI people no longer existed because they are invisible or erased from all aspects of modern U.S. society including the media. Only 34 percent of non-Natives believed AI people encountered a great deal of discrimination. Of those who lived near rural AI tribal lands, 56 percent believed more should be done to help AIs (Campisteguy *et al.*, 2018).

As part of a larger study, 342 AI adults responded to a telephone survey about their satisfaction with the quality of life and safety in rural U.S. American Indians reported discrimination in the following areas: 39 percent insensitive or offensive comments, 35 percent slurs, 33 percent paid or promoted equally, 31 percent job applications, 23 percent in clinical encounters, 15 percent avoided healthcare, 17 percent renting or buying a house, and 13 percent when either applying or attending college (Findling *et al.*, 2019; Blendon and Menschel, 2017). When interacting with the police, 47 percent who lived in majority-Native areas encountered discrimination as compared to 19 percent of those who lived in non-majority-Native areas. Forty-eight percent of AIs in majority-Native areas were more likely to report police used unnecessary force in contrast to the 25 percent who lived in non-majority-Native areas (Blendon and Menschel, 2019). The U.S. Commission on Civil Rights has held numerous hearings on the discrimination of AIAN in border towns surrounding reservations throughout the country. Incidents range from name calling at youth sports activities, denial of services in public places, to police brutality to failure to investigate AIAN murders (Woodard, 2016).

Harvey (2020) studied fatal encounters per population for AIs across the country from 2000 to 2017 and found AIANs had almost a 3 to 1 ratio comparative to the number of fatal encounters per population for white individuals. When analyzing gender statistics, AI males had more than 4 times the number of fatal encounters per population as the white population and AI women more than 2 times the number of per-population fatal encounters. Edwards *et al.* (2019) estimated the risk of being killed by police using force across social groups. American Indian and Alaskan Native men were nearly 1.2 and 1.7 times more likely to be killed by police over their life course than white men, whereas AIAN women were between 1.1 and 2.1 times more likely to be killed by the police than white women (Edwards *et al.*, 2019). Furthermore, from 1999–2017, law enforcement agencies failed to report 2,406 of the 4,821 AIANs murders to the FBI Uniform Crime System (Murder Accountability Project, 2019). Police-killings or jailhouse deaths of AIANs remain invisible as they are rarely covered in the top ten newspapers (Woodard, 2016).

MALTREATMENT IN INDIAN COUNTRY

American Indian and Alaska Native children, women, and men suffer violence at alarmingly high rates, especially if they live on reservations. American Indian and Alaskan Native children are abused at a rate of 15.2 cases per 1,000 AIAN children as compared to 8.2 cases per 1,000 for Whites (Statista Research Department, 2020). Exposure to violence in any form harms children but many AIAN children are polyvictimized by experiencing multiple forms of abuse including family violence, child physical and sexual abuse, community violence, and mental health disorders. Their exposure to multiple forms of violence puts them at higher risk for serve lifelong problems with physical health, posttraumatic stress disorder (PTSD), mental health disorders, suicidality, eating disorders, substance abuse, and sexual behavior. The AIAN PTSD rate of 22 percent (Dorgan *et al.*, 2014) is higher than the rate of 11 percent in children and adolescents diagnosed with a conduct disorder (Bernhard *et al.*, 2018).

Rosay (2016) studied intimate partner and sexual violence in 2,473 AIAN women and 1,505 AIAN men who were affiliated or enrolled with a tribe or village and lived in Indian Country during the past year. Of the respondents, 84 four percent of AIAN women experienced some form of violence during their lifetime as compared to 71 percent of White women. In the past year, 39.8 percent of AIAN women had endured violence in contrast to 23.3 percent of White women. Eighty-one percent AIAN men experienced violence in their lifetime as compared to 64 percent Non-Hispanic White men. During the past year, 34.6 percent of AIAN men suffered from violence in contrasted to 25.7 percent White men. Most of AIAN victims, 97 percent women and 90 percent men experienced violence by an interracial perpetrator. Whereas 35 percent AIAN women and 33 percent AIAN men were abused by intraracial perpetrators (Rosay, 2016). Both AIAN women and men were frequently unable to obtain the necessary medical and legal assistance because of issues such as poverty, previous child abuse, and jurisdiction issues. The impact of sexual assault is especially significant to AIAN women because the long-term consequences can include the physical effects of pregnancy or sexually transmitted diseases, economic instability of homelessness and unemployment, and psychological and emotional disorders such as post-traumatic stress, depression, severe distress, suicidal thoughts, and suicidal attempts especially if the first assault occurred before the age of 16 (Begay and Zandamela, 2018). Further, AIANs are more likely to be diagnosed with traumatic brain injury from violence. In a study by Linton and Kim (2014), they detected over 32 percent of AIAN women and over 46 percent of AIAN men experienced violent brain injuries which puts them at a higher risk of developing Alzheimer's and other dementia than the general population.

Elder abuse is a growing social issue in the AIAN population because it impacts the health and rights of elders to live safely in their home and free from violence. Jervis *et al.* (2017) studied 50 urban (South Central Metropolitan) and 50 rural (Northern Plains' reservations) AI elders' perceptions of mistreatment by family and found that 16 percent had been treated badly and 76 percent discussed cases where others had experienced abuse. Fifty-four percent in the Northern plains and 28 percent in South Center were at risk for abuse, neglect, and exploitation (Cox and Jervis, 2018; Jervis *et al.*, 2014). The AIAN elders described their mistreatment as financial exploitation, neglect, lack of respect, psychological abuse, and physical abuse. They believed the causation of maltreatment was related to problematic drinking and culture loss of traditional values (Jervis *et al.*, 2017).

Spiritual and cultural are additional forms of abuse not usually considered by the general population. Spiritual abuse occurs when AIAN elders are denied access to ceremonies, traditional healing or healers, or having traditional regalia removed from their possession without their permission (Cox and Jervis, 2018). Whereas cultural abuse is viewed as attacking someone for their identity, background, or beliefs (Jump, 2018). Furthermore, AINA may use different words or terms to identify the way to treat elders and elder abuse. Traditionally, AIAN elders were treated with respect because they passed down the tribal culture, knowledge, wisdom, and experience to the next generation. American Indian elders believe that being disrespectful, not honoring elders and their place in history, and treating them less than human is a form of abuse (Hudson *et al.*, 1998). When interviewing AIAN elders regarding potential abuse, nurse practitioners and nurses should use the terms disrespect to describe abuse and bothering when addressing sexual abuse (Baker-Demaray, 2005).

Health care providers in Tribal health clinics are encountering elder abuse among older AIAN adults. In a study of 23 phone calls and 90 online surveys with Tribal health clinic providers, only 54 percent routinely screened for elder abuse and only three clinics use an elder specific screening tool. Seventy percent of the providers reported they had already intervened with elder abuse cases, 70 percent AIAN elders experienced financial exploitation, 60 percent neglect or emotional abuse, and 43 percent physical abuse. Many of the providers reported a lack of protocols for managing cases of elder abuse, little training, and lack of information on accessing community services and support, if available (Crowder *et al.*, 2019).

Several resources are available to tribal leaders and healthcare providers to learn how to address violence in the tribal community. The StrongHearts Toolkit provides resources and information on domestic violence and healthy relationships (StrongHearts Native Helpline, 2020). The National Indian Country Clearinghouse on Sexual Assault is a one-stop, comprehensive resource for material on sexual violence in Indian Country (NICCSA, 2020). Reclaiming What Is Sacred: Addressing Harm to Indigenous Elders and Developing a Tribal Response to Abuse in Later Life identifies issues related to AIAN elder abuse and strategies that can be developed to promote balance and prevent harm to older adults in the community (Litton and Ybanez, 2017). The National Indigenous Women's Resource Center provides resources for individuals working on issues of violence against AIAN women on domestic violence, teen dating violence, sexual assault, and more (NIWRC, 2020).

MISSING, MURDERED OR TRAFFICKED AMERICAN INDIAN AND ALASKAN NATIVES

Despite the ongoing crisis of missing, murdered, or trafficked AIAN, there continues to be a lack of comprehensive state and federal data because of poor record-keeping, racial misclassification, and adverse relationships between tribal governments and county law enforcement (Ortiz, 2020). Even with the underreporting and inconsistent documentation, in 2018 there were 7,497 AIAN juveniles under the age of 18 years old and 2,417 AIANs over the age of 18 who were missing. The numbers included women, men, girls, and boys; however, while the data was separated by race, it was not broken down by gender (NCIC, 2020) so statistics on missing AIAN men and boys was not available. American Indian and Alaskan men may also be vulnerable if they suffer from addictions, sexual and cultural abuse, and absent parents and their disappearances may be delayed because of the belief they can care for themselves (Hilleary, 2019; Fonseca, 2020).

Brave Heart Society and Sovereign Bodies Institute are conducting longitudinal studies that examine the scope and severity of missing, murdered, and sex trafficked AIAN women and children. In the Northern Plains region, the authors found that from 1900 to 2019, there were 411 missing and murdered Indigenious women and girls (MMIWG) with 69 percent disappearing since 2000 in North Dakota, South Dakota, Montana, and Nebraska. Of these MMIWG cases 62 percent were missing, 29 percent were murdered, and 9 percent were unknown. The AI women and children represented 41 tribal nations and they were missing from 142 locations, and 59 percent resided on reservations or rural areas. Four in five MMIWG cases occurred in counties near or intersecting with the Keystone XL pipeline; more than one-third of cases were misclassified without a thorough investigation; over three-fourths were not entered into the federal database; and one in every two white male killers were not charged or convicted (Spotted Eagle *et al.*, 2019).

Sovereign Bodies Institute (SBI) recorded nearly 4,000 sex trafficking cases in the U.S. and Canada, of which over half of these cases involved sex trafficking or survival sex work and at least 10 percent experienced sexual violence. Almost all the MMIWG victims sex trafficked suffered from other forms of violence; nearly half experienced domestic violence or sexual assault, 14 percent were homeless, and 14 percent died in police custody (Spotted Eagle *et al.*, 2019). Traffickers pursue AIAN women and children because of the high rates of poverty in tribal communities, homelessness, runaways, chemical dependency, experience of previous abuse, lack of resources and/or support systems. They control AIAN women and children by inflicting sexual, emotional, or mental abuse; enabling addiction(s); and withholding money or identification (National Congress of American Indians Policy Research Center, 2016). Farley et al. (2011) surveyed 105 AIAN women who were subjected to commercial sexual exploitation in Minnesota. When review the health consequences of trafficking: 92 percent had been raped, 84 percent had been physically assaulted, 79 percent were sexually abused as children with an average of four perpetrators, 72 percent suffered traumatic brain injuries, and 52 percent had post-traumatic stress disorder.

According to the National Crime Information Center, there are over 1,400 unsolved cases of missing and murdered AIANs in the U.S. (United States Department of the Interior, 2020, July 27). Several legislative initiatives were implemented in 2019 and 2020 to address the violence against AIANs and unresolved cases. The Operation Lady Justice Task Force, a multi-agency task force was developed to collect and manage data across jurisdictions; establish protocols for new and unsolved cases; establish multi-jurisdictional cold case teams; improving the response to investigative challenges; and provide clarity on the roles, authorities, and jurisdiction among agencies (The White House, 2019, November 26). Congress passed two legislative bills to stop the violence and address issues related to missing and murdered AIANs. S. 227 Savanna's Act requires the Department of Justice to increase coordination between federal and tribal agencies, improve access to law enforcement databases, review, revise, and develop law enforcement and justice protocols to address missing or murdered Native American (Congress.gov, 2020, March 11a). S. 982 Not Invisible Act of 2019 increases intergovernmental coordination to identify and combat violent crime within Indian country and of Indians (Congress.gov, 2020, March 11b). Proclamation 10026 declares May 5, 2020 as Missing and Murdered American Indian and Alaska Natives Awareness Day and requests all federal, state, tribal, and local governments to increase awareness of the missing and murdered AIANs. Additionally, seven Missing and Murdered Native American Cold Case offices were opened across the country to reduce the staggering number of violent crimes committed against AIANs and close longstanding cold cases and child abductions (Federal Register, 2020, May 8). Several resources are available for rural nurse practitioners and nurses and the AIAN community to address AIAN abuse and human trafficking. For example, rural nurse practitioners and nurses can complete *SOAR Preventing Human Trafficking Training for Native Communities to understand the issues surround human trafficking and its impact on Native populations* (TRAIN, 2020). Additional, they can utilize the *MMIWG2 Organizing and MMIP Toolkit* (Aqpik Apok *et al.*, 2020), *Combating Trafficking Native Youth Toolkit on Human Trafficking* (ACF and ANA, 2017), Special Collection: *Missing and Murdered Indigenous Women and Girls* (NIWRC, 2020), and *Tribal Community Response When a Woman is Missing: A Toolkit for Action* (NIWRC, 2018) to educate their healthcare team and collaborate with interprofessional agencies and community members to address the issues of AIAN missing, murdered, and human trafficking in their communities.

AMERICAN INDIAN AND ALASKAN NATIVE SOCIAL DETERMINANTS OF HEALTH

Historical and Intergenerational Trauma

When examining the health disparities in this population, it is important to recognize how many of these issues stem from generational and historical trauma, a concept that became publicized in the mid-1990s (Brave Heart, 1995). Brave Heart (1999) describes historical trauma as the massive cumulative emotional and psychological wounding of an individual or generation caused by a traumatic experience or event. American Indian and Alaskan Natives' historical trauma began in 1492 with the start of the European colonization. The effects of colonization are still experienced today including loss of life (genocide), land, language, culture, and identity. Furthermore, historical trauma has been linked to health disparities including depression, suicide, anxiety, eating disorders, commercial tobacco use, lack of contraceptive use, substance misuse, family violence, and incarceration (Yellow Horse Brave Heart, 2003; Subia Bigfoot, Lamb and Delmar, 2018; Gone *et al.*, 2019; Hoss 2019; Skewes and Blume, 2019).

Adverse Childhood Experiences

American Indians and Alaskan Natives are documented as being adversely affected by Adverse Childhood Experiences (ACE). ACE experiences include abuse (physical, emotional, sexual, mental), neglect (physical, emotional), family challenges (mental illness, incarcerated relatives, addiction, and divorce), injury (traumatic brain injury, fractures, burns), maternal health (unintended pregnancy, complications, fetal death) infectious disease (HIV, STDs), chronic disease (cancer, diabetes), and opportunity (education, occupation, income) (Association of American Indian Physicians, 2020). The ACE score is based on the number of challenges an individual experiences growing up. Higher ACE scores means the individual had more adverse experiences and he or she is at greater risk for poor health outcomes (Kenny and Singh, 2016; Warne *et al.*, 2017). Warne *et al.* (2017) compared ten categories of ACEs between AI and non-AIs. Overall, AIs had a higher total number of ACEs when compared to non-Natives. They had a higher prevalence of ACEs in the areas of abuse, neglect, and household dysfunction than non-Natives. Additionally, AIs and non-Natives with six or more ACEs had significantly increased risks for depression, anxiety, PTSD, severe alcohol misuse, and smoking when compared to individuals with no ACE scores (Warne *et al.*, 2017).

Boarding Schools

Prior to colonialization, tribal nations assumed responsibility of educating the children, teaching them survival and social skills, traditional values, and relations. In the late 1800s, the U.S. government signed a treaty with American Indians agreeing that in exchange for giving up their land (millions of acres), the federal government would fully operate and fund schools for AIAN students. From the late 1800s to the 1920s, the federal government opened residential boarding schools on and off the reservation, often contracting with religious denominations to provide the education. In the1890s Richard Pratt introduced the philosophy to "kill the Indian, save the man" into the boarding school education (Churchill, 2004). In the late 1920s, states assumed control of AI education after the federal government's approach was physically and emotionally damaging students. American Indian or Alaskan Native children were forced to assimilate to European ways, and it was the beginning phase of stripping them of their cultural identity and the only way of living they had ever known (Adams, 1995; Child, 1995; Trafzer *et al.*, 2006). Nearly 83 percent of AIAN school-age children were enrolled in boarding schools by 1926 (National Native American Boarding School Healing Coalition, n.d.). By 1928, the U.S. Government Meriam Report was released and provided evidence the boarding schools were completely inadequate in the areas of education, nutrition, overcrowding, medical services, student labor, and quality of teachers. Some boarding schools closed and the government built day schools on the reservations (Catwhipple, 2017; Schrank, 2016) but states remained in control of the curriculum, policies, and how AI children were taught; the federal government's only involvement was through financial support (McCoy, 2004).

In the 1960s, the Kennedy Report noted that AI children had high rates of illiteracy and were dropping out of school at disproportionately higher rates, with the public-school system ignoring their needs and culture (Special Subcommittee on Indian Education, 1969). In 1972, the Indian Education Act (Pub. L. No. 92-318) was enacted and recognized the unique educational and cultural academic needs, addressed educational needs from pre-school to graduate-level education, provided additional grant funding to schools serving AI children, and required input by parents (McCoy, 2004). During the same time, Tribal members visited the Indian boarding schools and demanded changes. Tribal members worked with the BIA to develop and implement new polices for the education and treatment of AIAN students. Most of the boarding schools closed (Dixon and Trafzer, 2006, Lajimodiere, 2020) and those that remained open, emerged as new contemporary off-reservation boarding schools that focus on academics, Native culture, and sports. Although some may not agree, Dixon and Trafzer (2006) report that AIAN students attend off-reservation boarding schools because of positive experiences of relatives; structure, curriculum, or philosophy; access to special colleges, universities, or trade schools; or personal reasons.

Bureau of Indian Education

The Bureau of Indian Education (BIE) system was established to meet the federal government's commitment to providing quality education opportunities from early childhood through life in accordance with the tribe's needs for cultural and economic well-being. The BIE serves over 47,000 AIAN students (NWEA, 2018) and supports a total of 183 elementary, secondary, residential, and peripheral dormitories on 64 reservations across 23 states. Fifty-nine schools are operated directly by the BIE and 124 are operated by local tribal school boards and superintendents (Pinto, 2020). Additionally, the BIE funds two post-secondary schools and administers grants for 33 tribally controlled colleges and universities and two tribal technical colleges (BIE, 2020). The BIE manages a school system of 169 elementary and secondary schools and 14 dormitories providing education services to an estimated 46,000 individual American Indian and Alaska Native students in 23 states, as well as operates two post-secondary schools and administers grants for 29 tribally controlled colleges and universities and two tribal technical colleges.

Tribal Colleges and Universities (TCUs) started in the 1960s and their missions were tied to their tribal nation's culture, language, and history. The TCUs are open to all racial and ethnic groups, and they must maintain a 51 percent enrollment of AIAN students to receive federal funding. Currently, 16 states have 37 Tribal Colleges and Universities (TCU) with more than 75 campuses, which typically provide educational opportunities in remote, rural regions that would not otherwise provide access to higher education (Lindquist, 2018); Sanders and Van Alstine Makomenaw, 2018). Most TCUs are two-year institutions and offer certificate or associate degrees, but others offer degrees from bachelor's to doctoral (Sanders and Van Alstine Makomenaw, 2018). Courses are designed from an AIAN perspective, helping to keep retention levels high. Tribal colleges or universities have been designated land grant institutions by Congress in recognition of the ties between the colleges, tribal lands, and local economic development (HAC, 2013).

Educational Attainment

Ninety percent of the AIAN students attend public schools, while 8 percent attend BIE schools (NCAI, 2020). In 2017, the status dropout rate for one race AIAN's youth was highest (10.1%) of all ethnic groups (5.4%). Dropout rates were higher for AINA males (11.6%) versus AINA females (McFarland *et al.*, 2019a). The average graduation rate for AIANs enrolled in public schools was 72 percent as compared to 89 percent for the White population. The highest percentage was 92 percent for AIANs in New Jersey, while South Dakota had the lowest percentage at 50 (McFarland *et al.*, 2019b). It is important to note that these percentages are from public high schools; however, BIE high school graduation rates were much lower at 53 percent and the students had poorer educational outcomes (Camera, 2015).

Seventeen percent of AINAs enroll in college or universities after high school as compared to 60 percent of the U.S. general population. In 2017, Tribal Colleges and Universities (TCUs) had 483 applications with a 90.3 percent acceptance rate, 16,621 enrolled students, and 290 (16.3%) graduates (Data USA: Tribal Colleges, 2020). According to the Office of Minority Health in 2017, 19.6 percent AIAN age 25 had at least a bachelor's degree, in comparison to 35.8 percent of whites. Of the AIAN population, 6.8 percent had completed an advanced graduate or professional degree, as compared to 13.8 percent of the white population (OMH, 2018).

INDIAN GAMING AND EMPLOYMENT

Rural reservations are often the poorest places in the United States (RHO, 2010). Many AIAN living on reservations lack employment opportunities, and for some tribes, there are limited opportunities for economic development which would create new jobs (HAC, 2010). In 1988, the Indian Gaming Regulatory Act (IGRA) was implemented as a way for tribes to achieve economic self-sufficiency on reservations by owning and operating casinos, bingo halls, and other forms of Indian gaming (NIGC, 2015). The National Indian Gaming Commission oversees the regulation of 520 gaming establishments operated by 247 tribes across 29 states (Harris, 2018[Is the pub date 2018, or 2019?]). Consistent with the IGRAs requirements, tribal governments invest the net gaming revenues in programs that improve the tribal welfare, but Indian gaming revenues vary substantially from tribe to tribe and location of casinos (Akee *et al.*, 2014).

In the more remote rural areas, fewer visitors travel to the casinos which results in lower net gaming revenues than those located closer to urban and higher populated areas (HAC, 2013). Some tribal governments provide a percentage of their gaming revenues to enrolled members (Akee *et al.*, 2015), but it is a myth that all tribes provide monthly checks to their enrolled members or Natives are millionaires from casino revenues (Lindquist, 2016). For many tribes, Indian gaming revenues addresses the unacceptable living conditions, but the accumulated economic and social deficits on reservations are so large that even if the income growth continues, it will take decades for AINA to close the financial gap with average Americans (Akee *et al.*, 2015; Akee and Taylor, 2014; Conner and Taggart, 2013).

In 2006–2018, American Indians residing on reservations had an unemployment rate of 11.4 percent which is higher than the 6.6 percent for AIAN not residing on Native lands or 4.4 percent of the general population. Fifty-two percent of AIANs who resided on reservations were employed or seeking employment as compared to 63.6 percent of those who did not live on reservations or 62.8 percent of the total population (U.S. Bureau of Labor Statistics, 2019).

American Indians and Alaskan Natives employed on reservations frequently earn below poverty wages and have few or no benefits. The median income on a reservation is $29,097 (Muhammad *et al.*, 2019) as compared to the national income of $40,315 for all AI/AN households living off-reservation and $57,652 nationally (United States Census Bureau, 2018b). As a result, AIAN living on reservations are disproportionally dependent on income from Social Security payments, Supplemental Security Income, and public assistance (HAC, 2013).

POVERTY ON RURAL RESERVATIONS

Poverty rates are high among AIAN families who live on rural reservation areas. According to the 2018 United States Census Data, AIANs had the highest persistent poverty rate by race at 25.4 percent as compared to 8.1 percent national poverty rate. However, unemployment and poverty rates vary regionally and within tribal areas. For example, Pine Ridge Reservation in South Dakota is one of the most impoverished reservations. Of female-headed households with children under 18 years old, 64 percent live below poverty level (U.S. Department of Commerce, 2018).

HOUSING AND HOMELESSNESS ON TRIBAL LANDS

The AIAN population who live on tribal reservations and surrounding communities continues to rapidly grow. Approximately 70 percent of homes on AIAN tribal land are owner-occupied as compared to 66.9 percent across the nation. On tribal lands, homeownership is different because often the tribe or government owns the property instead of individual tribal members (HAC, 2013). Thus, mortgage lending on tribal land is uncommon occurrence because lenders cannot foreclose on the land and resell it; for example, in 2015 only 822 of more than 44,000 loans to AIANs were to individuals on tribal lands (HAC, 2013; Bowman and Krueger, 2017).

Home renting is less common on tribal land than nationally; however, there remains a high demand for rental units as there is a major shortage of adequate, affordable rental properties on tribal lands. Private rental development is limited on tribal lands, so renters do not receive a high return on their investment. As a result, there are many rental supply issues across tribal lands. For example, at Rosebud Reservation in South Dakota, there were 816 occupied rental properties in 2010 with a waiting list of over 400 individuals (HAC, 2013). The waiting list for tribal lands is long and sometimes AIAN wait months to years for a home (Pindus *et al.*, 2017).

Forty percent of housing on tribal lands is considered substandard as compared to 6 percent of the general population. Rates change depending on tribal lands but overall, 5.8 percent of AIAN households lacked complete indoor plumbing compared to 0.3 percent of white households and 6.6 percent had incomplete kitchen deficiencies in comparison to 1.7 percent of white family units (Pindus *et al.*, 2017). In a 2019 study, Harvard researchers interviewed 1,405 adults, regarding satisfaction with the quality of life and safety in rural United States. Two percent of the participants were AIAN and more than one in five experienced housing problems with pests, bugs, or wild animals (36%), phone service (28%), electricity (27%), the safety of their drinking water (26%), mold or other environmental problems (23%), or inadequate heating or cooling (22%) (Blendon and Menschel, 2019). Inequities in healthcare and housing infrastructure continue to put AIANs at higher risk for the spread of the coronavirus. Handwashing and social distancing prevent the spreading of the contagion during this coronavirus pandemic; however, many tribal homes lack complete indoor plumbing and access to portable water for handwashing (Rodriguez-Lonebear *et al.*, 2020).

Overcrowded homes are common on tribal lands because families will not turn away others who need a place to live; however, it also highlights the major shortages of safe, affordable housing. Of the homes on tribal lands, 8.8 percent are crowded compared to 3 percent nationally. These crowded conditions lead to substandard living conditions that are linked to the spread of diseases transmitted in crowded spaces (HAC, 2013).

HOMELESS ON TRIBAL LANDS

Homelessness in Indian Country is frequently hidden because it takes the form of doubling up in the homes rather than allowing others to live on the street. According to Pindus *et al.* (2017) between 42,000–85,000 Indigenous people would be homeless in tribal lands if they did not double up and live with relatives or friends. Nineteen percent of the household heads reported they had more household members than could live comfortably in their home and 17 percent had others living with them because they did not have another place to stay. Eighty percent of the doubled-up respondents wanted to have their own home. The Minnesota Homeless on America Indian Reservations study, 89 percent of the doubled-up respondents lived, or couch surfed in two-plus homes during the previous year, while 49 percent lived in four-plus homes during the past year (Aman *et al.*, 2020).

American Indians and Alaskan Natives are significantly undercounted in the U.S. Census so it is difficult to obtain accurate homelessness counts although, these counts are critical to receive the support needed to assist AIAN homeless secure safe, permanent housing. To address these issues, Housing Assistance Council and the Corporation for Supportive Housing developed the Conducting Homeless Counts on Native American Lands: A Toolkit to conduct homeless counts on tribal lands (Oberdorfer *et al.*, 2013).

BROADBAND INTERNET

Of the 882,702 households, 88.6 percent had computers and 79.2 percent had broadband internet (United States Census Bureau, 2018b, Table S0201). Major gaps exist in the availability for broadband internet between tribal areas versus non-tribal areas. The Federal Communications Commission (FCC, 2019) has been working to minimize the discrepancy, but challenges persist including expense, vast and rugged terrain of the land, the complexity of gaining access to tribal lands through appropriate channels, lack of infrastructure necessary to support installation, and low population areas coupled with low-income residents (FCC, 2019). Some states are dedicating legislative funding to help meet the needs of underserved and unserved communities. For example, in 2014, the state of Minnesota began its Border-to-Border grant program in collaboration with the Department of Employment Economic Development (DEED). In 2019, Bois Forte Reservation, located in northeastern Minnesota, received $1.24 million from the grant program, along with local matching funds, to upgrade broadband internet to 10 unserved and 468 underserved locations throughout their rural tribal lands (MN DEED, 2019).

FOOD DISTRIBUTION PROGRAM ON INDIAN RESERVATIONS

The USDA estimated that 11.1 percent (14.3 million) of US households were food insecure at least some time during 2018 and had difficulty providing enough food for all their members due to a lack of resources. Rates of food insecurity were substantially higher than the national average for households with incomes near or below the federal poverty line (Coleman-Jensen *et al.*, 2019). Supplemental Nutrition Assistance Program (SNAP) provides funding to 15 nutrition assistance programs including breakfast and school lunch; Women, Infants, and Children (WIC); adult and child daycare; and food distribution (USDA FNS, 2020). The Food Distribution Program on Indian Reservations (FDPIR), more commonly known to AIAN as "commodities", is a federally funded program providing additional or alternative food source to SNAP (Warne and Lajimodiere, 2015; USDA FNS, 2018, April).

As of 2020, there are approximately 286 tribes receiving FDPIR benefits through 102 Indian Tribal Organizations or three state agencies (USDA Food and Nutrition Service, 2020). Each month, eligible participants can select from over 100 products based on the Dietary Guidelines for Americans 2015–2020 and MyPlate (U.S. Department of Health and Human Services and U.S. Department of Agriculture, 2015). Families can choose fresh produce instead of canned or frozen fruits or vegetables. In addition, traditional foods are also available including wild rice, bison meat, salmon, cornmeal, and catfish. Nutrition education grants are available for food distribution agencies to provide nutrition education including individual counseling, cooking demonstrations, nutrition classes and recipes that contribute to a healthy diet (USDA FDPIR, 2020).

AMERICAN INDIAN RURAL HEALTH CHARACTERISTICS

Coronavirus Disease 2019 Impact on Tribal Lands

Coronavirus Disease 2019 (COVID-19) breached the US borders in January 2020. While this pandemic impacted the world, like many times throughout history, AIAN people are disproportionately affected by the virus but they are not reflected in the counts. In May nearly half of the states that released racial demographic data did not explicitly include AIAN in their breakdowns but instead lumped them under the "Other" category (Doshi *et al.*, 2020; Nagle, 2020). The failure of states to provide inclusive data limits data-informed policy making and prioritized resource distribution to tribes (Doshi *et al.*, 2020). When COVID-19 incidence was studied in 14 states, Arrazola *et al.* (2020) found mortality was 1.8 times higher for AIAN than among non-Hispanic Whites. Further, mortality was higher among AIAN males and persons aged

20–49 years. The results from this study are important and need to be considered when planning and implementing prevention and medical strategies because the COVID-19 virus is exposing every disparity tribal nations continue to grapple with from economics to housing to healthcare (Arrazola *et al.*, 2020; Kakol *et al.*, 2020).

The primary source of tribal nations' income was stopped with the closure of casinos resulting in billions of dollars lost revenue (Meister Economic Consulting, 2020; Mineo, 2020). Tribal gaming revenues are equivalent to state tax revenues so when the casinos had to unexpectedly close, tribal nations lost large sources of income. Without the tribal gaming/casino revenue they were unable to deliver essential services such as health, education, transportation, and public safety (Doshi *et al.*, 2010; Mineo, 2020).

Coronavirus Aid, Relief, and Economic Security (CARES) Act was signed into Public Law 116-136 on March 27, 2020 and provided $2 trillion in economic relief (Congress.gov, 2020c). The money was slated to help small businesses; American families and workers; preserve jobs; and aid state, local and tribal governments (U.S. Department of Treasury, 2020a). The CARES Act included Title VI, Coronavirus Relief Fund (CRF) to provide financial relief by April 27, 2020 to states, tribes, and local governments for the increased costs associated with the COVID-19 public health emergency. Of the $150 billion allotted to the CRF, $8 billion was allotted to tribal governments. Statutory guidelines were developed that outlined eligible and ineligible expenditures for the states, tribes, and local governments but it was revised multiple times. The Treasury Department disbursement deadline of April 27, 2002 was met for states and local governments but the first distribution for tribes did not start until May 5, 2020.

The $8 billion fund for tribal governments was split into two portions, 60 percent was to be distributed immediately to address health and human services costs and other costs directly related to COVID-19 and allocated based on population, and 40 percent based on tribal expenses (Springer, 2020). The Treasury Department requested tribes submit information including figures on enrolled members of the tribe, to calculate how the money should be divided. The information provided by the tribes was disregarded, the Treasury Department used specific geographic location population data from the Department of Housing and Urban Development's Indian Housing Block Grant program to determine funding levels (Cochrane and Walker, 2020; Springer, 2020). Not all tribes have designated reservations or service areas, so their population counts were recorded as zero and they received only the minimum funding, whereas other tribes had more enrolled members than were counted. After repeated requests to the Treasury Department to revise the formula, some tribes filed lawsuits over the counting issues because the payments were not reflective of the number of tribal citizens or tribal needs. The second distribution of funds was started on June 12, 2020 and was based on tribal employees and tribal government expenditures. The final distribution payment was made on June 17, 2020 after Judge Amit P. Mehta of the United States District Court for the District of Columbia decided the funding needed to be distributed because the tribes had waited over 80 days when the funds were meant for immediate distribution (Allis and Desiderio, 2020). The payments to tribes increased but still lack transparency on how the amounts were determined for tribes (Cochrane and Walker, 2020). According the U.S. Department of Treasury website, as of June 17, 2020, all payments based on employment and expenditure data, other than payment of amounts allocated to Alaska Native corporations, have been made (U.S. Department of Treasury, 2020a).

In addition to the devastating economic disaster, many tribal nations have multiple risk factors that increase the likelihood of contracting the virus. American Indian and Alaskan Natives suffer from higher rates of co-morbidities such as diabetes and heart disease, live in remote communities, have less access to clean water and healthcare, live in multigenerational homes with many people, and are at or below poverty guidelines. The Navajo (Diné) Nation, located in Arizona, Utah, and New Mexico, made national headlines as they suffered the greatest impact of COVID-19 in the U.S. (Silverman *et al.*, 2020). At one point, the Navajo Nation, had the highest infection rate in the country with 2,300 cases per 100,000 as compared to New York (1,806 per 100,000) and New Jersey (1,668 per 100,000), which were the "hot spots" in the U.S. (Silverman *et al.*, 2020). The Navajo people experience many of the risk factors listed above, but the three most significant factors contributing to their vulnerability to the virus are the multigenerational homes, the remoteness of the communities (more people shopping at limited grocery stores), and up to 40 percent of the residents not having indoor plumbing (Silverman *et al.*, 2020).

To exacerbate the vulnerability to the infection, tribal nations were faced with critical shortages of hospital beds, Personal Protective Equipment (PPE), testing kits, and disinfecting supplies. Michael Toedt, Indian Health Services (IHS) Chief Medical Officer reported 37 ICU beds, 81 ventilators and just over 1,200 hospital beds were available for 2.5 million people (as cited in Cancryn, 2020). These numbers included IHS facilities and tribal health systems. In addition to a critical shortage of hospital beds and ventilators, PPE was so desperately needed, tribal nations were putting out requests on social media for homemade masks to protect their community members. Initially, the states were provided with a limited number of testing kits and were then tasked with distributing the kits. Tribal nations were given minimal kits or none (Doshi *et al.*, 2020; Hilleary, 2020).

Many tribes took their communities' health into their own hands by implementing strict curfews, stay-at-home orders, and closing the borders of their reservation to minimize the spread. In early April 2020, two South Dakota tribes (Cheyenne River Sioux and Oglala Sioux) initiated stay-at-home orders for their respective reservations despite the state not implementing the same mitigation strategy. In addition, the tribes incorporated check points onto their tribal lands, preventing non-residents from entering unless they were essential employees or obtained travel permits from the tribe. Residents could leave the reservation for essential activity only and the travel did not involve entering "hot spots". The governor of South Dakota, Kristi Noem, threatened legal action if the checkpoints were not removed (Carlisle, 2020). As sovereign nations, the tribes had the authority to protect their communities. In June 2020, the Cheyenne River Sioux and Oglala Sioux tribes filed a lawsuit against President Donald Trump, White House officials, and leadership in the Department of Interior and Bureau of Indian Affairs. The tribes claimed the federal government was attempting to coerce and threaten financial retribution if the checkpoints were not removed (Associated Press, 2020).

Cheyenne River Sioux tribe was a model community for how it handled the coronavirus pandemic and kept its community members safe. Tribal leaders began emergency preparedness meetings in February when the threat of the virus was first known. The tribe inventoried supplies, hospital beds, and medical staff. When it was apparent, they could not adequately care for their 6,000 residents if they all became sick, safety measures were deployed. The tribe employed 30 new police officers to help with public safety, curfew enforcement, and assistance with delivering supplies since there are limited transportation options available. In addition, the tribe prepared a building for individuals to self-quarantine if they became sick with the coronavirus; developed a roster of all the elders in the community; and called to check on them daily as well as administering to their needs such as food and assistance with electricity bills. They enlisted the support of local ranchers to donate thousands of pounds of beef and pork, so if there was a food shortage, they were well prepared. As of the end of May 2020, only one person in the community had tested positive for the coronavirus, and that individual was quarantined (Pfankuch, 2020). Historically known as a community-focused population, it is not surprising that there were no issues with compliance of any implemented mitigations to protect all residents on the reservation, both Native and non-Native.

MENTAL AND BEHAVIORAL HEALTH

In 2018, 4.5 percent of AIANs over the age of 18 reported serious psychological distress (NCHS, 2018a, Table A-8a). They were almost twice as likely to experience the feeling that everything is an effort all or most of the time, as compared to the White population (NCHS, 2018b, Table A-7a). American Indians and Alaskan Natives communities have endured generations of historical trauma which eroded their family structure, tribal structure, and spiritual relations. It has shaped their identity, relationship skills, personal behavior, transmission of traditions and values, and attitudes and beliefs about their future. The stress of these traumas combined with the continued discrimination and racism toward AIANs contributes to the rates of high rates mental illness in AIAN communities and can result in substance misuse, anxiety, depression, and suicide (Willis *et al.*, 2016).

Opioid Epidemic

According to the Centers for Disease Control (CDC), of the 70,237 drug overdose deaths, approximately 47,600 involved opioids (Wilson *et al.*, 2020). Every racial, economic, and age group has been impacted which in 2017 led the Department of Health and Human Services to declare the opioid epidemic a public health emergency. While the opioid epidemic is a multifaceted problem that crosses all aspects of life, the rates of drug usage and overdoses in rural areas and reservations are rising and surpassing rates in urban areas (Mack *et al.*, 2017). In 2018, AIAN populations had the second highest overdose rates from all opioids (14.2 deaths/100,000 population), second to White, non-Hispanic at 18.6 deaths/100,000. The AIAN population also had the second highest overdose deaths rates from heroin, 5.1/100,000 and third highest from synthetic opioids 7.3/100,000 (Wilson *et al.*, 2020).

Additionally, some Indian Health Services (IHS) hospitals are placing AI patients at risk for opioid abuse and overdoses because providers are not following prescription and dispensing protocols. In 2019, a Health and Human Services (HHS) Office of Inspector General audited 25 Indian Health Services (IHS) hospitals and identified major deficiencies in five because there was a lack of compliance with policies and procedures for prescribing and dispensing opioids, and they lacked adequate cybersecurity and IT services. The results of the chart audit demonstrated that each hospital met or exceeded the CDC recommendation of prescribing no more than 90 morphine milligrams equivalents per day. At one IHS hospital, the daily dosage was more than four times the recommended amount (Cheidi, 2019).

American Indian tribes took the lead to address the opioid crisis on rural reservations. Tribes from 28 states along with over 600 cities and counties filed a federal lawsuit against Purdue's Sackler Family for aggressively marketing OxyContin, a painkiller drug responsible for addiction, overdose, and death that has damaged millions of lives and families (Fonseca, 2019; Ellis and Schuman, 2019). Every aspect of AIAN Tribal communities is negatively impacted by the opioid epidemic, including healthcare, law enforcement, social services, children, multigeneration families, homes, and employment. Tribal communities are already impoverished, and they do not have the funding to provide the additional resources needed to prevent and treat this epidemic. The Tribal Opioid Response Resource Toolkit was developed to provide tribes and healthcare providers the materials, tools, resources, and links to support them as they try to implement interventions to address the epidemic within their tribal communities (NIHB, 2020).

Alcohol Misuse

Alcohol is the most used drug by AIANs and as a result, the rate of substance dependence or abuse is higher among Native Americans than any other group. The 2018 National Survey on Drug Use and Health results revealed that one in six AIAN adolescents, age 12–17 was involved in underage drinking, the highest rate of alcohol used of all racial/ethnic groups and 22 percent of AIAN adults participated in binge drinking during the past month (Hardey *et al.*, 2020). Nearly one in five AINA young adults, age 18–25 years, have a substance use disorder, including 11 percent with illicit drugs and 10 percent with alcohol (Kaliszewski, 2020). American Indians with an alcohol use disorder was 7.1 percent which is higher than 5.4 percent for the total population (Hardey *et al.*, 2020). Contributing factors to the high risk of addiction is historical trauma, violence, poverty, high levels of unemployment, ACEs, discrimination, racism, stereotypes, myths, lack of health insurance, and low levels of attained education (Szalavitz, 2015; Kaliszewski, 2020; Kurup, 2020).

The "Firewater Myth" is the belief that AIANs have specific biological and genetic vulnerability to the effects of alcohol and associated problems (Gonzalez *et al.*, 2019; Gonzalez and Skewes, 2018; Kurup, 2020). The "Firewater Myth" is from a racist belief that was fueled from colonialism and while genetics play a role in the risk for alcohol abuse disorder, there is no evidence that AINA are more biologically susceptible to alcohol use disorders (Szalavitz, 2015; Gonzaler and Skewes, 2018). However, for AIAN college students who drink, their belief in biological vulnerability impacts the strategies utilized to moderate alcohol use and avoiding alcohol-related harm (Gonzalez *et al.*, 2019; Gonzalez and Skewes, 2018).

In 2018, 13 percent of AIANs age 12 and older were classified as needing substance abuse treatment, however, only 3.5 percent received treatment at a specialty facility (Kaliszewski, 2020; SAMHSA, 2019, Table 5.38B). Barriers to AIANs receiving treatment were transportation issues, lack of health insurance, poverty, and a shortage of treatment centers (Kaliszewski, 2020). Treatment programs that incorporate cultural traditions, spirituality, provide a holistic, well-rounded approach to substance abuse. As a way to provide holistic treatment, tribes are implementing Tribal Healing to Wellness Courts which assimilates substance abuse treatment with the criminal justice system to provide substance-abusing offenders judicially supervised treatment and transitional services through the use of intense supervision, sanctions and incentives and drug testing in a non-punitive setting (Kurup, 2020). When traditional healing approaches such as powwows, drum circles, and sweat lodges are incorporated into the treatment plans, AINA have better outcomes (Kaliszewski, 2020).

Suicide

American Indians and Alaskan Natives continue to have the highest rates of suicide than any other racial/ethnic group in the U.S. In 2015, 18 states were part the National Violent Death Reporting System (NVDRS) study and Leavitt *et al.* (2018) found that AIAN suicide rates were 21.5 which was more than 3.5 times higher than those for White decedents. More than 35.7 percent of the AIAN decedents were aged 10–25 in contrast to 11.1 percent of Whites. When compared with Whites, 69.4 percent AIAN lived in rural areas and were more than twice as likely to have a family member or friend commit suicide. Twenty-eight percent of the descendants reported alcohol abuse issues and 49 percent used alcohol within hours of their death (Leavitt *et al.*, 2018).

From 2009–2018, AIAN the suicide rate was higher at 22.1 per 100,000 than 14.2 per 100,000 for the US population. When reviewed by age, AIAN suicide rates peaked during adolescence and young adulthood and then declines which is different than the pattern for the US population. The suicide rates for AIAN men, 28.0 per 100,000, was three times the rate for AIAN women, 8.0 per 100,000. A higher percentage of AIAN adults reported past-year serious thoughts of suicide (5.8%), a past-year suicide plan (1.6%) or a past year suicide attempt (1.0%) (Education Development Center, 2020).

The higher AIAN suicide rates have been linked to the higher rates of poverty, substance abuse, unemployment, historical trauma, and violence. Further, the geographic isolation makes it difficult to access mental health services that may or may be offered in rural settings (Dastagir, 2019). Culturally competent suicide prevention strategies need to be integrated into the provision of healthcare especially if mental health services are limited or nonexistent in rural settings. Rural Nurse Practitioners and nurses can utilize the multiple resources available on the Indian Health Services website to promote community education and awareness efforts, implement interventions and postvention services (IHS, n.d.b). Additionally, the Mental Health Technology Transfer Center Network (MHTTC) hosts free monthly webinars for behavioral health professionals (MHTTC, 2020).

Dementia and Alzheimer Disease

Dementia itself is not a disease but instead is an umbrella term that includes the diagnoses of Alzheimer's, vascular dementia, or non-specific dementia (CMS, 2016). It is projected the number of individuals identifying only as AIAN age 65 years and older will grow from 235,000 in 2010, to 918,000 in

2050, increasing the proportion of older adults from 10 percent to 16.8 percent (Vincent and Velkoff, 2010). In a longitudinal study conducted by Mayeda *et al.* (2016), the average annual rate of dementia was 26.6 cases per 1,000 for Blacks, 22.2 cases per 1,000 for AIAN, 19.6 cases per 1,000 for Latinos and Pacific Islanders, 19.3 cases per 1,000 for Whites and 15.2 cases per 1,000 for Asian Americans. The researchers projected that among the Native elders who reach age 65 dementia-free, 35 percent will develop dementia in the next 25 years (Mayeda *et al.*, 2016)

The escalating incidence in dementia indicated the need for increased education and outreach efforts to improve community awareness and understanding of dementia on rural reservations. Native experts and leaders assisted in the development of the landmark document, The *Healthy Brain Initiative Road Map for Indian Country*. This document is a tool and guide for tribal leaders and encompasses eight public health strategies that integrates community strength by including traditional practices, resilience, and existing services. As a greater emphasis is placed on dementia, the Native community needs to recognize it as a chronic disease, provide early diagnosis and treatment options, utilize culturally appropriate screening tools, collect accurate data on incidence and prevalence, and provide family support (Alzheimer's Association and Centers for Disease Control and Prevention, 2019).

The impact of dementia is multigenerational as elders living with this chronic condition gradually need additional help with daily cares with the progression of the disease. In Native communities, family members frequently are the caregivers for elders diagnosed with dementia, yet they may be unprepared or untrained for this role. The Savvy Caregiver in Indian Country program was developed to help caregivers acquire the knowledge, skills, and attitudes for the new role they are undertaking. Additionally, they learn strategies for managing client behavior, managing daily life, day-to-day management skills, and family resources of care. The Native elder diagnosed with dementia will never return to the person he or she used to be as a mother or father. To avoid frustration, family caregivers need to let go of their expectations based on who the person used to be and what they were able to do as a healthy parent (NICA, 2013).

Depression

In 2017, 16 percent of AIAN adolescents aged 12–17 had a major depressive episode as compared to 14 percent of the White population. Eight percent of AIAN age 18 or older experienced a major depressive episode with severe impairment (NIMH, 2019). Twenty-two percent of AIAN women self-reported postpartum depression symptoms which was significantly higher than other ethnic and racial groups (Bauman *et al.*, 2020). If adults are diagnosed with chronic disease(s), their risk for depression is much higher, approximately between 25–33 percent (Goldberg, 2017). Little is known about the prevalence of depression in older AIANs, but the diagnosis can be complicated because multiple chronic diseases can cause, hide, or worsen the disease. Depression is a common comorbidity among individuals diagnosed with diabetes and it reduces quality of life while increasing morbidity, mortality, and healthcare costs (Bell *et al.*, 2005). With the projected increase in the aging AIAN population, along with the forecasted increase diagnosis of multiple chronic diseases, rural health care providers need to address the growing mental health issues in Indian Country.

CHRONIC HEALTH CONDITIONS AND MORTALITY

Chronic diseases are long-term medical conditions that generally worsen over time and frequently older adults are diagnosed with one or more chronic diseases especially as they age (CDC, 2019, August 17b). Adamsen *et al.* (2018) conducted a national survey of 14,632 AIAN elders aged 55 and older. The researchers found that 89.7 percent were diagnosed with at least one of ten chronic diseases; 69.8 percent had two or more; and 45.2 percent had three or more. The three most common chronic diseases were high blood pressure (58.9%), diabetes (53.9%), and arthritis (47.2%) (Adamsen *et al.*, 2018). Chronic diseases significantly impact the mortality and disabilities of individuals as noted in 2017, cardiovascular disease, cancer, unintentional injuries, and diabetes were the leading causes of AIAN deaths (See Table 9.2 for Leading Causes of Death for AIAN and White Populations) (Heron, 2019).

Cardiovascular Disease

The Strong Heart Study (SHS) has been tracking Cardiovascular Disease (CVD) and associated risk factors among AIs on reservations since 1988 and is considered the most comprehensive resource on the subject. The largest epidemiological study ever of American Indians, the SHS offers the advantage of including multiple communities, 13 tribes in three geographic areas. The SHS incorporates extensive physical measurements, interviews regarding risk behavior and dietary intake, and recent genetic sequencing. The research findings and development of educational materials contributes to the overall understanding of disease pathways and genetics of CVD (Strong Heart Study, 2017). The *Strong Heart Study* is especially important as cardiovascular continues to be the leading cause of death for AIAN and the seventh cause of death is cerebrovascular disease (See Table 9.2) (Heron, 2019, June). Rural nurse practitioners and nurses can use the SDPI *Healthy Heart Project HH Toolkit* as a resource to educate AIAN patients on topics such as high blood pressure, high cholesterol, and smoking (IHS, n.d.c. *Heart Healthy Toolkit*).

TABLE 9.2. 2017 Deaths and percentage of total deaths for leading causes of death, by Native American and White Populations.

Leading Causes of Death	AIAN Rank	AIAN Deaths	AIAN Deaths	White Rank	White Deaths	White Percentage of all Deaths
All causes		19,198			2,179,857	
Cardiovascular disease	1	3,472	18.1	1	508,485	23.0
Malignant neoplasms (cancer)	2	3,257	17.0	2	465,679	21.3
Accidents (unintentional injuries)	3	2,229	11.6	4	137,029	5.7
Diabetes mellitus	4	1,114	5.8	7	55,116	3.0
Chronic liver disease and cirrhosis	5	1,047	5.5	11	30,223	1.4
Chronic lower respiratory diseases	6	939	4.9	3	139,833	6.0
Cerebrovascular disease (stroke)	7	737	3.8	5	110,038	5.2
Intentional self-harm (suicide)	8	602	3.1	9	38,106	1.8
Influenza and pneumonia	9	391	2.0	8	43,397	2.0
Alzheimer disease	10	376	2.0	6	101,876	4.3
Nephritis, nephrotic syndrome, and nephrosis (kidney diseases)	11	333	1.7	10	35,191	1.7
Septicemia	12	295	1.5	12	30,198	1.4
Assault (homicide)	13	266	1.4	20	5,747	0.3
Essential hypertension and hypertensive renal disease	14	190	1.0	14	24,465	1.1

Cancer

Cancer rates vary among the AIAN tribes and geographic regions because of differing traditions and behaviors that influence disease risk. From 2012–2016 for all sites, the five most common cancers for AIANs were lung, colon and rectum, kidney, liver, and stomach. Similarly, the five highest mortality incidences for AIANs were lung, colon and rectum, liver, kidney and renal pelvis, and stomach cancers (Siegel *et al.*, 2019, Table 9). Breast cancer is the most common cancer among AIAN women. From 2012–2016 the overall incident rates for breast cancer increased by 0.8 percent per year for AIAN women in contrast to the 0.5 percent for Whites. For AIAN women the incidence and mortality rates for breast cancer were 94.7 and 14.6 as compared to White women, respectively 130.8 and 20.3 (American Cancer Society, 2019). Fifty-one percent of AIAN women over the age of 40 had mammogram screening in contrast to 65.8 percent for White women (NCHS, 2019 Table 33). The incidence of prostate cancer for AIAN men was 73.1 and 101.7 for White men, whereas the mortality rate was 19.1 for AIAN men and 101.7 for White men (Siegel *et al.*, 2019, Table 9). To prevent cancer and eliminate the associated burdens in the Native community, the American Indian Cancer Foundation (2019) developed multiple culturally tailored infographics, toolkits, and webinars. Rural nurse practitioners and nurses can use these educational resources for the prevention, early detection, treatment, and survivor support (AICAF, 2019).

Diabetes Mellitus

American Indians and Alaskan Natives on average tend to have the highest diabetes rate than any other U.S. racial group (CDC, 2017a). In 2019, 23.5 percent of AIAN were diagnosed with diabetes as compared to 8.6 percent of White adults (NCHS, 2018c, Table A-4a.). The death rate of AIANs from diabetes was 15.1 in contrast to 7.4 for Whites. The *Special Diabetes Program for Indians* (SDPI) was developed in 1997 to address the epidemic of type 2 diabetes. In 2020, 301 AIAN communities in 35 states received SDPI funding to focus on treatment and prevention interventions in Native communities (IHS SDPI, 2020 June). These communities are encouraged to apply for CDC Recognition and offer the National Diabetes Prevention Program for reimbursement and long-term sustainability (CDC, 2019, July 9c).

To prevent diabetes and implement lifestyle changes in AIAN communities, nurse practitioners and nurses can use prevention strategies outlined in the Diabetes Prevention Program Toolkit (CDC, 2019, July 9b). They can also implement segments of the Native Wellness Diabetes Program to promote health and prevent type 2 diabetes among AIAN youth and families. The Native Wellness Program offers the *Eagle Books Toolkit for Families, Classrooms, and Communities* and all materials can be downloaded from the CDC website which includes beautifully illustrated novels, guides for educators and communities, educational tools, games and activities that promote health in AINA youth (CDC, 2016a). Additionally, teachers and nurses can collaborate to teach the Health Is Life in Balance Diabetes Education in Tribal Schools (DETS) K–12 curriculum to grades K–12. The lesson plans are based on health, Type 1 and Type 2 diabetes, science, community knowledge, and civic responsibility (CDC, 2016b). Free continuing education webinars on diabetes-related topics are provided for clinicians on the IHS website (IHS, n.d.d. CME/CE Online Education).

As a co-author and daughter of a Bureau of Indian Affairs Law Enforcement Officer, I have had the unique opportunity to live on the Turtle Mountain Band of Chippewa, Spirit Lake Nation, Standing Rock Sioux, Rosebud Sioux, Red Lake Nation, and Bois Forte Band of Chippewa Indian Reservations for the first 25 years of my life. The health disparities described in this section were not only seen on each reservation, but they are also current issues within my own family. The life-altering, long-term effects of diabetes are seen daily in rural reservation communities. Amputation of lower extremities is a common occurrence and creates fear and anxiety when American Indians are diagnosed with diabetes (Wilkie-Condiff, 2009; Carson *et al.*, 2015). Dialysis centers may not be available on the reservation and can require two or more hours of driving time to access the closest available. Considering the financial and transportation issues many AIAN face, this creates additional hardships to complying with prescribed dialysis. Because so many relatives have been down the road of amputation, AIANs see this as their fate as well. Their history and experience with healthcare providers and late access to healthcare may exacerbate their lack of trust, and therefore may be unlikely to follow the medical advice of following a healthy diet and implementing exercise. It is important to provide culturally relevant education regarding changes in diet and exercise and providing adequate resources and support groups to address concerns (Purnell and Fenkl, 2019).

Obesity

Obesity rates for AIANs are 50 percent more likely to be higher than Whites. Slattery *et al.* (2010) studied 11,293 Native Americans (Alaska and Navajo) for associations among body mass index, waist circumference, and health indicators. Of the population studied, 34 percent were overweight, and 47.1 percent were obese. Waist circumference was greater than 102 cm for 41.7 percent of men and 88 cm for 78.3 percent of women. American Indian and Alaskan Natives younger than 30 years old were three times more likely to perceive their health as being fair or poor when their BMI results were 35 or greater. The associations between previously diagnosed medical conditions were stronger for AIAN men than women. Men were 75 percent more likely to have two or more medical conditions when they had of 35 kg/m^2, whereas only 36 percent of women had two or more conditions. The association between high blood pressure, high cholesterol, and prior history of gall bladder disease, arthritis, and diabetes were much higher for men than women. American Indian and Alaskan Natives with higher BMI levels also reported fewer hours of vigorous exercise and more hours of watching television.

Between 2011–2014, Gibbs *et al.* (2016) studied 1,256 Native American Tribal College students and found 33 percent were overweight and 35 percent were obese. The researchers also studied the subjects' perception of weight by gender. Males were more likely to underestimate their weight than females. Additionally, most of the subjects did not meet the recommendations for fruit intake (78.7%), vegetable intake (96.6%), and/or physical activity (65.5%). Keith *et al.* (2017) conducted a qualitative study to explore the barriers and strategies for healthy food choices with 20 Native American tribal college students. The barriers to healthy choices were related to taste, food gathering and preparation, and difficulty identifying healthy food choices. Positive strategies included taste, cultural traditions and practices, and personal motivation.

Bullock *et al.* (2017) examined the Indian Health Service National Data Warehouse data for the prevalence of obesity and overweight in AIAN children. The sample included 184,000 AIAN children aged 2 to 19 years who had body mass index data for annually for 2006 to 2015. In 2015, the prevalence of overweight and obesity in AIAN children aged 2 was 18.5 percent to 19 years old at 29.7 percent. American Indian and Alaskan Native boys had higher obesity prevalence at 31.5 percent than girls at 27.9 percent. The prevalence of overweight and obesity was higher for youth aged 12 to 19 years than younger children (Bullock *et al.*, 2017).

Traditional and Commercial Tobacco

Traditional tobacco has been used by AI for centuries and it is viewed as a sacred and powerful medicine to be used only in ceremonies and prayers. The preparation and use of traditional tobacco differ across tribes and regions. The variances are due to the different teachings and preparation of tobacco for specific ceremonial or sacred rituals. As a medicine, traditional tobacco is used in a prescribed way to promote spiritual, emotional, mental, and physical guidance. It can also be used as a gift to the Creator or another person, place, or being. When asking an AI person for help, guidance, or protection, it is a sign of respect to give a small gift of traditional tobacco (Keep It Sacred, 2015a). Traditional and commercial tobacco differ in the way they are planted, grown, harvested, prepared, and used. Commercial tobacco is produced for recreation use by companies, contains chemical additives such as nicotine and is associated with death and disease (Keep It Scared, 2015b).

Commercial tobacco use is the leading preventable cause of disease, disability, and death, however, AIAN adults have the highest cigarette smoking rate at 22.6 percent in contrast to 13.7 percent of adults of all racial and ethnic groups. The 2019 National Youth Tobacco Survey data revealed that AIAN high school students smoking rate was 16.2 percent as compared to 5.8 percent overall. Of AIAN middle school students, 3.7 percent were smoking cigarettes in contrast to 2.3 percent of all middle schoolers. Forty percent of percent of AINA high schoolers and 16.1 percent of AINA middle schoolers were e-cigarette users which is higher than the general population, respectively 27.5 percent among high schoolers and 10.5 percent among middle schoolers. An estimated 55.6 percent of AIANs wanted to quit smoking compared to 67.5 percent Whites (CDC, 2019, November 25d; U.S. Department of Health and Human Services, 2014; Wang *et al.*, 2019). Clinicians can use *The Tobacco Cessation within American Indian and Alaskan Native Communities Toolkit* (Rhodes *et al.*, n.d.) or In a Good Way: Indigenous Commercial Tobacco Control Practices (Slobig *et al.*, 2017) to implement tribally based strategies to reduce commercial tobacco use in tribal communities.

AMERICAN INDIAN AND ALASKAN NATIVE HEALTH CARE

Insurance Coverage

American Indian and Alaskan Natives (AIAN) continue to have lower rates of insurance coverage than the non-Hispanic White population which is a significant barrier to their obtaining the much-needed healthcare. In 2018, 51.3 percent of AIAN, alone or in combination with another race, had private health insurance coverage. Forty-three percent relied on Medicaid or public assistance coverage, and 14.9 percent did not have health insurance coverage. These percentages compare with non-Hispanic Whites by 75.4 percent, 33.7 percent, and 5.9 percent respectively (United States Census Bureau, 2018a, B02010).

Indian Health Service

The Indian Health Service (IHS) was established in 1955 to meet the federal treaty obligations to provide health services to federally recognized American Indian and Alaskan Native tribes (Sequist *et al.*, 2011). Under the Indian Self-Determination and Education Assistance Act, Public Law 93-638, Indian Tribes and Tribal Organizations have the option to (1) administer programs and services the IHS would provide or (2) assume control over health care programs and services that IHS would provide (Warne, 2011; IHS, n.d.e). Twelve area offices provide oversight to 170 IHS and tribally managed hospitals, health centers, health stations, school health centers, and youth regional treatment centers (IHS, 2020). Approximately 2.56 million AIANs are provided comprehensive primary care, some specialty services, and prescription drug coverage. Purchased/Referred Care (PRC), formerly known as Contract Health service, funds provide services not routinely available within the facilities, including subspecialty and hospital care. However, these funds are extremely limited, to be used only as a last resort, and only available to those residing on the reservation with approval. The IHS is authorized to collect revenue from external sources including Medicare, Medicaid, and private insurers when patient care is delivered within IHS facilities (Sequist *et al.*, 2011).

Indian Health Services funding is appropriated by Congress each fiscal year. This appropriation is severely underfunded as it only serves 50 percent of the healthcare needs of the AIAN population (Dorgan, 2019). In 2017 the IHS budget appropriation was $5.0 billion for the annual IHS per patient spending was only $4,079 which was much lower than the $9,726 U.S. National Health Expenditure per person (IHS, 2020). If the service demands exceed available funds, services are prioritized or rationed (Artiga *et al.*, 2013; Dorgan, 2019).

Most of the AIAN receiving IHS service primarily live on reservations and rural communities in 37 states. There are many challenges to IHS institutions providing and improving healthcare for rural and remote Native populations. Access to care can be limited due to geographic isolation, physician recruitment, and limited access to secondary and tertiary specialized care (Sequist *et al.*, 2011). The IHS system has been damaged with cases of insufficient staffing, poor management, changing and inconsistent leadership, incompetence of professional staff, second-rate medical practice, corruption, medical staff lacking credentials, transferring incompetent staff from one facility to another, poor coordination with local partners, sexual harassment and child sexual abuse (Cheidi, 2019; Dorgan, 2019; Weaver and Frosch, 2020). Furthermore, diverse healthcare professionals frequently display unconscious bias toward AIAN patients. Research has demonstrated with unintentional bias, some healthcare providers make treatment decisions based on their cultural, racial biases and stereotypes of underrepresented groups which perpetuates health inequities (Dorgan, 2019; Marcelin *et al.*, 2019).

AMERICAN INDIAN AND ALASKAN NATIVE NURSING WORKFORCE

The first record of American Indian nursing reaches as far as the late 1800s. These nurses were true pioneers of their time, facing racism, discrimination, and attempts to rid them of their cultural identity, yet they persevered to obtain a nursing degree. Many of these nurses continued to make significant contributions to their communities and the nursing profession (Charbonneau-Dahlen and Crow, 2016). While there is a long history of AI in nursing, there continues to be a disproportionate representation in the workforce. In 2010, The Institute of Medicine released a report titled "The Future of Nursing: Leading Change, Advancing Health"; recommendations included improving the diversity of the nursing workforce as a critical factor in meeting population health needs (Institute of Medicine, 2011). This is especially relevant in North Dakota where all four of the AI reservations are in health professional shortage areas and are among the most underserved populations in the state (Center for Rural Health, 2019). Health Resources and Services Administration (HRSA) established the Nursing Workforce Diversity (NWD) program to provide federal grant funding to nursing programs seeking to increase the number of nurses from disadvantaged backgrounds, including ethnic and racial minorities (HRSA, 2020).

For decades, colleges and universities have been doing their part to recruit, retain and graduate American Indian nurses. With poor social determinants of health and varying disparities, including health, financial and educational, recruiting is not easy task to accomplish. As described in the Education section, American Indian students, particularly those coming from rural reservation communities, face greater academic challenges in the college and university setting. To be successful, these students will likely need support from the application process through to graduation and beyond. It is also helpful for them to have an environment that supports their cultural identity. Recruitment can also be challenging with a limited number of American Indian nurses and faculty. To recruit and retain American Indians in nursing, an international award-winning documentary titled Essence of Healing: The Journey of American Indian Nurses was produced in 2016. The documentary highlights the journeys of 14 American Indian nurses and provides details into their journeys from why they became nurses to the challenges of nursing education and where they are now (Heuer *et al.*, 2016).

Nursing programs have established programs of support to increase the number of American Indian nursing students. The program with the longest and most successful history of graduating American Indian nurses, from BSN to MSN, is the RAIN (Recruitment and Retention of American Indians in Nursing) program at the University of North Dakota (UND) (UND RAIN, 2020). RAIN has been providing culturally supportive academic monitoring, advisement, mentoring, and tutoring American Indian nursing students since 1992 and supported 235 graduates with a bachelor's in nursing (Charbonneau-Dahlen and Crow, 2016; UND RAIN, 2020). As a graduate of UND's master's in nursing program, co-author Dr. Wilkie used some of her experiences with RAIN to develop Niganawenimaanaanig (an Ojibwe word translating to "we take care of them") at Bemidji State University in Minnesota when the university was awarded a $2 million HRSA NWD in 2017 (Wilkie, 2020a). To have the greatest success in retaining and graduating American Indian students, it is vital to have a program that embraces students' cultural identity and provide a community of support, including academic, social, cultural, and financial (Wilkie 2020b).

Currently there are almost 200 nursing positions available in IHS and the job vacancies vary from clinical nurse, OB, emergency room, urgent care, post-anesthesia care unit, community health, and nurse practitioner. Many of these positions are located in rural reservation communities like Crownpoint, Zuni, and Shiprock, NM; Rosebud, Wakpala, Sisseton, and Pine Ridge, SD; Chinle and Whiteriver, AZ; and Fort Yates and Belcourt, ND (IHS, n.d.). Indian Health Service offers competitive salaries, loan repayment programs, and being AIAN is not a requirement to be employed though Indian preference is given. For students, scholarship and internship/externships opportunities are available (IHS, n.d.h).

OPPORTUNITIES FOR NURSE PRACTITIONERS AND NURSES

When working in rural areas with the AIAN populations, nurses and nurse practitioners can learn about their culture, traditions, and the numerous contributions they made to the disciplines of sign language, sports, transportation, music, governmental structure, agriculture, conservation, astrology, engineering, and medicine (Brown, 1975; Keoke and Porterfield, 2003). In the area of medicine, pre-Columbian AI's had complex medical practices that combined the knowledge and usage of drugs with physical and psychological treatments. According to Moerman (2009), AIs used over 2,700 plants for medicinal uses that included analgesics, narcotics, cathartics, febrifuges, contraceptives, gastrointestinal aids, hypotension, sedatives, and psychotherapy (Brown, 1975; Moerman, 2009). Many of the tribes performed arthrocentesis, surgical and wound debridement, orthopedic techniques, thoracentesis, and trephination (Smith, 2017). Further, there are hundreds of AI interventions that have been integrated into the daily lives of Americans, such as syringes, rubber and cotton for surgical use, baby bottles, and mouthwash (Kiger, 2019; Schilling, 2017). By having an increased understanding of AI contributions to modern-day life, nurse practitioners and nurses can gain a deeper appreciation of the tribal cultures.

When providing care to the AIAN population, non-Native nurse practitioners and nurses can conduct a self-assessment of biases, either conscious or unconscious, that are derived from stereotypes that facilities the continuation of health inequities (Marcelin *et al.*, 2019). By dispelling negative stereotypes held by healthcare providers, it allows them to build trust, respect, and understanding with the Native population (Mitchell-Brown, 2020).

Lowe and Struthers (2004) developed the Native American Nursing Conceptual Framework which represents the seven dimensions of caring, traditions, respect, connection, holism, trust, and spirituality. Each dimension is essential to the practice of nursing in Native American culture. Non-Native nurses can use this framework to serve as a cultural foundation in practice, to support personal and professional growth, guides research in health-related studies, and guides the development of cultural appropriate nursing and healthcare resources (Lowe and Nichols, 2014).

While the rurality of some reservation communities may be a deterrent for employment, there are numerous benefits that are available as well. Becoming a welcomed member into an Indigenous community allows for a unique and intimate look into the culture, values, traditions, and practices. When non-Native healthcare providers dedicate their services to improving the quality of life of Indigenous people and communities, they become aware of the best practices in Indian country while also practicing holistically. Community members begin to open more, sharing more of their authentic selves, and the true beauty of the AIAN culture is learned by the healthcare providers. These opportunities also permit healthcare providers to learn more about the support for families and availability of community resources. The nurse practitioners and nurses also learn about the generosity and kindheartedness of the Native people to others.

SUMMARY

Rural nursing in AIAN communities presents atypical challenges and disparities for healthcare providers. This population has endured genocide and racism since the Europeans first arrived. In present day, these populations still encounter systemic oppression and racism through every facet of daily living, including from the federal government. American Indians and Alaskan Natives suffer from higher rates of chronic diseases and mental health issues compared to other races and ethnicities. Residing in remote, and sometimes desolate areas of the U.S., often adds to the challenges in providing adequate services to these communities.

This chapter focused on rural nursing in AIAN areas with specific examples and data provided from North and South Dakota and Minnesota. While not all rural areas have the same unique differences, the traditional cultural beliefs of family and community-focused living are similar. American Indians and Alaskan Natives have survived on these values and this way of living for hundreds of years. The grim history and traumatic experiences have shaped this population and negatively impacted physical and mental health for generations. However, it is also important to recognize that the resilience and instinct to protect loved ones have positively affected their lives as well. The most recent example being the way the Cheyenne River Sioux and the Navajo nation deviated from their states' leadership, developing their own tribal nation policies to protect community members and mitigate the novel coronavirus pandemic. This leadership style represents the natural community-centered thinking of AIAN people as compared to the egocentric actions of the majority.

By fully engaging in the Indigenous culture on rural reservations, non-Native nurse practitioners and nurses can build relationships with tribal members in which they gradually become respected and welcomed members of Indigenous communities. Although there continues to be a great need for AIAN nurses because they can connect western medicine and AIAN holistic views to provide culturally appropriate care for Native patients. Educational support programs to empower AIAN students academically while preserving and enhancing cultural identity have helped to increase the number of Indigenous nurses in recent years. However, there will always be a need for non-Native nurses and healthcare providers to be allies and advocates for AIAN people in the arenas of clinical practice, education, research, and policy.

REFERENCES

Adams, D. W. (1995). *Education for Extinction American Indians and the Boarding School Experience 1875–1928*. Lawrence: University Press of Kansas.

Adamsen C., S. Schroeder, S. LeMire and P. Carter (2018). Education, income, and employment and prevalence of chronic disease among American Indian/Alaska Native elders. *Preventing Chronic Disease, 15*(E37), 1–9. 170387. https://doi.org/10.5888/pcd15.170387

Administration for Children and Families [ACF] and Administration for Native Americans [ANA] (2017). *Combating trafficking Native youth toolkit on human trafficking.* https://www.acf.hhs.gov/sites/default/files/otip/native_youth_toolkit_on_human_trafficking.pdf

Akee, R. K. Q., K. A. Spilde, and J. B. Taylor. (2015). The Indian Gaming Regulatory Act and its effects on the American Indian economic development. *The Journal of Economic Perspectives, 29*(3), 185–208. DOI: 10.1111/ssqu.12009

Akee, R. K. Q. and J. B. Taylor. (2014). Social and economic change on American Indian Reservations: A databook for the US Census and American community survey, 1990–2010. Sarasota, FL: https://static1.squarespace.com/static/52557b58e4b0d4767401ce95/t/5379756ce4b095f55e75c77b/1400468844624/AkeeTaylorUSDatabook2014-05-15.pdf

Allis, K. and D. Desiderio. (2020, July 9). U.S. Treasury's upcoming coronavirus relief fund report. Native American Finance Officers Association and National Congress of American Indians. http://www.ncai.org/Covid-19/administrative/7_9_20_Letter_on_Treasury_CRF_Reporting_-NCAI_-_NAFOA-.pdf

Alzheimer's Association and Centers for Disease Control and Prevention. (2019). *Healthy Brain Initiative, Road Map for Indian Country*. Chicago, IL: Alzheimer's Association. https://www.cdc.gov/aging/healthybrain/pdf/HBI-Road-Map-for-Indian-Country-508.pdf

Aman, J., Pendleton, V., Martin Rogers, N., Bosch, W. and Decker Gerrard, M. (2020). *Homelessness on American Indian reservations. Key findings from 2018 Minnesota reservation homeless study*. Wilder Research. http://mnhomeless.org/minnesota-homeless-study/reports-and-fact-sheets/2018/2018-homeless-reservations-4-20.pdf

American Cancer Society [ACS]. (2019). *Breast Cancer Facts and Figures 2019–2020.* Atlanta: American Cancer Society, Inc.

American Indian Cancer Foundation [AICAF]. (2019). *AICAF Resources*. Infographics, Toolkits, Webinars. https://www.americanindiancancer.org/resources/

Andrews, J. D. (2013). Native Americans. Cultural, ethnic, and religious reference manual for healthcare providers. (4th ed., pp. 269–286). Kernersville, NC: JAMARDA Resources, Inc.

Aqpik Apok, C., S. Baker, G. Balandran, B. Bar Heels, M. Benally, T. Carpenter, C. Deford, D. Ewenin, A. Fisher, A. Fixico, D. Green, L. Hayes, C. Horn, R. Ibarra, *et al.* (2020, May 5). MMIWG2 Organizing and MMIP Toolkit. https://2a840442-f49a-45b0-b1a1-7531a7cd3d30.filesusr.com/ugd/6b33f7_2585fecaf9294450a5955 09cb701e7af.pdf

Arrazola, J., M. *et al.* (2020). COVID-19 mortality among American Indian and Alaskan Native persons—14 States. *Morbidity & Mortality Weekly Report, 69*, 1853–1856. DOI: http://dx.doi.org/10.15584/mmwr.mm6949a3.

Artiga, S., R. Arguello, and P. Duckett. (2013, October). Health coverage and care for American Indians and Alaska Natives. Executive Summary, Issue Brief. *The Kaiser Commission on Medicaid and the Uninsured.* https://www.kff.org/wp-content/uploads/2013/10/8502-health-coverage-and-care-for-american-indians-and-alaska-natives.pdf

Associated Press. (2020, June 24). South Dakota tribe sues feds to keep COVID-19 checkpoints. *Rapid City Journal.*

https://apnews.com/article/9b9fd6f0bd1d4d944ae3b35015d76f05

Association of American Indian Physicians. (2020). Aces toolkit. Strengthening our Native communities: How understanding adverse childhood experiences can help. https://www.aaip.org/programs/aces-toolkit/

Austin, B. (2019). Languages of the people forever: Bay Mills spins thread typing Ojibwa Communities together. In B. Shreve (Ed), *Language revitalization at tribal colleges and universities* (pp.122–126). Tribal College Press.

Bailey, S.J., *et al.* (2019). Rural Native and European American custodial grandparents: Stressors, Resources and Resilience. *Journal of Cross-Cultural Gerontology, 34*, 131–148. https://doi-org.ezproxy.lib.ndsu.nodak.edu/10.1007/s10823-019-09372-w

Baker-Demaray, T. B. (2005). Perceptions of elder abuse among Native American seniors, *Master's Thesis*, University of North Dakota.

Barry-Bratcher, S. (2019, May 8). The Native American Church: Ancient tradition and modern controversy. *Medium.* https://medium.com/@siobhanbarry/the-native-american-church-ancient-tradition-and-modern-controversy-ca2ed9bf879f

Bartlett, F. (2018). *The way of the Medicine Wheel. Integrating modern medicine and ancient wisdom to reshape the future of healthcare, healing, and happiness.* Medicine Wheel Wellness.TM

Bauman, B. L., *et al.* (2020, May 15). Vital Signs: Postpartum depressive symptoms and provider discussions about perinatal depression—United States, 2018. *Morbidity and Mortality Weekly Report, 69*(19), 575–581. http://dx.doi.org/10.15585/mmwr.mm6919a2

BBC develops Montana's first language app. (2013, May 15). *Tribal College: Journal of American Indian Higher Education, 24*(4). https://tribalcollegejournal.org/bcc-develops-montanas-first-native-language-app/#:~:text=The%20BCC%20Blackfeet%20Culture%20and,available%20to%20Apple%20iPhone%20users.

Becenti, A. and B. Gladue. (2018). Tribal Best Practices, A toolkit with best practices, research, and resources. *National Indian Child Welfare Association.* https://www.nicwa.org/wp-content/uploads/2019/01/Fam-Engagement-Toolkit-2018.pdf

Begay, C. and T. Zandamela. (2018, January). Sexual assault among Native American women living on reservations in the United States. *Ballard Brief*, Ballard Center. http://ballardbrief.org/uploaded/sexual-assault-on-native-american-reservations-in-the-us.pdf

Bell, J. (2017, December 6). Mass incarceration: A destroyer of people of color and their communities. *HUFFPOST*. https://www.huffpost.com/entry/mass-incarceration-a-dest_b_578854

Bell, R. A., *et al.* (2005). Prevalence and correlates of depressive symptoms among rural older African Americans, Native Americans and Whites with diabetes. *Diabetes Care, 28*(4), 823–829. https://doi.org/10.2337/diacare.28.4.823

Bernhard, A., *et al.* (2018). Association of trauma, posttraumatic stress disorder and conduct disorder: A systematic review and meta-analysis. *Neuroscience and Biobehavioral Reviews, 91*, 153–169. https://doi.org/10.1016/j.neubiorev.2016.12.019

Blackfeet Community College Develops Montana's First Language App. (2019). In B. Shreve (Ed), *Language revitalization at tribal colleges and universities* (pp. 138). Tribal College Press.

Blendon, R. and R. L. Menschel (2017). *Discrimination in America: Experiences and views of Native Americans*. NPR, Robert Wood Johnson, Harvard T.H. Chan School of Public Health. https://cdn1.sph.harvard.edu/wp-content/uploads/sites/21/2017/11/NPR-RWJF-HSPH-Discrimination-Native-Americans-Final-Report.pdf

Bowman, J. and T. Krueger. (2017, Fall). Helping Native Americans become homeowners through Section 184. *Rural Voices Meeting Native American Housing Needs, Housing Assistance Council, 21*(3), 1–39. Retrieved from: file:///F:/7-9-20/2020%20AI%20Rural%20Nursing%20Book%20Chapter/AI%20Housing/rv-fall-2017.pdf

Boyer, P. (2019). Native languages and Tribally controlled colleges: Giving voice to Native Nations. In B. Shreve (Ed), *Language revitalization at tribal colleges and universities* (pp. 94–100). Tribal College Press.

Brave Heart, M. Y. H. (1995). *The return to the sacred path: Healing from historical trauma and historical unresolved grief among the Lakota* (Doctoral dissertation). Smith College School for Social work, Massachusetts, USA. https://doi.org/10.1080/00377319809517532

Brave Heart, M. Y. H. (1999). Oyate Ptayela: Rebuilding the Lakota Nation through addressing historical trauma among Lakota parents. *Journal of Human Behavior and the Social Environment, 2*(1/2), 109–126. https://doi-org.ezproxy.lib.ndsu.nodak.edu/10.1300/J137v02n01_08

Brayboy, D. (2017). Two Spirits, one heart, five genders. Indian Country Today. https://indiancountrytoday.com/archive/two-spirits-one-heart-five-genders-9UH_xn-bfVEWQHWkjNn0rQQ

Brown, J.W. (1975). Native American contributions to science, engineering, and medicine. *Science, 189*(4195), 38–40. https://doi.org/10.1126/science.189.4196.38

Brown, J.E. and E. Cousins. (2001). *Teaching spirits Understanding Native religious traditions*. New York: Oxford University Press.

Bullock, A., *et al.* (2017). Obesity and overweight in American Indian and Alaskan Native children, 2006–2015. *AJPH Research, 107*, 1502–1507. https://doi.org/10.2015/AJPH.2017.303904

Bureau of Indian Education [BIE]. (2020). *Bureau Highlights. BIE Funding*. U.S. Department of Internal Affairs. BH-95. file:///D:/7-19-20/2020%20AI%20Rural%20 Nursing%20Book%20Chapter/fy2020_bib_bh095.pdf

Camera, L. (2015, November 6). Native American students left behind. Native youth post the worst achievement scores and lowest graduation rates of any student subgroup. *U.S.News*. https://www.usnews.com/news/articles/2015/11/06/native-american-students-left-behind

Campisteguy, M. E., J. Messenger Heilbronner, and C. Nakamura-Rybak. (2018, June). Reclaiming Native truth, research findings: Compilation of all research. *First Nations Development Institute and Echo Hawk Consulting*, Denver, Colorado. https://rnt.firstnations.org/wp-content/uploads/2018/06/FullFindingsReport-screen.pdf

Cancryn, A. (2020, March 20). Exclusive: Emergency coronavirus funds for American Indian health stalled. *Politico*. https://www.politico.com/news/2020/03/20/coronavirus-american-indian-health-138724

Carlisle, M. (2020, May 9). South Dakota gov. Demands tribes remove COVID-19 checkpoints. *Time*. https://time.com/5834749/south-dakota-governor-native-american-tribes-coronavirus/

Carson, L. D., *et al.* (2015). American Indian diabetes beliefs and practices: Anxiety, fear, and dread in pregnant women with diabetes. *Diabetes Spectrum, 28*, 4, 258–263. https://doi.org/10.2337/diaspect.28.4.258

Catwhipple. (2017, August 10). A brief history of American Indian boarding schools. *The Circle of News*. http://thecirclenews.org/news/education/a-brief-history-of-american-indian-boarding-schools/

Center for Disease Control and Prevention [CDC]. (2016a). Toolkits for families, classrooms, and communities. https://www.cdc.gov/diabetes/ndwp/eagle-books-toolkit/planning-guides/toolkit_for_families.html

Center for Disease Control and Prevention [CDC]. (2016b). Diabetes education in tribal schools DETS curriculum. Native Diabetes Wellness Program. https://www.cdc.gov/diabetes/ndwp/eagle-books-toolkit/planning-guides/dets_curriculum.html

Centers for Disease Control and Prevention [CDC]. (2017a). *Native Americans with diabetes, Better diabetes care can decrease kidney failure*. https://www.cdc.gov/vitalsigns/pdf/2017-01-vitalsigns.pdf

Centers for Disease Control and Prevention [CDC]. (2017b). *CDC and Indian country working together*. https://www.cdc.gov/chronicdisease/pdf/CDC-indian-country.pdf?s_cid=bb-NCCDPHP-OD-Indian_Working_Together

Centers for Disease Control and Prevention [CDC]. (2019a). *HIV and American Indians and Alaska Natives*. https://www.cdc.gov/hiv/group/racialethnic/aian/index.html

Center for Disease Control and Prevention [CDC]. (2019, July 9c). *American Indian/Alaska Native communities prevent Type 2 Diabetes*. Native Diabetes Wellness Program. https://www.cdc.gov/diabetes/ndwp/prevent-type-2/index.html

Center for Disease Control and Prevention [CDC]. (2019, July 9d). *American Indian/Alaskan Natives and Tobacco Use*. Smoking and Tobacco Use. https://www.cdc.gov/tobacco/disparities/american-indians/index.htm

Center for Disease Control and Prevention [CDC]. (2020). *National Center for Injury Prevention and Control.* Web-based Injury Statistics Query and Reporting System (WISQARS). https://www.cdc.gov/injury/wisqars/index.html

Center for Rural Health. (2019, November). *North Dakota health professional shortage areas.* University of North Dakota School of Medicine and Health Sciences. https://ruralhealth.und.edu/assets/2783-12669/nd-hpsa.pdf

Centers for Medicare and Medicaid Services [CMS]. (2016). *Emerging LTSS issues in Indian Country: Alzheimer's and Dementia.* Retrieved from: https://www.cms.gov/Outreach-and-Education/American-Indian-Alaska-Native/AIAN/LTSS-TA-Center/pdf/CMS-319_LR-BP-MiniTopics_Alzheimers-and-Dementia.pdf

Charbonneau-Dahlen, B. and K. Crow. (2016). A brief overview of the history of American Indian Nurses. *Journal of Cultural Diversity, 23*(3), 79–90.

Cheidi, J.M. (2019, July). *IHS needs to improve oversight of its hospitals' opioid prescribing and dispensing practices and consider centralizing its information technology functions.* A-18-17-111400. Department of Health and Human Services Office of Inspector General. https://oig.hhs.gov/oas/reports/region18/181711400.pdf

Child, B.J. (1995). *Boarding School Seasons, American Indian Families 1900–1940.* Lincoln: University of Nebraska Press.

Churchill, W. (2004). *Kill the Indian, Save the man: The genocidal impact of American Indian residential school.* San Francisco: City Lights Books.

Cochrane, E. and M. Walker. (2020, June 19). Tribes in a battle for their share of virus stimulus money. *New York Times.* https://www.nytimes.com/2020/06/19/us/politics/tribes-coronavirus-stimulus.html

Coleman-Jensen, A., *et al.* (2019, September). Household food security in the United States. A report summary from the Economic Research Service, United States Department of Agriculture. https://www.ers.usda.gov/webdocs/publications/94849/err270_summary.pdf?v=3775.2

Congress.gov. (2016). Public Law 114-157, 114th Congress. H.R.4238 — 114th Congress (2015–2016), H.R.4238 — To amend the Department of Energy Organization Act and the Local Public Works Capital Development and Investment Act of 1976 to modernize terms relating to minorities. https://congress.gov/114/plaws/publ157/PLAW-114publ157.pdf

Congress.gov. (2018, July 7). Public Law 115-196, 115th Congress. S.1091- 115th Congress (2017–2018). Supporting Grandparents Raising Grandchildren Act. *Congress.gov.* https://www.congress.gov/bill/115th-congress/senate-bill/1091

Congress.gov. (2020, March 11a). S.227 - Savanna's Act, 116th Congress (2019–2020). https://congress.gov/bill/116th-congress/senate-bill/227

Congress.gov. (2020, March 11b). S. 982 - Not Invisible Act of 2019. 116th Congress (2019–2020). https://www.congress.gov/116/bills/s982/BILLS-116s982es.pdf

Congress.gov. (2020, March 27c). H.R.748 – CARES Act. 116th Congress (2019–2020). https://www.congress.gov/bill/116th-congress/house-bill/748

Conner, T. W. and W. A. Taggart. (2013). Assessing the impact of Indian gaming on American Indian Nations: Is the house winning? *Social Science Quarterly*, 1–29. https://doi.org/10.1111/ssqu.12009

Connolly, M., *et al.* (2019). Identification in a time of invisibility for American Indians and Alaska Natives in the United States. *Statistical Journal of the IAOS*, 35, 71–89. https://doi.org/10.3233/SJ1-190495

Cox, D. W. and L. L. Jervis. (2018). American Indian perspectives, challenges, and approaches to elder abuse. In P. B. Teaster and J. E. Hall (Eds). *Elder Abuse and the public's health* (pp. 93–124). New York, NY: Springer Publishing Company.

Cross, S., A. Day, and P. Farrell. (2011). American Indian and Alaskan Native Grandfamilies: The impact on child development. In M. C. Sarche, P. Spicer, P. Farrell, and H. E. Fitzgerald (Eds.), *American Indian and Alaska Native children and mental health: Development, context, prevention, and treatment* (p. 43–62). Santa Barbara: ABC-CLIO, LLC.

Crotwell Pullis, B., *et al.* (2019). Veteran's health. In M. A. Nies and M. McEwen (Eds.), *Community/Public Health Nursing Promoting the Health of Populations* (p. 430–469).

Crowder, J., *et al.* (2019). Elder abuse in American Indian communities: An integrative review. *Journal of Forensic Nursing, 15*(4), 250–258. https://doi.org/10.1097/JFN.0000000000000259

Dastagir, A. E. (2019, June 22). Suicide rate for Native American women is up 139%. *USA Today*. https://www.usatoday.com/story/news/nation/2019/06/21/suicide-rate-native-american-indian-women-men-since-1999/1524007001/

DataUSA: Tribal Colleges. (2020). *Tribal Colleges*. https://datausa.io/profile/university/33

Dean, R. A. (2003). Native American humor: Implications for transcultural care. *Journal of Transcultural Nursing, 14*(1), 62–65.

Dewees, S. and B. Marks. (2017). *Twice Invisible: Understanding Rural Native American. Research Note #2*. First Nations Development Institute. https://usetinc.org/wp-content/uploads/bvenuti/WWS/2017/May%202017/May%208/Twice%20Invisible%20-%20Research%20Note.pdf

Dixon, P. and C. E. Trafzer (2006). The places of American Indian boarding schools in contemporary society. In, C.E. Trafzer, J.A., Keller, and L. Sisquoc (Eds.), *Boarding School Blues Revisiting American Indian Education Experiences*. pp. 232–242). Lincoln: University of Nebraska Press.

Dorgan, B. L., *et al.* (2014). *Attorney General's Advisory Committee on American Indian/Alaska Native Children Exposed to Violence: Ending violence so children can thrive*. Office of Juvenile Justice and Delinquency Prevention, Office of Justice Programs, U.S. Department of Justice. https://www.justice.gov/sites/default/files/defendingchildhood/pages/attachments/2014/11/18/finalaianreport.pdf

Dorgan., B. L. (2019). *The girl in the photograph. The true story of a Native American child, lost and found in America*. New York: Thomas Dunne Books.

Doshi, S., *et al.* (2020, June 18). *The COVID-19 response in Indian Country, A Federal failure*. Center for American Process. https://www.americanprogress.org/issues/green/reports/2020/06/18/486480/covid-19-response-indian-country/

Douglas, L. (2011, August 12). Open doors to safety NHCADSV. http://opendoorsnh.blogspot.com/2011/08/generational-poverty-and-trauma.html

Dwyer-Lindgen, L., *et al.* (2017). Inequalities in life expectancy among US counties, 1980 to 2014. Temporal Trends and Key Drivers. *JAMA Internal Medicine, 177*(7), 1003–1011. https://doi.org/10.1001/jamainternmed.2017.0918

Education Development Center (2020). American Indian and Alaska Native Populations. Suicide Prevention Resource Center. *SAMHSA*. http://www.sprc.org/scope/racial-ethnic-disparities/american-indian-alaska-native-populations

Edwards, F., L. Hedwig, and M. Espositó. (2019, August 20). Risk of being killed by police use of force in the United States by age, race-ethnicity, and sex. *PNAS, 116*(34), 16793–16798. https://www.pnas.org/content/pnas/116/34/16793.full.pdf

Ellis, R. and M. Schuman. (2019). Hundreds of cities, counties and Native American tribes filed federal lawsuit against Sackler family over opioid crisis. *CNN Health.* https://www.cnn.com/2019/03/24/health/sackler-lawsuit/index.html

Farley, M., *et al.* (2011). Garden of Truth: The Prostitution and Trafficking of Native Women in Minnesota. St. Paul, MN: William Mitchell College of Law. www.prostitutionresearch.com/pdfs/Garden_of_Truth_Final_Project_WEB.pdf.

FBI.gov. (2018). Full-time Law Enforcement Employees by State by State, Tribal, and Other Agencies, 2018 Crime in the United States. Retrieved from: https://ucr.fbi.gov/crime-in-the-u.s/2018/crime-in-the-u.s.-2018/tables/table-81/table-81.xls/view

Federal Communications Commission. (2019). 2019 Broadband Deployment Report (FCC19-44). https://www.fcc.gov/reports-research/reports/broadband-progress-reports/2019-broadband-deployment-report

Federal Register. (2020, May 8). Title 3 Proclamation 10026 of May 5, 2020 *Missing and Murdered American Indians and Alaskan Natives Awareness Day, 85*(90), 27633–27635. https://www.govinfo.gov/content/pkg/FR-2020-05-08/pdf/2020-10076.pdf

Findling, M. G., *et al.* (2019). Discrimination in the United States: Experiences of Native Americans. *Health Services Research, 54*, 1431–1441. http://doi.org/10.1111/1475-6773.13224

Foley, R., *et al.* (2020, May 27a). Social media toolkit, developing a social media strategy to combat the HIV epidemic in Indian Country. *National Indian Health Board.* https://www.nihb.org/docs/05272020/350753_NIHB%20Social%20Media%20Toolkit_May21_Proof2.pdf

Foley, R., *et al.* (2020, May 27b). A toolkit for advancing the uptake and use of PrEP in Indian Country. National Indian Health Board. https://www.nihb.org/docs/05272020/347597_NIHB%20PrEP%20Toolkit_Apr21a_Proof3.pdf

Fonseca, F. (2019, July 23). Hospitals are putting Native American Patients at risk for opioid abuse, audit says. *USA Today.* https://www.usatoday.com/story/news/nation/2019/07/22/opioid-crisis-hospitals-put-native-americans-risk-abuse-overdose-audit/1794592001/

Fonseca, F. (2020, January 27). Are missing and murdered Indigenous men being ignored? Movement to highlight missing Native women expands to males. https://indiancountrytoday.com/news/are-missing-and-murdered-indigenous-men-being-ignored-ziGPw9BtNEibjhG0wXZtDw

Four Arrows, and D. Narvaez. (2015). A more authentic baseline. In N. McCrary and

W. Ross (Eds.), Working for social justice inside and outside the classroom: A community of teachers, researchers, and activists (pp. 93–112). In series, Social justice across contexts in education (S. J. Miller and L. D. Burns, Eds.). New York, NY: Peter Lang.

Frosch, D. (2015). Federal panel reviewing Native American sentencing. *The Wall Street Journal*. https://www.wsj.com/articles/federal-panel-reviewing-native-american-sentencing-1429608601

Garroutte, E. M., *et al.* (2014). Religio-Spiritual participation in two American Indian populations. *Journal for the Scientific Study of Religion, 53*(1), 17–37.

Garrow, C., K. Cordero, and L. van Schilfgaarde. (2018). Tribal Healing to Wellness Courts: Case Management. West Hollywood, California: Tribal Law and Policy Institute. Retrieved from: http://www.wellnesscourts.org/files/HTWC%20Case%20Management.pdf

Gibbs, H. D., C. Pacheco, and H. Yeh. (2016). Accuracy of weight perception among American Indian tribal college students. *American Journal of Preventive Medicine, 51*(5), e139-e-244. http://doi.org/10.1016/j.amepre.2016.06.002

Gilio-Whitaker, D. (2019, July 7). 4 facts about Native American reservations. *ThoughtCo*. https://www.thoughtco.com/facts-about-native-american-reservations-4082436

Gill, J. H. (2002). *Native American Worldviews: An introduction* (*philosophy of religion*). New York: Humanity Books.

Golberg, J. (2017, February 2). Dealing with chronic illnesses and depression. *WebMD*. https://www.webmd.com/depression/guide/chronic-illnesses-depression#2

Gone, J. P., *et al.* (2019). The impact of historical trauma on health outcomes for indigenous population in the USA and Canada: A systematic review. *American Psychologist, 74*(1), 20–35. https://doi.org/10.1037/amp0000338

Gonzalez, V. M., *et al.* (2019). Endorsement of the "firewater myth" affects the use of the protective behavioral strategies among American Indian and Alaska Native students. *Addictive Behaviors, 93*, 79–85. https://doi.or/10.1016/j.addbeh.2019.01.027.

Gonzalez, V. M. and M. C. Skewes. (2018). Association of belief of the "Firewater Myth" with strategies to avoid alcohol consequences among American Indian and Alaska Native college students who drink. *Psychology of Addictive Behaviors, 12*(4), 401–409. http://dx.doi.org/10.1037/adb0000.367

Grayshield, L., *et al.* (2015). Understanding and healing historical trauma: The perspectives of Native American elders. *Journal of Mental Health Counseling, 37*(4), 295–307.

Greenfeld, L. A. and S. K. Smith. (1999). American Indians and crime. Bureau of Justice Statistics. U.S. Department of Justice, Office of Justice Programs. NCJ 173386. https://bjs.gov/content/pub/pdf/aic.pdf

Grover, K. (2014, Summer). Nation to Nation: Treaties between the United States and American Indian Nations. *Magazine of Smithsonian's National Museum of the American Indian, 15*(2). https://www.americanindianmagazine.org/story/nation-nation-treaties-between-united-states-and-american-indian-nations

Hardey, S., *et al.* (2020, January 2). *Risks of alcoholism among Native Americans*. American Addiction Centers. https://americanaddictioncenters.org/alcoholism-treatment/native-americans

Harris, M. (2019, September 12). 2018 Indian Gaming Revenues of $33.7 Billon Show a 4.1% Increase. https://www.nigc.gov/news/detail/2018-indian-gaming-revenues-of-33.7-billion-show-a-4.1-increase

Harvard University. (2020). First encounters: Native Americans and Christians. Historical Perspectives, *The Pluralism Project*. https://pluralism.org/files/pluralism/files/first_encounters-_native_americans_and_christians_0.pdf

Harvey, M. (2020). *Fatal encounters between Native Americans and the police*. CSWEP Summer 2019 Economics Fellow. The Center for Indian Country Development. https://www.minneapolisfed.org/~/media/assets/articles/2020/fatal-encounters-between-native-americans-and-the-police/fatal-encounters-between-native-americans-and-the-police_march-2020.pdf?la=en

Health Resources and Services Administration [HRSA]. (2020). Nursing workforce diversity (NWD) program. https://www.hrsa.gov/grants/find-funding/hrsa-17-063

Hemmilä, A. (2016). Ancestors of two-spirits: Historical depictions of Native North American gender-crossing women through critical discourse analysis. *Journal of Lesbian Studies, 20*(3–4), 408–426. https://doi.org/10.1080/10894160.2016.1151281

Heron, M. (2019, June 24). Deaths: Leading causes for 2017. National Vital Statistics Reports, *U.S. Department of Health and Human Services. 68*(6), 1–77. https://www.cdc.gov/nchs/data/nvsr/nvsr68/nvsr68_06-508.pdf

Heuer, L. (Executive Producer), and C. Muggerud. (Executive Producer), *Essence of Healing: The Journey of American Indian Nurses*. (2016). United States: KAT COMMUNICATONS.

Heuer, L., *et al.* (2017). *Youth education and employment survey results, hope project: Four Winds*, Fort Totten, North Dakota, North Dakota State University. Research at CCCC. American Indian Youth Hope for Education and Employment. http://www.littlehoop.edu/research.html

Hilleary, C. (2019, September 30). Are missing and murdered Indigenous men in the U.S. being ignored? https://www.voanews.com/usa/are-missing-and-murdered-indigenous-men-us-being-ignored

Hodge, D. R. and R. J. Wolosin. (2015). Addressing the spiritual needs of American Indians: Predictors of satisfaction, *Social Work in Health Care, 54*(2), 118–133. http://doi.org.10.1080/00981389.2014.971213

Hoss, A. (2019). Federal Indian law as a structural determinant of health. *Journal of Law, Medicine, and Ethics, 47*(S4), 3–42. https://doi.org.10.1177/1073110519898041

Housing Assistance Council [HAC]. (2010). Native American Lands. Retrieved from: http://ruralhome.org/storage/documents/ts2010/ts-report/ts10_native_lands.pdf

Housing Assistance Council [HAC]. (2013). Housing on Native American Lands, *Rural Research Report*. 1–11. http://www.ruralhome.org/storage/documents/rpts_pubs/ts10_native_lands.pdf

Hudson, M. F., *et al.* (1998). Elder abuse: Two Native American views. *The Gerontologist, 38*(5), 538–548. https://doi-org.ezproxy.lib.ndsu.nodak.edu/10.1093/geront/38.5.538

Indian Country Media Network [ICTMN] Staff. (2014). *Muscogee (Creek) Nation Launches App to Help Preserve Language*. The University of Arizona Native Nations Institute. https://nnigovernance.arizona.edu/muscogee-creek-nation-launches-app-help-preserve-language

Indian Health Service [HIS]. (n.d.a). *HIV/AIDS training kit and guide*. HIV/AIDS https://www.ihs.gov/hivaids/trainingkit/

Indian Health Service. [IHS]. (n.d.b) *Resources for providers*. Suicide Prevention and Care. https://www.ihs.gov/suicideprevention/providerresources/

Indian Health Service [IHS]. (n.d.c). *Healthy Heart Toolkit*. SDPI Healthy Heart Project Toolkit, SDPI Toolkits. https://www.ihs.gov/sdpi/sdpi-toolkits/healthy-heart-program-toolkit/

Indian Health Service [IHS]. (n.d.d). *CME/CE online education*. Training. Division of Diabetes Treatment and Prevention (DDTP). https://www.ihs.gov/diabetes/training/cmece-online-edu/

Indian Health Service [IHS]. (n.d.e). *Tribal Self-Governance Program, What Is the Tribal Self-Governance Program*? Laws and Regulations. https://www.ihs.gov/SelfGovernance/aboutus/

Indian Health Service [IHS]. (n.d.f). *Diabetes Prevention Program Toolkit*. SDPI Toolkits. Special Diabetes Program for Indians (SDPI). https://www.ihs.gov/sdpi/sdpi-toolkits/diabetes-prevention-program-toolkit/

Indian Health Service [IHS]. (n.d.g). Job opportunities. https://www.ihs.gov/nursing/jobops/

Indian Health Service [IHS]. (n.d.h). Student opportunities. https://www.ihs.gov/nursing/studentops/

Indian Health Service [IHS]. (2017). *A quick look*. https://www.ihs.gov/sites/newsroom/themes/responsive2017/display_objects/documents/factsheets/QuickLook.pdf

Indian Health Service [IHS]. (2019, October). Disparities. https://www.ihs.gov/newsroom/factsheets/ihsprofile/

Indian Health Service [IHS]. (2020, April). *IHS Profile, Based on 2015–2019 data*. https://www.ihs.gov/newsroom/factsheets/ihsprofile/

Indian Health Service Special Diabetes Program for Indians [IHS SDPI]. (2020, June). *Special Diabetes Program for Indians 2020 Grant Programs*. Indian Health Service, Division of Diabetes Treatment and Prevention. https://www.ihs.gov/sites/sdpi/themes/responsive2017/display_objects/documents/factsheets/FactSheet_SDPI2020byState_508c.pdf

Indigenous Corporate Training, Inc. (2016, January 26). Indigenous Peoples Worldviews vs. Western Worldviews. Working Effectively with Indigenous Peoples®. https://www.ictinc.ca/blog/indigenous-peoples-worldviews-vs-western-worldviews

Institute of Medicine. (2011). *The future of nursing: Leading change, advancing health*. Washington, DC: The National Academies Press. https://doi.org/10.17226/12956

Jacobs, S., W. Thomas, and S. Lang. (1997). *Two-Spirited People Native American Gender Identity*. Chicago, Illinois: University of Illinois.

Jervis, L. L., *et al.* (2014). Assessment of elder mistreatment in two American Indian Samples: Psychometric characteristics of the HS-EAST and the Native Elder life-financial exploitation and neglect measures. *Journal of Applied Gerontology, 33*(3), 336–356. https://doi.org/10.1177/0733464812470748

Jervis, L. L., W. Sconzert-Hall, W. and the Shielding American Indian Elders Project Team (2017). The conceptualization of mistreatment by older American Indians, *Journal of Elder Abuse and Neglect, 29*(1), 43–58. https://doi.org/10.1080/08946566.2016.1249816

Jocks, C. (2019, May 28). *Native American religions*. Encyclopedia Britannica, Inc. https://www.britannica.com/topic/Native-American-religion

John, S. (2018). From warrior to soldier? Lakota Veterans on military valor. In J. S. Wendt (Eds.), *Warring over Valor: How Race and Gender Shaped American Military Heroism and Twenty-First Centuries*. New Brunswick: Rutgers University Press.

Jump, L. (2018, August 6). What is cultural abuse? *Indian Country Today*. https://indiancountrytoday.com/opinion/what-is-cultural-abuse-J_Nwyq6xs0iTzb5qwfWuow

Kakol, M., D. Upson, and A. Sood. (2020). Susceptibility of Southwestern American Indian tribes to Coronavirus Disease 2019 (COVID-19). *The Journal of Rural Health*, 1–3. https://doi.org/10.1111/jrh.12451

Kalbfleisch, P. J. (2009). Effective health communication in Native populations in North America. *Journal of Language and Social Psychology, 28*(2), 258–173.

Kaliszewski, M. (2020, February 19). *Alcohol and drug abuse among Native Americans*. American Addictions Centers. https://americanaddictioncenters.org/rehab-guide/addiction-statistics/native-americans

Keep It Sacred. (2015a). *Traditional Tobacco*. National Native Network. OneUpWeb. https://keepitsacred.itcmi.org/tobacco-and-tradition/traditional-tobacco-use/

Keep It Sacred. (2015b). *Traditional vs Commercial Tobacco*. National Native Network. OneUpWeb. http://keepitsacred.itcmi.org/tobacco-and-tradition/traditional-v-commercial/

Kenny, M. K. and G. K. Singh. (2016). Adverse childhood experiences among American Indian/Alaskan Native children: The 2011–2012 National Survey of Children's Health, *Scientifica*, 14 pages. DOI:/10.1155/2016/7424239.

Keoke, E. D. and K. M. Porterfield. (2003). *American Indian contributions to the world: 15,000 years of inventions and innovations*. New York: Checkmark Books.

Kiger, P. J. (2019, November 18). 10 Native American inventions commonly used today. *History*. https://www.history.com/news/native-american-inventions

Kurup, N. (2020, July 12). American spirit: Alcohol abuse in US highest among Native Americans but there is hope with spiritual treatment. *Meaww*. https://meaww.com/american-spirit-native-americans-alcohol-substance-abuse-spiritual-treatments-firwater-myth-culture

Lang, S. (2016). Native American men-women, lesbians, two-spirits: Contemporary and historical perspectives. *Journal of Lesbian Studies, 20*(3–4), 299–323. https://doi-org.ezproxy.lib.ndsu.nodak.edu/10.1080/10894160.2016.1148966

Lajimodiere, D. K. (2020, July 15). Native American boarding schools. *MN OPEDIA*. https://www.mnopedia.org/native-american-boarding-schools

Leavitt, R. A., *et al.* (2018, March 18). Suicides among American Indian/Alaska Natives—National violent death report system 18 states, 2003–2014. *Morbidity and Mortality Weekly Report, 67*(18), 237–242. http://dx.doi.org/10.15585/mmwr.mm6708a1

Lee, T. H. (2014). 7 most popular Native American languages in U.S. *Indian Country Today.* https://indiancountrytoday.com/archive/7-most-popular-native-american-languages-in-u-s-F8_vHNtMYEGWyW2Pm001RA

Liebler, C. and M. Zacher. (2013). American Indians without Tribes in the 21st Century. *Ethnic and Racial Studies*, 36(11), 1910–1934. https://doi.org/10/1080/01419870.2012.692800

Lindquist, C. (2019). American Indian voice: A national perspective. In *Overcoming Educational Racism in the Community College: Creating Pathways to Success for Minority and Impoverished Student Populations*, Angela Long (Ed.). Virginia: Stylus, pp. 127–140.

Linton, K. and B. Kim. (2014). Traumatic brain injury as a result of violence in Native American and Black communities spanning from childhood to other adulthood. *Brain Injury, 28*(8), 1076–1081. https://doi.org/10.3109/02699052.2014.901558

Litton, L.J. and V. Ybanez. (2017). *Reclaiming What is Sacred: Addressing Harm to Indigenous Elders and Developing a Tribal Response to Abuse in Later Life*. National Clearinghouse on Abuse in Later Life (NCALL). https://safehousingpartnerships.org/sites/default/files/2017-01/TLS-FINAL.pdf

Lowe, J. and L. A. Nichols. (2014). Utilisation of a Native American nursing conceptual framework: Implications for practice and research. *The Australian Journal of Advanced Nursing. 31*(2), 13–22. https://www.ajan.com.au/archive/Vol31/Issue2/2Lowe.pdf

Lowe, J. and R. Struthers. (2004). A conceptual framework of nursing in Native American culture. *Journal of Nursing Scholarship, 33*(3), https://doi.org/10.1111.j.1547-5069.2001.00279.x

Luna-Firebaugh, E. (2007). *Tribal policing, Asserting sovereignty, seeking justice*. Tucson: The University of Arizona Press.

Mack, K. A. C. M. Jones, and M. F. Balesteros. (2017, Summer). Illicit drug use, illicit drug use disorders, and drug overdose deaths in metropolitan and nonmetropolitan areas—United States. *MMWR Surveillance, 66*(No. SS-19), 1–12. http://dx.doi.org/10.15585/mmwr.ss6619a1external icon

Marcelin, J. R., *et al.* (2019). The impact of unconscious bias in healthcare: How to recognize and mitigate it. *The Journal of Infectious Disease, 229*(Suppl 2), S62–S73. https://doi.org/10.1093/infdis/jiz214

Mala Lindquist, C. (2016). Very good medicine: Indigenous humor and language. Tribal College of *Journal of American Indian Higher Education.*

Mayeda, E. R., *et al.* (2016). Inequalities in dementia incidence between six racial and ethnic groups over 14 years. *Alzheimer's and Dementia, 12*(3), 2016–224. https://doi.org/10.1016/j.jalz.2015.12.007

McCarty, T. L., S. E. Nicholas, and L. T. Wyman. (2015). 50(0) years out and counting: Native American Language education the four Rs. *International Multilingual Research Journal, 9*(4), 227–252. https://doi.org/10.1080/19313152.2015.1091267

McCoy, M. (2004). *Trailblazing Indian education.* The Native American Rights Fund Indian Education Legal Support Project. http://www.narf.org/wordpress/wp-content/uploads/2015/01/purple.pdf

McFarland, J., *et al.* (2019a). *Trends in High School Dropout and Completion Rates in the United States: 2019* (NCES 2020-117). U.S. Department of Education. Washington, DC: National Center for Education Statistics. https://nces.ed.gov/pubs2020/2020117.pdf

McFarland, J., *et al.* (2019b). *The Condition of Education 2019* (NCES 2019-144). U.S. Department of Education. Washington, DC: National Center for Education Statistics. https://nces.ed.gov/pubs2019/2019144.pdf

Meister Economic Consulting. (2020, June 2). *Coronavirus impact on tribal gaming.* http://www.meistereconomics.com/coronavirus-impact-on-tribal-gaming

Mental Health technology Transfer Center Network (MHTTC). (2020). *Mental Health Webinar Series*. American Indian and Alaska Native MHTTC Navigation. https://mhttcnetwork.org/centers/national-american-indian-and-alaska-native-mhttc/webinars

Mineo, L. (2020, May 8). For Native Americans, the COVID-19 is "the worst of both worlds at the same time." *The Harvard Gazette*. https://news.harvard.edu/gazette/story/2020/05/the-impact-of-covid-19-on-native-american-communities/

Minnesota Department of Employment and Economic Development [MN DEED] (2019). *Broadband Grant Program.* 2019 Grantees. https://mn.gov/deed/programs-services/broadband/grant-program/

Minton, T. D. and M. Cowhig. (2017). *Jails in Indian Country, 2016*. NCJ 250981. Bureau of Justice Statistics, U.S. Department of Justice. Retrieved from: https://www.bjs.gov/content/pub/pdf/jic16.pdf

Mitchell-Brown, F. (2020). Enhancing cultural competency: A phenomenological study. *Journal of Nursing Education, 59*(9), 485–492. https://doi.org/10.3928/01484834-20200817-02

Moerman, D. E. (2009). *Native American medicinal plants: An ethnobotanical dictionary*. Timber Press.

Moss, M. P. (2016). *American Indian health and nursing*. New York: Springer Publishing Company.

Muhammad, D. A., R. Tec, and K. Ramirez. (2019, November 18). Racial Wealth Snapshot: American Indians/Native Americans. National Community Reinvestment Coalition. https://ncrc.org/racial-wealth-snapshot-american-indians-native-americans/

Murder Accountability Project. (2019, March 14). *Half of Native American homicides not reported to FBI.* http://www.murderdata.org/2019/03/half-of-native-american-homicides-are.html

Muscogee (Creek) Nation. (2016). The Muscogee (Creek) Nation. Culture and History. https://www.mcn-nsn.gov/services/mvskoke-language-program/

Mwaniki, A. (2018, March 26). *US Counties with the Shortest Life Expectancy*. WorldAtlas, https://www.worldatlas.com/articles/us-counties-with-the-shortest-life-expectancy.html

Nagle, R. (2020, April 24). Native Americans being left out of US coronavirus data and labeled as "other." *The Guardian*, https://www.theguardian.com/us-news/2020/apr/24/us-native-americans-left-out-coronavirus-data

National Native American Boarding School Healing Coalition. (n.d.). US Indian

Boarding School History. https://boardingschoolhealing.org/education/us-indian-boarding-school-history/

National Congress of American Indians Policy Research Center. (2016, Spring). Human and sexual trafficking: Trends and responses across Indian Country. *Tribal Insights Brief*, NCAI Policy Research Center. http://www.ncai.org/policy-research-center/research-data/prc-publications/TraffickingBrief.pdf

National Center for Health Statistics [NCHS]. (2018a). Table A-8a. Age-adjusted percentages (with standard errors) of feelings of nervousness, feelings of restlessness, and serious psychological distress among adults aged 18 and over, by selected characteristics: United States, 2018. Summary Health Statistics: National Health Interview, 2018. U.S. Department of Health and Human Services, Centers for Disease Control and Prevention. https://ftp.cdc.gov/pub/Health_Statistics/NCHS/NHIS/SHS/2018_SHS_Table_A-8.pdf

National Center for Health Statistics [NCHS]. (2018b). Table A-7a. Age-adjusted percentages of feelings of sadness, hopelessness, worthlessness, and that everything is an effort among adults aged 18 and over, by selected characteristics: United States, 2018. Summary Health Statistics: National Health Interview, 2018. U.S. Department of Health and Human Services, Centers for Disease Control and Prevention. https://ftp.cdc.gov/pub/Health_Statistics/NCHS/NHIS/SHS/2018_SHS_Table_A-7.pdf

National Center for Health Statistics [NCHS]. (2018c). Table A-4a. Age-adjusted percentages of selected diseases and conditions among adults aged 18 and over, by selected characteristics: United States, 2018. Summary Health Statistics: National Health Interview, 2018. U.S. Department of Health and Human Services, Centers for Disease Control and Prevention. https://ftp.cdc.gov/pub/Health_Statistics/NCHS/NHIS/SHS/2018_SHS_Table_A-4.pdf

National Center for Health Statistics [NCHS]. (2019). Table 33. Use of mammography among women aged 40 and over, by selected characteristics: United States, selected years 1987–2015. *Health, United States*, 2018. Hyattsville, MD. https://www.cdc.gov/nchs/data/hus/hus18.pdfmer

National Center for Veterans Analysis and Statistics [NCVAS]. (2020, May). American Indian and Alaskan Native Veterans: 2017. https://www.va.gov/vetdata/docs/SpecialReports/AIAN.pdf

National Congress of American Indians [NCAI]. (2019). Data disaggregation, the Asterisk Nation. NCAI Policy Research Center. http://www.ncai.org/policy-research-center/research-data/data

National Congress of American Indians [NCAI]. (2020, February a). Tribal Nations and United States, An introduction. http://www.ncai.org/tribalnations/introduction/Indian_Country_101_Updated_February_2019.pdf

National Congress of American Indians [NCAI]. (2020, February b). Tribal jurisdiction: Civil/criminal. Tribal Nations and the United States, An introduction (p. 29). http://www.ncai.org/tribalnations/introduction/Indian_Country_101_Updated_February_2019.pdf

National Congress of American Indians Policy Research Center. (2016, Spring). Human and sex trafficking: Trends and responses across Indian Country. *Tribal Insights*

Brief. https://www.ncai.org/policy-research-center/research-data/prc-publications/TraffickingBrief.pdf

National Crime Information Centers (NCIC). (2020, January). 2018 National Crime Information Center's missing person and unidentified person statistics. A compilation of statistics from the National Crime Information Center's (NCIC's) missing person and unidentified person statistics pursuant to the Requirements of the Crime Act of 1990, Pub. L. No. 101–647, 104 Stat. 4789. https://www.fbi.gov/file-repository/2018-ncic-missing-person-and-unidentified-person-statistics.pdf/view

National Indian Child Welfare Association [NICWA]. (2018). Setting the record straight: The Indian Child Welfare Act, Fact Sheet. A publication of the National Indian Child Welfare Association. https://www.nicwa.org/wp-content/uploads/2018/10/Setting-the-Record-Straight-2018.pdf

National Indian Council on Aging [NICA]. (2013). *The Savvy Caregiver n Indian Country Trainer's Manual.* National Minority Aging Organization Technical Assistance Center for the Development of Dementia Care Resources for American Indians and Alaska Natives. https://www.nicoa.org/elder-resources/savvy-caregiver/

National Indian Country Clearinghouse Sexual Assault [NICCSA]. (2020). Victims with unique considerations. https://www.niccsa.org/victims-w-unique-consideration/

National Indian Gaming Commission [NIGC]. (2015). Indian Gaming Regulatory Act. https://www.nigc.gov/general-counsel/indian-gaming-regulatory-act

National Indian Health Board [NIHB]. (2020). Tribal opioid response resource toolkit. https://www.nihb.org/behavioral_health/tribal_opioid_response_resources.php

National Indigenous Women's Resource Center [NIWRC]. (2020). *Resources.* https://www.niwrc.org/resources

National Indigenous Women's Resource Center [NIWRC]. (2018, October 16). Tribal community response when a woman is missing: A toolkit for action. https://www.niwrc.org/resources/tribal-community-response-when-woman-missing-toolkit-action

National Indigenous Women's Resource Center [NIWRC]. (2020). Special collection: Missing and murdered Indigenous women and girls. https://www.niwrc.org/resources/special-collection-missing-murdered-indigenous-women-girls

National Institute of Mental Health [NIMH]. (2019). Major depression definitions. Statistics. Mental Health Information. https://www.nimh.nih.gov/health/statistics/major-depression.shtml#part_155032

Native American Program of Legal and Services of Oregon [NAPLSO], The Indigenous Ways of Knowing Program at Lewis and Clark College, Basic Rights Oregon and the Western States Center. (2013). *Tribal Equity Toolkit 2.0: Tribal Resolutions and Codes to Support Two Spirit and LGBT Justice in Indian Country.* https://graduate.lclark.edu/live/files/15810-tribal-equity-toolkit-20

Notah, T. (2017, May 24). Navajo Nation school focuses on language revitalization. *Indian Country Today.* https://indiancountrytoday.com/archive/navajo-nation-school-focuses-on-language-revitalization-VP5ms8NNJEiIY_Oo8cq9aA

NWEA. (2018, August). Bureau of Indian education report on student achievement and growth: 2014–2015 to 2016–2017. *NWEA Research.* https://www.bie.edu/sites/default/files/documents/idc2-089257.pdf

Oberdorfer, E., J. Anderson, and L. C. D. Rhea. (2013). Conducting homeless counts on Native American lands: A toolkit. Housing Assistance Council and the Corporation for Supportive Housing. http://www.ruralhome.org/storage/documents/rpts_pubs/na_homeless_count_toolkit.pdf

Office of Minority Health [OMH]. (2018, March 28). *Profile: American Indian/Alaskan Native*. U.S. Department of Health and Human Services. https://www.minorityhealth.hhs.gov/omh/browse.aspx?lvl=3andlvlid=62

Ortiz, E. (2020, July 30). Lack of awareness, data hinders cases of missing and murdered Native American women, study finds. A new report documents more than 2,300 missing Native American Women and girls in the U.S., underscoring the reasons behind the lack of awareness and scrutiny in these cases. U.S. News. https://www.nbcnews.com/news/us-news/lack-awareness-data-hinders-cases-missing-murdered-native-american-women-n1235233

Payne, R. K. (2019). A framework for understanding poverty—A cognitive approach (6th Ed.), Highlands, Texas: aha! Process, Inc.

Pettit, K. L. S., *et al.* (2014). Continuity and Change: Demographic, Socioeconomic, and Housing Conditions of American Indians and Alaska Natives. *U.S. Department of Housing and Urban Development.* https://www.huduser.gov/portal/publications/pdf/housing_conditions.pdf

Pfankuch, B. (2020, May 24). Beyond the checkpoints: How a S.D. Native American tribe is protecting its people from COVID-19. *Keloland Media Group.* https://www.keloland.com/news/healthbeat/coronavirus/beyond-the-checkpoints-how-a-s-d-native-american-tribe-is-protecting-its-people-from-covid-19/

Pindus, N., *et al.* (2017). Housing needs of American Indians and Alaskan Natives in tribal areas: A report from the assessment of American Indian, Alaska Native, and Native Hawaiian housing needs. *U.S. Department of Housing and Urban Development*, Office of Policy Development and Research. https://www.huduser.gov/portal/sites/default/files/pdf/HNAIHousingNeeds.pdf

Pinto, A. (2020, July 15). American Spirit: Why school dropout rates among Native American students are higher than any other ethnic group. Meww. https://meaww.com/american-spirit-native-american-school-drop-out-rates-high-than-any-ethnic-group-education-issues

Portman, T. A. A. and M. T. Garrett. (2006). Native American healing traditions. *International Journal of Disability, Development and Education, 53*(4), 453–469.

Probst, J. C., *et al.* (2004). Person and place: The compounding effects of race/ethnicity and rurality on health. *American Journal of Public Health, 94*(10), 1695–1703. https://doi-org/10.1080/10349120601008647

Randall, L. L. and B. Muneta (2000). Spirituality among American Indians in health and disease: Culturally appropriate recommendations for health care providers. *Home Health Care Management Practice, 12*(5), 25–30.

Rodriquez-Lonebear, D., *et al.* (2020). American Indian reservations and COVID-19 correlates of early infection rates in the pandemic. *Journal of Pub-*

lic Health Management and Practice, 26(4), 371–377. https://doi-org/10.1097/PHH.0000000000001206

Rosay, A. B. (2016, June). Violence against American Indian and Alaska Native women and men. NCJ Number: 249822. *NIJ Journal 277*, 38–45. https://www.ncjrs.gov/pdffiles1/nij/249822.pdf

Rural Home Organization [RHO]. (2010). Native American land. http://ruralhome.org/storage/documents/ts2010/ts-report/ts10_native_lands.pdf

Saenz, M. (2020). Federal and state recognized tribes. National Conference of State Legislatures. https://www.ncsl.org/research/state-tribal-institute/list-of-federal-and-state-recognized-tribes.aspx

Salazar, M. (2016). State Recognition of American Indian Tribes. National Conference of State Legislatures. https://www.ncsl.org/research/state-tribal-institute/state-recognition-of-american-indian-tribes.aspx

SAMHSA. (2019, August). Classified as Needing Substance Use Treatment and Receipt of Substance Use. Treatment at a Specialty Facility in Past Year among Persons Aged 12 or Older, by Demographic Characteristics: Numbers in Thousands and Percentages, 2017 and 2018. Table 5.38A, 190415. *Center for Behavioral Health Statistics and Quality. Results from the 2018 National Survey on Drug Use and Health: Detailed Tables. Prevalence Estimates, Standard Errors, P Values, and Sample Sizes.* https://www.samhsa.gov/data/report/2018-nsduh-detailed-tables

Sandefur, G. D. (1989). American Indian reservations: The first underclass area? *Focus 12* (Summer, No. 1), 37–41. https://www.irp.wisc.edu/publications/focus/pdfs/foc121f.pdf

Sanders, D., and M. Van Alstine Makomenaw. (2018). Tribal College Pathways. In Brayboy B. (Author) and Minthorn R. and Shotton H. (Eds.), *Reclaiming Indigenous Research in Higher Education* (pp. 107–123). London: Rutgers University Press.

Sawyer, W. (2019, December 19). Youth confinement: The whole pie 2019. Prison Policy Initiative. https://www.prisonpolicy.org/reports/youth2019.html

Schilling, V. (2017, July 13). 10 Native interventions and innovations that changed the world. *Indian Country Today,* https://indiancountrytoday.com/archive/10-native-inventions-and-innovations-that-changed-the-world-M0ZwDx1Ku0mQvn4Jn0KP4Q

Schrank, A. (2016, February 26). Today's remaining Native American boarding schools are a far cry from history. *Wyoming Public Media.* https://www.wyomingpublicmedia.org/post/todays-remaining-native-american-boarding-schools-are-far-cry-their-history#stream/0

Schultz, M. and M. Kroeger. (1996). *Contrasting Values.* Teaching and learning with Native Americans: A handbook for non-Native American adult educators. Four Winds Walk in Balance on Mother Earth Curriculum Guide for the Arizona Adult Literacy and Technology Resource Center, Inc. Western/Pacific LINCS. http://literacynet.org/lp/namericans/

Selden, D. and M. Martens. (2008). Basic Indian Law Research Tips—Part 1: Federal Indian Law. https://www.narf.org/nill/resources/federal_indian_law_research_guide.pdf

Sequist, T. D., T. Cullen, and K. J. Acton. (2011). Indian Health Service innovations have helped reduce health disparities affection American Indian and Alaskan Native people. *Health Affairs, 30*(10). https://doi.org/10.1377/hlthaff.2011.0630

Siegel, R., K. D. Miller, and A. Jemal. (2019). Cancer statistics, 2019. *CA Cancer J Clin, 69*, 7–34. http://doi.org/10.3322/caac.21551

Silverman, H. *et al.* (2020). Navajo Nation surpasses New York state for the highest COVID-19 infection rate in the US. CNN. https://www.cnn.com/2020/05/18/us/navajo-nation-infection-rate-trnd/index.html

Sitting Bull College. (2020). Native American Studies/Lakota Dakota Language. https://sittingbull.edu/2101-2/

Skewes, M. C. and A. W. Blume. (2019). Understanding the link between racial trauma and substance use among American Indians. *American Psychology, 74*(1), 88–100. http://doi.org/10.1037/amp0000331

Slate, C. (2019). Finding a place for Navajo: English must be restricted if Native language is to survive. In B. Shreve (Ed), *Language revitalization at tribal colleges and universities* (pp. 38–45). Tribal College Press.

Slattery, M. L., *et al.* (2010). Associations among body mass index, waist circumference, and health indicators in American Indian and Alaska Native Adults. *American Journal of Health Promotion, 24*(4), 246–253. https://doi-org/10.4278/ajhp.080528-QUAN-72

Slobig, Z., Martínez, *et al.* and C. Matter. (2017, September). *In a good way: Indigenous commercial tobacco control practices.* Clear Way Minnesota, Truth Initiative and Blue Cross and Blue Shield of Minnesota. https://docs.google.com/viewerng/viewer?url=http%3A//keepitsacred.itcmi.org/wp-content/uploads/sites/5/2015/02/InAGoodWay_finalWeb-1.pdf&hl=en

Smith, C. (2017, January 10). Native American history: A tale of medicine. *The Differential*, The University of Arizona College of Medicine—Phoenix Student Publication. http://www.thedifferentialdx.com/native-american-history-a-tale-of-medicine/

Special Subcommittee on Indian Education. (1969). *Indian education: A national tragedy—A national challenge*. Committee on Labor and Public Welfare United States Senate. Report No. 91-501. (ED034625) ERIC. https://files.eric.ed.gov/fulltext/ED034625.pdf

Spotted Eagle, F., *et al.* (2019, November). Zuya Wicayuonihan honoring warrior women. A study on missing and murdered Indigenous women and girls in states impacted by the Keystone XL pipeline. https://2a840442-f49a-45b0-b1a1-7531a7cd3d30.filesusr.com/ugd/6b33f7_27835308ecc84e5aae8ffbdb7f20403c.pdf

Springer, T. J. (2020, April 16). Highlights of the CARES Act—Tribal Governments, *News and Resources, Quarles and Brady*, LLP. https://www.quarles.com/publications/highlights-of-the-cares-act-tribal-governments/

Statista Research Department. (2020, January 16). Child abuse rates in the United States in 2018, by race/ethnicity of the victim. https://www.statista.com/statistics/254857/child-abuse-rate-in-the-us-by-race-ethnicity/

Strong Heart Study. (2017). *About strong heart study.* Center for American Indian health Research—College of Public Health, University of Oklahoma Health Sciences Center. https://strongheartstudy.org/About

StrongHearts Native Helpline. (2020). Resources. https://www.strongheartshelpline.org/resources

Subia BigFoot, K. Lamb, and M. Delmar. (2018, November). Honoring children: Treating trauma and adverse childhood experiences in American Indian and Alaska Native communities, Culturally enhanced treatment for ACEs. *Adult Development and Aging News*, American Psychological Association. https://www.apa.org/pi/families/resources/newsletter/2018/11/native-american-trauma

Sullivan, L. (2003). *Native religions and cultures of North America: Anthropology of the scared.* Bloomsbury.

Sweeney, T. (2020, January 30). Indian entities recognized by and eligible to receive services from the United States Bureau of Indian Affairs. *Department of Interior, 85*(20). 5462–5467. https://www.govinfo.gov/content/pkg/FR-2020-01-30/pdf/2020-01707.pdf

Szalavitz, M. (2015, October 2). No, Native Americans aren't genetically more susceptible to alcoholism. *Time to retire the "firewater" fairytale*. The Verge. https://www.theverge.com/2015/10/2/9428659/firewater-racist-myth-alcoholism-native-americans

Taylor, R. (2019, September 23). 6 Native leaders on what it would look like if the US kept its promises. *Vox*. https://www.vox.com/first-person/2019/9/23/20872713/native-american-indian-treaties

Taylor, C.F., and W. C. Sturtevant. (1992). The Native Americans the Indigenous people of North America. Smithmark Publishing, Inc.

The White House. (2019, November 26). President Donald J. Trump is committed to supporting and protecting Native American women and children across the country. Law and Justice. https://www.whitehouse.gov/briefings-statements/president-donald-j-trump-committed-supporting-protecting-native-american-women-children-across-country/

Thornton, R. (1997). Tribal membership requirements and the demography of "old" and "new" Native Americans. *Population Research and Policy Review, 16*, 33–42.

Tighe, S. (2014). "Of course we are crazy": Discrimination of Native American Indians through criminal justice. *Justice Policy Journal, 11*(1), 1–38. http://www.cjcj.org/uploads/cjcj/documents/tighe_discrimination_final_formatted.pdf

Trafzer, C. E., J. A. Keller, and L. Sisquoc. (2006). Introduction. Origin and development of the American Indian Boarding School Systems. In. C. E. Trafzer, J. A., Keller, and L. Sisquoc (Eds.), *Boarding School Blues Revisiting American Indian Education Experiences*. University of Nebraska Press.

Training and Technical Assistance Center [TRAIN]. (2020). *SOAR for Native communities*. SOAR Online. https://www.train.org/main/course/1088753/

Tribal Court Clearinghouse (n.d.). Tribal Courts. A project of the tribal law and policy institute. https://www.tribal-institute.org/lists/justice.htm#CFR%20Courts

University of North Dakota Recruitment and Retention of American Indians into Nursing [UND RAIN]. (2020). Recruitment and Retention of American Indians into Nursing. https://cnpd.und.edu/rain/

United States Census Bureau. (2018a). American Indian and Alaska Native Alone or In Combination with One or More Other Races. American Community Survey. Table:

B02010. https://data.census.gov/cedsci/table?q=B02010&hidePreview=false&tid=ACSDT1Y2018.B02010&vintage=2018

United States Census Bureau. (2018b). Selected population profile in the United States. 2018: ACS-1Year Estimates Selected Population, Survey/Program: American Community Survey, Table ID: S0201. https://www.census.gov/acs/www/data/data-tables-and-tools/data-profiles/2018/

United States Census Bureau. (2018). American Indian and Alaska Native alone or in combination with one or more other races. American Community Survey. Table: B02010. https://data.census.gov/cedsci/table?q=B02010&hidePreview=false&tid=ACSDT1Y2018.B02010&vintage=2018

United States Department of Justice. (2019, July). *Tribal crime data-collection activities, 2019*. NCJ 252983. https://www.bjs.gov/content/pub/pdf/tcdca19.pdf

United States Department of the Interior. (2020, July 27). Trump administration establishes the first Cold Case Task Force Office for missing and murdered American Indians and Alaskan Natives. Seven offices being established across the country to handle cold cases in Indian Country. https://indiancountrytoday.com/the-press-pool/trump-administration-establishes-the-first-cold-case-task-force-office-for-missing-and-murdered-american-indians-and-alaska-natives-r5iRqHdmfEqtv-jO-v1JwA

U.S. Bureau of Labor Statistics. (2019, October). Labor force characteristics by race and ethnicity, 2018. *BLS Report 1082*. https://www.bls.gov/opub/reports/race-and-ethnicity/2018/pdf/home.pdf

U.S. Department of Agriculture [USDA]. (2020, January). *Food distribution Program on Indian Reservations*. Food and Nutrition Service, Nutrition Program Fact Sheet. https://fns-prod.azureedge.net/sites/default/files/resource-files/fdpir-program-fact-sheet-2020-for%20website.pdf

U.S. Department of Agriculture Food and Nutrition Service [USDA FNS]. (2018, April). *Commodity supplemental food program*. Food and Nutrition Service, Nutrition Program Fact Sheet. https://fns-prod.azureedge.net/sites/default/files/csfp/programFactSheet-csfp.pdf

U.S. Department of Agriculture Food and Nutrition Service [USDA FNS]. (2020, April 20). *Indian Tribal Organization*. https://www.fns.usda.gov/fdpir/indian-tribal-organization

U.S. Department of Commerce. (2018). *My Tribal Area: Pine Ridge Reservation*. https://www.census.gov/tribal/?aianihh=2810

U.S. Department of Education, National Center for Education Statistics. (2019). *The Condition of Education 2019* (NCES 2019-144), Public High School Graduation Rates. https://nces.ed.gov/pubs2019/2019144.pdf

U.S. Department of Interior. (2020). *Budget justification and performance information. Fiscal year 2021. Bureau of Indian Education*. The United States Department of the Interior. https://www.doi.gov/sites/doi.gov/files/uploads/fy2021-budget-justification-bie.pdf

U.S. Department of Health and Human Services and U.S. Department of Agriculture. (2015, December). 2015–2020 Dietary Guidelines for Americans. 8th Edition. https://health.gov/sites/default/files/2019-09/2015-2020_Dietary_Guidelines.pdf

U.S. Department of Health and Human Services. (2014, January). *The Health Consequences of Smoking—50 Years of Progress: A Report of the Surgeon General*. Atlanta: U.S. Department of Health and Human Services, Centers for Disease Control and Prevention, National Center for Chronic Disease Prevention and Health Promotion, Office on Smoking and Health. https://www.ncbi.nlm.nih.gov/books/NBK179276/pdf/Bookshelf_NBK179276.pdf

U.S. Department of Health and Human Services (2018, April). *Indian Health Service Disparities*. https://www.ihs.gov/newsroom/factsheets/disparities/

U.S. Department of the Treasury. (2020a). *The CARES Act Work for all Americans*. https://home.treasury.gov/policy-issues/cares

U.S. Department of the Treasury. (2020b). *The CARES Act provides assistance to workers and their families*. https://home.treasury.gov/policy-issues/cares/assistance-for-american-workers-and-families

U.S. Department of Veteran Affairs. (2020). Rural Veterans Health Care Challenges. Rural Veterans. https://www.ruralhealth.va.gov/aboutus/ruralvets.asp

U.S. Treasury. (2020, May 5). Coronavirus Relief Fund, Allocations to Tribal Governments. https://home.treasury.gov/system/files/136/Coronavirus-Relief-Fund-Tribal-Allocation-Methodology.pdf

Utacia Krol, D. (2017, May 11). Life expectancy falling in US—But in Tribal communities, not so much. https://indiancountrytoday.com/archive/life-expectancy-falling-in-us-but-in-tribal-communities-not-so-much-nh_16pV-I0i_cY8vNKmGgA

VA-Center for Applied Systems Engineering. (2016). Memorandum of Understanding Annual Report Fiscal Year 2015. Department of Veterans Affairs and Indian Health Service. https://www.ruralhealth.va.gov/docs/2015_VA-IHS_Report.pdf

Vincent, G. and V. A. Velkoff. (2010, May). The next four decades: The older population in the United States: 2010 to 2050. Population estimates and projections. https://www.census.gov/prod/2010pubs/p25-1138.pdf

Wang, T. W., *et al.* (2019, December 6). Tobacco product use and associated factors among middle and high school students—United States, 2019. Morbidity and Mortality Weekly Report (*MMWR*), *68*(12), 1–22. http://dx.doi.org/10.15585/mmwr.ss6812al

Warne, D. (2011). Policy issues in American Indian health governance. *Journal of Law, Medicine, and Ethics, 39*(1_suppl), 42–45. https://doi-org/10.1111/j.1748-720X.2011.00564.x

Warne, D., *et al.* (2017). Adverse childhood experiences (ACE) among American Indians in South Dakota and associations with mental health conditions, alcohol use, and smoking, *Journal for Poor and Underserved, 28*, 1559–1577. https://doi-org/10.1353/hpu.2017.0133

Warne, D. and D. Lajimodiere. (2015). American Indian health disparities: psychosocial influences. *Social and Personality Psychology Compass, 9/10*. 567–579. https://doi-org/10.1111/spc3.12198

Weaver, C. and D. Frosch. (2020, February 13). U.S. Indian Health Service doctor indicted on charges of sexual abuse. https://www.pbs.org/wgbh/frontline/article/u-s-indian-health-service-doctor-indicted-on-charges-of-sexual-abuse/

Weiser, K. (2020, February). Native American religion. Legends of America. https://www.legendsofamerica.com/na-religion/

Wigington, P. (2019, March 16). Native American Two Spirit. *ThoughtCo.* https://www.thoughtco.com/native-american-two-spirit-4585024

Wilkie, M.L. (2020a). Empowered by cultural identity and catalyzed by resilience: A path to support American Indian nursing student success. *Creative Nursing, 26*(1), 43–47.

Wilkie, M. (2020b). *Niganawenimaanaanig Nursing Program*, Bemidji State University. https://www.bemidjistate.edu/academics/departments/nursing/programs/niganawenimaanaanig/

Wilkie-Condiff, M. L. (2009). *Organ donation and transplantation: The lived experience of American Indians* (Doctoral dissertation). University of Minnesota School of Nursing, Minneapolis.

Willis, D. J. (2016). Ethnicity and health in America Series: Stress in the Native American community. Ethnicity and Health in America Series. American Psychology Association. https://www.apa.org/pi/oema/resources/ethnicity-health/native-american/stress

Wilson, N., *et al.* (2020). Drug and opioid-involved overdose deaths—United States, 2017–2018. *MMWR Morbidity and Mortality Weekly Report, 69*, 290–297. DOI: .http://dx.doi.org/10.15585/mmwr.mm6911a4.

Wiltz, T. (2016, March 4). American Indian girls often fall through the cracks. *Stateline,* The Pew Charitable Trusts. https://www.pewtrusts.org/en/research-and-analysis/blogs/stateline/2016/03/04/american-indian-girls-often-fall-through-the-cracks

Wise, M. and S. R. Kostelecky. (2018). Respecting the language: Digitizing Native American language materials. *Digital Library Perspectives, 34*(3), 200–214. https://doi-org/10.1108/DLP-02-2018-0006

Woodward, S. (2016). The police killings No one is talking about. A special investigation. https://inthesetimes.com/features/native_american_police_killings_native_lives_matter.html

Wyman, L. T., T. L. McCarty, and S. E. Nicholas. (Eds.). (2014). Indigenous youth and multilingualism: Language identity, ideology, and practice in dynamic cultural worlds. New York: Routledge.

Yellow Horse Brave Heart, M. (2003). The Historical Trauma response among Natives and its relationship with substance abuse: A Lakota illustration, *Journal of Psychoactive Drugs, 35*(1), 7–13, https://doi.org/10.1080/02791072.2003.10399988

Zornosa, L. (2020, November 7). CNN election night graphic deemed Native Americans "something else". *The Forum,* © 2020 Los Angeles Times, Distributed by Tribune Content Agency, LCC. https://epaper.inforum.com/html5/reader/production/default.aspx?pubname=&edid=35cadb28-9993-4ed4-915c-fbc8e59ba201

CHAPTER 10

Health Challenges Faced by Immigrant Populations in Rural Areas

Joy Elwell

Objectives:

1. Discuss the challenges that communication presents to immigrant populations in rural settings.
2. Discuss the complexities involved in health insurance coverage and payment as they apply to immigrant populations in rural settings.
3. Discuss the impact implicit bias and racism have on the health of immigrant populations living in rural settings.

Discussion Questions:

1. Your rural health clinic is the closest primary care office for an immigrant community but is located three miles from the nearest bus stop. What creative solution could you design and implement to facilitate this population to access your clinic?
2. A newly settled immigrant family comes to your rural health clinic. While the children are covered by Medicaid, the parents are not. The mother has insulin-dependent diabetes and the father has hypertension. How could you help the parents obtain the healthcare they need?
3. When you refer patients for specialized procedures, you find that specialists are not following the latest evidence-based practice guidelines for your patients who are immigrants. Further, these patients report back to you that they do not want to go to the specialists anymore because they feel they are treated disrespectfully. You suspect implicit bias and racism are involved. To best advocate for your patients and make the specialists aware of behaviors they may not realize they are engaging in, how would you open a dialogue with the specialists to address this?
4. Describe three positive attributes of rural AIAN people and communities.

INTRODUCTION

With the exception of Indigenous peoples, the United States is a nation of immigrant populations. Immigrations to the New World began with the Viking explorations, in the early 1000s and remains of at least one settlement exist in Newfoundland, Canada (Ingstad and Ingstad, 2000). Immigrations to what is now the United States of America began in 1607, in Jamestown, Virginia (Corbett, et al., 2015). Succeeding waves of immigrations followed, and continue to the present day. Health challenges face immigrant populations, regardless of where they settle, be it in urban, suburban, or rural settings. Rural healthcare poses challenges to all populations. Resources, or the lack thereof, are potentiated for immigrant populations. Rural status confers higher risk for poor outcomes for most healthcare use measures, independent of poverty and healthcare supply.

SIGNIFICANCE OF THE PROBLEM

In a nation of nearly 329 million people (U.S. Census, 2020), immigrant populations are estimated to comprise nearly 14 percent of the overall population. According to the American Community Survey (2018), more than 44.7 million immigrants lived in the United States, about one in seven U.S. residents.

As immigrant populations move to rural communities, their health needs are intensified, potentially resulting in poor health outcomes. Healthcare providers and institutions, as well as communities and local, state, and federal agencies are challenged to address these needs.

SPECIFIC ISSUES AND THEIR IMPACT ON HEALTH OF IMMIGRANT POPULATIONS IN RURAL SETTINGS

Communication

Communication challenges exist when immigrants, particularly those who are from non-English speaking populations, enter any new community. According to Evans, Keys, and Meltzer (2016) language barriers may prevent immigrants from interfacing with clinical institutions. Even when they do, difficulties with verbal and written communication can result in poor health outcomes. This challenge intensifies in rural communities where resources for translation are not readily available. Table 10.1 illustrates a breakdown of languages other than English spoken at home by immigrant populations.

Every aspect of health and its attendant challenges is affected by the ability to send and receive communication in one's first language. Many factors influencing health outcomes are tied to communication. There are a multitude of examples of nuanced communications, including but not limited to those in this list:

- History taking
- Pre- and post-operative instructions
- Dietary instructions
- Medication reconciliation
- Insurance and payment information
- Exercise and activity instruction
- Growth and development information
- Family planning information

Errors in communication are frequent. In a study of 52 Spanish-speaking Latino patients in northern California, researchers found communication errors in fully half of the encounters, even when using professional interpretation

TABLE 10.1. Top Languages Spoken at Home, Population Ages 5 and Older, United States, 2018.

	Estimate	Share of All Speakers of Foreign Languages
Speak Language Other than English	67,259,000	100%
Spanish	41,460,000	62%
Chinese (including Mandarin, Cantonese)	3,472.000	5%
Tagalog (including Filipino)	1,760,000	3%
Vietnamese	1,542,000	2%
Arabic	1,259,000	2%
French (including Cajun)	1,232,000	2%
Korean	1,086,000	2%
Russian	919,000	1%
German	890,000	1%
Hindi	874,000	1%
Haitian	834,000	1%
Portuguese	816,000	1%
Amharic, Somali, or other Afro-Asiatic languages	582,000	1%
Yoruba, Twi, Igbo, other languages of Western Africa	582,000	1%
Italian	554,000	1%
Yiddish, Pennsylvania Dutch, other West Germanic languages	533,000	1%
Polish	509,000	1%

Source: Migration Policy Institute (MPI) tabulation of data from the U.S. Census Bureau 2018 American Community Survey (ACS), (Batalova, Blizzard, Bolter, 2020)

services. Seven percent of the errors were considered "moderately to highly clinically significant" (Napoles *et al.*, 2015). Extrapolating that statistic to the greater non-English speaking populations present across the U.S., it is clear the potential for communication errors resulting in poor health outcomes is considerable. With an estimated 67,259,000 non-English speaking individuals in the U.S., the resulting projected moderate-to-serious medical interpretation rate of 7% results in 4,708,130 potential poor health outcomes

Beyond the issue of accuracy, the issue of cost is also significant. Medical translation services are expensive. According to Jacobs *et al.* (2018) the cost of face-to-face interpreters can range from $45–$150 per hour, depending on how common or rare the needed language translation is. The cost of telephonic translation range between $1.25–$3.00 per minute, depending on the time of day and language requirement. Video remote interpretation costs range between $1.95–$3.49 per minute. The only states in which Medicaid provides reimbursement for medical translation services are District of Columbia, Hawaii, Idaho, Iowa, Kansas, Maine, Minnesota, Montana, New Hampshire, New York, Utah, Vermont, Virginia, Washington, and Wyoming (p. 73). Given the restricted amounts reimbursed by Medicare, Medicaid, and private insurers, deducting translation fees can make this service cost-prohibitive. For the uninsured, adding the cost of a translator to the cost of medical services can make medical services unaffordable.

Transportation

Transportation is a key factor in accessing healthcare services, including office visits, urgent and acute hospital care, physical therapy, mental health services, pharmacy, and nutrition. Even with the expansion of telehealth services as a result of the COVID-19 coronavirus pandemic health crisis, the ability to travel to certain services is crucial. In a study of 1,054 residents in rural Arizona, researchers found that there was a significant need for public bus service, as many residents did not own cars, and needed transportation for medical visits, and to obtain pharmaceuticals. While the study did not differentiate immigrants from citizens, 495 (78%) of the respondents indicated Spanish as their preferred language. It is plausible that a significant percentage of this group were immigrants. Eighty-four percent of the respondents stated they needed public bus service in order to access healthcare services (DelRio *et al.*, 2017).

HEALTH INSURANCE AND COSTS ASSOCIATED WITH HEALTHCARE SERVICES

Healthcare costs are significant and for all, but for individuals with chronic health conditions, healthcare services can be cost-prohibitive. Despite the pas-sage and implementation of the Patient Protection and Affordable Care Act, commonly referred to as the Affordable Care Act (ACA), or Obamacare, in 2010, which made health insurance coverage available to 23 million Americans who were previously uninsured, the cost of insurance remains out of reach for many. Further, the estimated 11.7 million undocumented immigrants are excluded from ACA coverage (Hall and Cuellar, 2016). The impact of this on accessing healthcare services is significant. One example is diabetes. Without regular testing and screening, access to insulin and supplies, the risk for morbidity and mortality associated with diabetes increases dramatically. The uninsured individual bears the full cost. Cefalu *et al.* (2018) discuss the precipitous increase in the price of insulin since 2002. This has important implications for those with this and other health conditions.

In their qualitative study of immigrants living in rural eastern Maryland, Sangaramoorthy, T. and Guevara, E. (2017) identified, in numerous interviews, that costs associated with healthcare were a significant barrier to access, leading this population to delay seeking care until it was "absolutely necessary". Unfortunately, delaying timely screenings and follow up appointments results in late detection of complications of an existing condition, or late detection of a new health condition.

Even for those immigrants who fit the criteria for health insurance coverage, actually obtaining coverage is not assured. In a study of 69,985 refugees resettled in various parts of the U.S., conducted in 2014, 41,684 of the refugees were settled within 28 states that had Medicaid expansion. The other 28,301 refugees (31% of the total) were settled within 23 states that did not have Medicaid expansion. (Agrawal and Venkatesh, 2016). Considering the many stressors that refugees face as newly immigrated residents, those who live in rural areas, will have their stress compounded by this barrier to access to healthcare.

IMPLICIT BIAS AND RACISM

Implicit attitudes are defined by Hall *et al.* (2016) as "thoughts and feelings that often exist outside of conscious awareness, and thus are difficult to consciously acknowledge and control". Everyone has implicit attitudes and these contribute to implicit bias. Implicit bias contributes to inequities and disparities in healthcare.

Racism, discrimination against, or prejudice towards a population or group due to their race or ethnicity, born out of implicit bias, has dangerous implications for the health and well-being of immigrant populations. Dayna Bowen Matthew (2018) developed her Structural Theory of Implicit Racial and Ethnic Bias in Healthcare. Her theory posits that implicit bias and unconscious racism exist in medicine, resulting in the limiting of resources for racial and ethnic minority populations. This is supported in a report by James *et al.* (2016), which concludes that racial disparities in healthcare access are found in rural communities, just as they are in urban settings. In a study of 152 African American women, Barcelona de Mendoza *et al.* (2018) identified and link between perceived racial discrimination and disease-associated genes, which supports the argument that racism is a risk for disease, to the posing a genetic risk. While this study addressed African American women, not immigrants, the study is about the effects of racism. For immigrants, coping with racism is yet an additional toxic stressor contributing to poor health outcomes.

CONCLUSIONS AND IMPLICATIONS

It is evident that immigrants face unique stressors and challenges to health when living in rural settings. Disparities and inequities are further exacerbated by being foreign-born. All of the social determinants of health are impacted by immigrant status.

There is an opportunity for healthcare systems, for legislative and for regulatory bodies, at the local, state, and federal levels to improve health outcomes among immigrant populations. Implementing local and state transportation policies to improve public transportation would not only benefit immigrant and native-born residents, but would also lessen the environmental impact of carbon emissions. Expanding English proficiency classes and making them available at different times to accommodate shift workers would benefit both immigrants and provide employment opportunities for teachers. Expanding Medicaid availability in all states would eliminate a barrier to access to healthcare services. Encouraging a national dialogue on implicit bias and systemic racism would help reduce their effects, which negatively influence every aspect of health in minority populations, regardless of country of origin.

REFERENCES

Agrawal, P., and A. K. Venkatesh (2016). Refugee resettlement patterns and state-level healthcare insurance access in the United States. *American Journal of Public Health, 106*, 662–663. doi:10.2105/AJPH.2015.303017.

Barcelona de Mendoza, V., *et al.* (2018). Perceived racial discrimination and DNA Methylation among African American women in the InterGEN Study. *Biological Research for Nursing 20*(2) 145–152.

Batalova J., B. Blizzard, and J. Bolter. (2020). Frequently requested statistics on immigrants and immigration in the United States. https://www.migrationpolicy.org/article/frequently-requested-statistics- immigrants-and-immigration-united-states.

Cefalu, W. T., *et al.* (2018). Insulin Access and Affordability Working Group: Conclusions and Recommendations. *Diabetes Care 41* (6) 1299–1311; DOI: 10.2337/dci18-0019.

Corbett, P. S., J. Janssen, J. M. Lund. 2015. *U.S. History.* Openstax.

DelRio, M., *et al.* (2017).Transportation matters: A health impact assessment in rural New Mexico. *Int. J. Environ. Res. Public Health, 14*(6), 629; https://doi.org/10.3390/ijerph140606293303983CED604426PQ/4?accountid=14518.

Hall, E. and N. G. Cuellar. (2016). Immigrant health in the United States: A trajectory toward change. *Journal of Transcultural Nursing, 27*(6), 611–626.

Ingstad, H., and A. Ingstad. (2000). The Viking discovery of America: *The excavation of a Norse settlement in L'Anse Aux Meadows, Newfoundland.* Breakwater Books.

Jacobs, B., *et al.* (2018). Medical interpreters in outpatient practice. *Annals of family medicine, 16*(1) 70–76.

James, C. V., *et al.* (2016). Racial/ Ethnic health disparities among rural adults—United States, *2012–2015 MMWR Surveillance Summaries 66*(23); 1–9.

Matthew, D. (2015). Toward Structural Theory of Implicit Racial and Ethnic Bias in Healthcare. *Health Matrix: Journal of Law-Medicine, 25*, 61–86.

Napoles, A. N., *et al.* (2015). Inaccurate language interpretation and its clinical significance in the medical encounters of Spanish-speaking Latinos. *Medicare Care, 53*(11) 940–947.

Sangaramoorthy, T. and E. Guevara. (2017). Immigrant health in rural Maryland: A qualitative study of major barriers to healthcare access. *Journal of immigrant minority health, 19*:939–946. DOI 10.1007/s10903-016-0417-z.

U.S. Census Bureau. 2020. U.S. and World Population Clock. https://www.census.gov/popclock/.

CHAPTER 11

Mental Health and Substance Use

Kathleen T. McCoy

Objectives:

1. Identification of challenges meeting mental health/substance use needs of patients in rural delivery systems.
2. Discussion of legal and technical issues/conflicts that may arise in rural settings related to mental health and substance use.
3. Outline of support services/resources meeting mental health and related substance use needs in rural areas.

Discussion Questions:

1. Provide two distinct social determinants of health influencing long-standing challenges in meeting mental health and substance use needs of rural populations.
2. Discuss ways communities can close gaps in mental health and substance use services secondary to lack of funding/adequate funding and distance issues.
3. To improve future rural community outcomes, outline three different ways rural communities can creatively practice preventative ways to reduce long-term trauma and effect reduction of illicit drug use in populations at risk.

INTRODUCTION

Rural settings possess a distinct constellation of advantages and challenges relevant to mental health and substance use. Most of these attributes falling, albeit broadly, into Distance, Access and Isolation categories being inherently related to social determinants of health. These three separate major areas of concern may overlap with one another, making it difficult to assess distinct issues. Further, challenges in rural populations are paradoxically advantages, depending upon how they are perceived and/or experienced.

SECTION I: ISSUES AND BACKGROUND

Mental health services are severely under resourced in both urban and rural areas. The issues of distance, access, and isolation are exacerbated in rural areas. Sadly, the COVID-19 pandemic has only increased the need for recognition, support for mental health services. Symptoms and manifestations of mental health conditions often are pervasive across diagnoses. Waiting periods of six months or more to see a mental health provider in urban areas is commonplace, often with tragic consequences. The wait is even longer or simply not available in rural settings. Mental health problems may present with a variety of symptoms and nurses and nurse practitioners practicing in rural areas need to develop a both a broad skill set and resources to support mental health. Mental health issues are not simply evidenced by psychiatric diagnoses, but also by drug overdoses, suicides, and increases in runaways which sadly result in increases in human trafficking.

DRUG OVERDOSES

The opioid crisis is second only to COVID-19, as America's contemporary health epidemics. Recent books and movies such as *Quinones's Dreamland, A True Tale of America's Opiate Epidemic, and Hillbilly Elegy: A Memoir of a Family and Culture in Crisis*, written by Vance, trace the foothold of the epidemic to its current black tar heroin market scheme, and the deterioration of Appalachian culture as related to the opioid culture among other influences (Vance, 2017; Quinones, 2019). Per Mack *et al.*, drug overdoses are a leading cause of American injury and death, with approximately 52,000 deaths in 2015 (Mack, 2019). Understanding distinct differences between illicit drug use, illicit drug use disorders, and overall drug overdose deaths in metropolitan and nonmetropolitan areas is important for informing public health programs, interventions, and policies. The reporting period of 1999–2015 for illicit drug use and drug use disorders during 2003–2014, and drug overdose deaths during 1999–2015 is reflected in the following data reported from the National Survey of Drug Use and Health (NSDUH) collection (Substance Abuse and Mental Health Services Administration [SAMHSA], 2019). Information was collected through face-to-face household interviews about use of illicit drugs, alcohol, and tobacco among noninstitutionalized U.S. civilian population aged

≥ 12 years. Residents of households and non-institutional group quarters (e.g., shelters, rooming houses, dormitories, migratory workers' camps, and halfway houses) and civilians living on military bases were respondents. NSDUH variables include sex, age, race/ethnicity, residence (metropolitan/nonmetropolitan), annual household income, self-reported drug use, and drug use disorders. The National Vital Statistics System Mortality (NVSS-M) data for U.S. residents from that time include information from death certificates filed in all states plus the District of Columbia. Cases were selected with an underlying cause of death based on drug overdose diagnostic criteria with NVSS-M variables including decedent characteristics (sex, age, and race/ethnicity) and information on intent (unintentional, suicide, homicide, or undetermined), location of death (medical facility, in a home, or other [including nursing homes, hospices, unknown, and other locations] and county of residence, metropolitan/nonmetropolitan), with metropolitan/nonmetropolitan status assigned independently to each group. Results: Both metropolitan and nonmetropolitan areas experienced significant increases from 2003–2005 to 2012–2014 in self-reported past-month use of illicit drugs. Prevalence was highest for large metropolitan areas compared with small metropolitan or nonmetropolitan areas throughout the study period with a notable past-month use of illicit drugs decline over the study period for the youngest respondents (12–17 years). Prevalence of past-year illicit drug use disorders among persons using illicit drugs (in the past year) varied by metropolitan/nonmetropolitan status. Changing over time, prevalence of past-year illicit drug use disorders across both metropolitan and nonmetropolitan areas revealed declines between 2003–2014. In 2015, an approximate 6:1 ratio of drug overdose deaths occurred in metropolitan areas: nonmetropolitan areas (metropolitan: 45,059; 7,345: nonmetropolitan). Drug overdose death rates (per 100,000 population) for metropolitan areas were higher than in nonmetropolitan areas in 1999 (6.4 versus 4.0), with converging 2004 rates. By 2015, the nonmetropolitan rate (17.0) was slightly higher, exceeding metropolitan rates (16.2). Interpretation: Drug use and subsequent overdoses continue as a critical and complicated public health challenge across metropolitan/nonmetropolitan areas. Declines in illicit drug use by youth and lower prevalence of illicit drug use disorders in rural areas during 2012–2014 are favorable reports; however, increasing drug overdose death rates in rural areas, now surpassing in urban areas, is concerning.

Necessary Public Health Actions include understanding the differences between metropolitan and nonmetropolitan areas in drug use, drug use disorders, and drug overdose deaths can help public health professionals to identify, monitor, and prioritize responses. Location of where people live and die from overdose could enhance specific overdose prevention interventions, such as training on naloxone administration/rescue breathing. Prescriber education is also needed. Prescribers on CDC's guidelines for prescribing opioids for chronic pain (Dowell *et al.*, 2016) and facilitating better access to Medication-Assisted Treatment (MAT) with methadone, buprenorphine, or naltrexone could benefit communities with high opioid use disorder rates. MAT training including dismantling stigma in regard to substance use is essential for communities to embrace and support new MAT systems and options available as well as promotion of the concept of addiction as an illness rather than as a moral deficit (Harvard Office of External Education, 2019). Because attitudinal learning takes the longest, systematic education and exposure to people living in rural communities must be organized and occur on multiple levels, and supported by community stakeholders, funding, and staff to ensure sustainability of both the education needed to enhance community uptake of these programs so those with SU conditions can presently thrive sooner and later.

SUICIDE

Rural Suicides

Depression and suicide are an increasing reality. U.S. suicides reported in 2015, were responsible for 44,193 deaths (CDC, 2018). As one of the top ten leading causes of death in the U.S, it is notable that suicide rates are higher in rural America than in urban America, with this gap growing steadily between 1999–2015. This gap widened more quickly after 2007, with White Non-Hispanics having the highest suicide rates in urban areas (metropolitan counties) and American Indian and Alaska Native Non-Hispanics having the highest rates in rural areas. While suicide is preventable with multiple, comprehensive suicide prevention strategies, measurement-based care implementation of screening for depression in primary care, distance links, crisis line management, response times, and innovative ways supported by adequate funding to increase access to healthcare and mental healthcare in rural counties must occur.

First responders also have higher risks for suicide and may dread responding to domestic calls related to violence, and/or motor vehicle accidents of friends, family, and acquaintances. Rural responders suffer doubly, first from the trauma of events and second in personal knowledge of victims. Training, debriefing, and reasonable time off to decompress or change roles are some strategies that can assist communities with a limited number of first responders to ensure their mental health as they are regularly exposed to tragedy and loss.

Agricultural Sector Suicide

"American Farmers ask for mental health help in the face of economic stress" states the Washington Examiner headline (Quinn, 2019). Farmers and agricultural workers are at elevated risk of suicide. Suicide data from the Georgia Violent Death Reporting System, 2008–2015 disclosed farmers who died from suicide were predominantly white, male, non-Hispanic, older, with half attaining a high school diploma and/or never marrying (Scheyett, Bayakly, Whitaker, & 2019). The most common means ware self-inflicted gunshot (75%), hanging (16%), and 25% reported concomitant relationship conflict and/or chronic pain/decreased function. Twelve percent were suffering financially and substance users were 11% with 21% of cases reporting previous suicidal threats, which families often discounted. Additionally, every factor contributing to the success of a farmer is outside of personal control of any farmer, reports Quinn (Quinn, 2019). Weather and the economy are unpredictable, indeed, at times volatile. The natural environment is isolated, the "law of the farm" requires relentless daily commitment to repeated mundane tasks, and unforgiving if neglected (Covey, 1994). Suicides among agricultural workers have been shown to be above other work sectors with a recent study urging suicide prevention programs to be explored for the agricultural industry (Ringgenberg *et al.*, 2018). With the agricultural sector being the industry that provides the bulk of American food sourcing, it would serve the nation to provide mental health support for farmers, their families, and farm workers.

HUMAN TRAFFICKING

In the December 2019 issue of *Nursing Clinics of North America*, it is reported that human trafficking is not limited to sex workers, and includes by definition, any worker retained against their will for labor/s. In rural settings it is highly likely that exploited workers may include agricultural workers (Costa *et al.*, 2019). Trafficking in persons may include secret movement of people with intent to smuggle them and is akin to modern-day slavery. Slavery can take several different forms, including sexual servitude and forced labor. It is difficult to accurately identify or predict which creates problems for law enforcement.

Human trafficking is the fastest-growing criminal industry globally, with an estimated 27 million people enslaved worldwide. Between 14,500 and 17,500 people are trafficked into the U.S. annually, and this is growing. The agricultural industry relies upon migrant and transitional workers and has been a long-standing haven for the plight of human devastation, bondage, etc., as portrayed in Steinbeck's original 1939 classic *The Grapes of Wrath* (Steinbeck, 2006). Human trafficking victims have been captured and transported into agricultural settings, especially older people, and may even include entire families, exploited for labor without regard to basic needs or human rights, but treated as objects to fulfill hard labor. Healthcare for these individuals is needed due to natural processes such as pregnancy, labor, and delivery, injury from accidents including but not limited to motor vehicles and/or heavy equipment, human frailty, poor housing, and weather-related incidents. Healthcare provid ers must be aware of the prospect that this population may present to healthcare settings, and be seeking care, and that not only care, but also recognition and effective reporting as recommended by various agencies is recommended.

Physician/Psychiatrist Decline Trends

The Affordable Care Act (ACA) and the Mental Health Parity and Addiction Equity Acts expanded behavioral health coverage to cover more citizens of the U.S. However, the psychiatric workforce of physicians is in the midst of a professional shortage, which is projected to worsen by 2025, with rural populations affected more greatly than metropolitan populations (University of Michigan Behavioral Health Workforce Research Center [UMBHWRC], 2018). In a study of this shortage, data were derived from the American Medical Association Masterfile, which includes private and publicly funded practices. In the U.S., there are approximately 41,133 psychiatrists practicing within 1,397 counties (of 44.4% total U.S. counties). There are 9,956 child and adolescent psychiatrists (CAPS) practicing in 828 counties (23% of U.S. county totals), 1,265 geriatric psychiatrists (GP) practice in 321 counties (10% of total counties), and 836 addictions psychiatrists actively practice in 230 total U.S. counties (UMBHWRC, p. 3,2018). Psychiatrist locations are primarily in the NE and in certain counties on the West Coast. The ACA expanded Medicaid to more recipients while also increasing mental health and substance use (SU) disorder management. The high demand for CAP, GP, and AP specialists is not matched by a proportionate to population need distribution nationwide.

With 20% of children possessing behavioral health disorders, 41 states have severe CAP shortages (1–17 CAPS/100,000 children), 9 states are high shortage states (18–46 CAPs/100,000 children) with one sole area, Washington, D.C., with a sufficient supply of > 47 CAPs/100.000 children). Fifteen percent of persons over age 60 suffer from a mental health disorder, and demand for the GP will increase by as much as 20% as the geriatric population expands due to baby boomers living extended lives. Over half of GP reside in only seven states, and only four states have not one board certified GP. With over

21.5 million U.S. citizens age 12 up sustain substance use (SU) disorders, only 0.9% of psychiatrists specialize in addictions, with most found in urban settings. Counties with greater representation of black, rural, uninsured citizens are less likely to have access to a SU facility accepting Medicaid. (UMBHWRC, p. 4–5, 2018). With U.S. population needs for mental healthcare increasing due to increasing violence, trauma-related sequelae, family disruptions, big weather, and usual genetic predisposition to mental illness, combined with a shrinking workforce access, thinking outside of the physician box, may hold many other viable options.

SECTION II: SOLUTIONS

Addressing the U.S. Rural Health Landscape

The Roundtable on the Promotion of Health Equity (2018) convened envisioning a strong, healthy, and productive rural society, with the capacity to cultivate human capital and equal opportunity. This recognizes that outcomes such as improved life expectancy, quality of life, and health for all are shaped by the interdependence of social, economic, environmental, genetic, behavioral, and healthcare factors, weaved together with national and community-based policies. Dependable resources are required to achieve the identified and optimal outcome, both locally and nationally. Conveners of the nation's experts in health disparities and health equity met with the goal of raising awareness and driving change. Created in 2007 to promote health equity and reduce rural health disparities by advancing the visibility of and understanding about the inequities in health and healthcare among racial and ethnic populations, amplifying research, policy, and community-centered programs, and catalyzing the emergence of new leaders, partners, and stakeholders. This workshop outlines a pragmatic approach to address the path to significant change in how rural mental health is approached nationally.

Integrative Care

Per SAMHSA-HRSA (n.d.), Integrative Care is defined as settings where people can receive, in the same setting, both primary and mental health care. Dual services can be provided in a variety of ways, not limited to face to face, visiting providers, or be digitally connected through the use of internet links such as telehealth. Home of the newest evidence-based resources, tools, and support for organizations working to integrate primary and behavioral healthcare, and funded through the Substance Abuse and Mental Health Administration grant award from the National Council for Behavioral Health, through the National Center for Excellence for Integrated Health Solutions (CIHS) grant award from the Substance Abuse and Mental Health Administration.

The publication Advancing Behavioral Health Integration within NCQA Recognized Patient-Centered Medical Homes (SAMHSA-HRSA, 2014) guides the development and operationalization of integrated care sites. A review of standards relating relate to integration of behavioral health and primary care includes six approaches: (1) Patient-centered access, (2) Team-based care, (3) Population health management, (4) Care management support, (5) Care coordination and transitions, and (6) Performance Measurement and Quality Improvement systems. These items provide an intent for a stepwise development of services with ultimate measurable outcomes for ready access to care across levels and its varied/broad nuances. The CIHS' Standard Framework for Levels of Integrated Healthcare helps primary and behavioral healthcare provider organizations improve outcomes by helping them understand where they are on the integration continuum. The federally supported plan for integrative healthcare through the establishment of medical homes is one step to bring mental health substance use care closer to those in non-suburban areas. The report of the University of Michigan Behavioral Health Workforce Research Center recommends a three-pronged approach to remediating the disproportionate distribution of U.S. psychiatrists: (1) Develop physician re cruitment programs to underserved, rural locations, (2) Strengthen psychiatric residency ties to training sites, and (3) Barrier removal for behavioral telehealth (UBHWRC, 2016).

The Role of Advanced Practice Providers

A broader view to enlightened solutions includes the burgeoning growth of non-physician advanced practice providers, who include Psychiatric Mental Health Nurse Practitioners (PMHNP). While the number of both primary care physicians and psychiatrists have been reducing for a few decades, in particular, pediatric psychiatrists, the Nurse Practitioner (NP) population, who are defined by populations served, is growing. The American Association of Nurse Practitioners (AANP) has over 104,000 members (AANP, 2019), to wit, the NP population in the U.S. exceeds 270,000 (2019) as captured in the AANP Statement on Texas Medical Center Survey on Future of Healthcare Workforce. Of these, Family NPs, Adult-Geriatric NPs, Adult-Geriatric Acute Care NPs, Pediatric NPs, and Pediatric Acute Care NPs can address aspects of mental health within their respective scopes of practice.

The PMHNP falls into two roles, the PMHNP (Adult), currently unavailable as a certification, and the PMHNP (Lifespan), which all programs have transitioned to. Per AANP NP Fact (2019) sheet: Respectively, the PMHNP (Adult): PMHNP (Lifespan) roles represent 2%:2.1% of the total NP 270,000 population, or approximately 5400:5670 certified professionals respectively. This number is a moving target as PMHNP programs continue to proliferate rapidly in meeting psychiatric mental health needs of the U.S. population. The unique PMHNP role is prepared to serve populations, across the lifespan, in all aspects of mental health prevention and care. Per the American Nurses Credentialing Center, *PMHNP Role Delineation Study* (2018) the PMHNP is able to diagnose, prescribe, and treat individuals, families and communities, including through the employment of psychotherapies (ANCC, 2018). Because the role encompasses, but is not limited to interviewing, psychotherapies, counseling, crisis intervention, assessment, biological therapies (medicine, etc.), the PMHNP has portability through most expected services that full service behavioral health practices/sites require. For example, PMHNPs servicing long-term care facilities can diagnose, prescribe, treat using biological approaches as well as psychosocial and psychotherapeutic implementation/s. Only psychiatrists and psychiatric mental health advance practice nurses (both NP and Clinical Nurse Specialist roles), and but in few limited states, psychologists, are prepared to both prescribe and treat with psychotherapies. For those in rural settings, this complement of services is a boon to any community. Additionally, PMHNPs are able to build programs and services to assist specific populations in matters of mental health. The PMHNP is prepared to practice in any setting, and in full practice authority (FPA) of practice based upon the state in which practice is occurring. The Nurse Practitioner role is the best kept secret in healthcare. To date, 21 of 50 states plus Washington, DC, and Guam have FPA, the number narrowing as individual states battle their way through legislative barriers imposed by other professions/industries not perceiving the clinical capacity or level of rigor present in education, both academic and clinical preparation of NPs health and economic value of Advance Practice Nurse FPA and legislators not grasping clinical capacity or level of rigor present in education (academic/clinical preparation) of NPs.

Making matters a bit complex are three retiring certification roles in advanced practice nursing in Psychiatric Mental Health. Between 2013 and 2016, the American Nurses Credentialing Center, the certification body for these roles, consolidated all advance practice mental health roles into the one "lifespan" Psychiatric Mental Health Nurse Practitioner (PMHNP). Ultimately, this role will be the only advance practice mental health role. There are currently other roles which can be continued, but no longer available to attain, with programs of study adapting to the single lifespan PMHNP role. One additional role, augmenting the work of all teams and patient outcomes is the Board-Certified Psychiatric Nurse, included in Table 11.1. These roles are important because these board-certified providers are currently in the workforce and providing valuable and exemplary service. See the represented numbers of all certified mental health nurses on the generalist and advance practice levels.

Generalist Psychiatric Nurses are required to attain a BSN, a certain number of hours and pass an ANCC board examination. Advanced Practice Nurses need to attain an MSN in the specialty scope of practice, be exposed to a minimum of two psychotherapy modalities during a minimum of 500 supervised clinical across the lifespan patient contact hours, plus pass the ANCC board certification examination. While 21 of 50 states have FPA, other states have restrictions on practice, which must be abided by, or amended. Expansion of nursing practice as well as other advanced practice professions has burgeoned, especially since NP practice has been established across the nation in the retail sector, now expanding outside of standalone and larger clinic affiliated settings such as hospitals.

TABLE 11.1. Current ANCC Certified Psychiatric Mental Health Certified Nurses.

Adult Psychiatric Mental Health Clinical Nurse Specialist: PMHCNS-BC	4,371
Child and Adolescent Psychiatric-mental Health Clinical Nurse Specialist: PMHCNS-BC	(renewal only)
Adult Psychiatric Mental Health Nurse Practitioner: PMHNP-BC	759
Psychiatric Mental Health Nurse Practitioner: PMHNP-BC	(renewal only)
Psychiatric Mental Health Nurse: RN-C	3,772 (renewal only)
Total: Certified Psychiatric Mental Health Advance Practice and Registered Nurse	10,373
Total: Advance Practice PMH Nurses (all 4 roles)	10,817
Total: PMHNP (both NP roles)	30,092

(ANCC, 2018)

Telehealth

Utilization of long-distance technological support systems, which includes, but is not limited to telephonic, smartphone use, apps and telehealth face-to-face encounters, widens the net of patient, family, and population care (Sturm & Varner, 2019). Not without challenges, the opportunity rises to meet needs that can be linked by support systems in organizations designed to incorporate such into services provided negating most travel and the myriad variables that often confound psychiatric mental health appointment fulfillment. Successful interstate telemental health has been captured well in the *Journal of the American Psychiatric Nursing Association* (*JAPNA*) article by Adams *et al.* (2018). PMHNPs and psychiatric nurses and team members can cross state lines and effectively provide care to patients, families, and populations in other states provided state requirements in both originating and receiving sites are fulfilled completely (Adams *et al.*, 2018).

One of the most fortuitous outcomes of telemental health is that limits placed upon advanced practice nurses, CNSs, and NPs, in one state, may not necessarily encumber them from practicing across state lines in Full Practice Authority, further benefiting hard-to-reach rural populations, and linking providers who themselves may be found in rural settings. The keys are distance technology support, an amenable accessible charting and billing/coding system, and a team that operates in the best interest of the patient population, and in concert.

Patient Navigators

Care providers, whether family members or assigned patient navigators, are utilized since the role of healthcare navigators rose to industry recognition following the Affordable Care Act's healthcare coverage expansion, according to HealthCare.gov and captured in Heath's 2017 column in Patient engagement HIT (Heath, 2017). The role has emerged and been finessed since its rudiments in the sponsor framework established by Alcoholics Anonymous Big Book, several generations later (Alcoholics Anonymous, n.d.). Informal sponsor/advocate/navigators now have formal status through CMS. In the southwest, patient navigators are known as promontoras, lay health workers. Per RIH (2019) lay health workers are most effective when they are members of the target population (Heath, 2019). These individuals best know the life lived of patients represented, or have similar physical/cultural characteristics, but are bonafide community members, not simply those who translate or have similar physical/cultural characteristics. Rural border communities may benefit from promotoras conducting health/home assessment and health hazard education, all of which play into mental health. Expansion of care workers into this role extends to more patient engagement, which leads to health seeking and health promoting behaviors within homes and a community, ultimately linking the community to services and means to improve social determinants of health, thereby strengthening the community from within.

REWARDS OF RURAL HEALTH MENTAL HEALTH AND SUBSTANCE USE CARE

Populations in rural settings are generally family based, and gen erationally bound, even if a family, or part of a family, relocates, it is not uncommon for these to return or visit often. The "grapevine" and oral traditions are living entities, with both formal and informal leaders, sharing information and resources generously. The barter system, as well as yard sales, is another dynamic source of trade and sourcing of nearly any type, including the rich agricultural product landscape or services, such as tree removal, dressing of game, or materials needed or desired (stones, planting soil). The internet and other digital means also bring people together who formally only made contact when they made journeys to town for supplies, etc. Rural populations can enjoy the peace and tranquility of the countryside, and have contact with the world external to their small towns if they choose to, and on their terms, for company or supplies/materials. Warm relationships between people, families, and churches can stay lively, or become discordant at any time; however, there are true benefits to keep the peace in small towns. Civil service employees such as police, utilities, and responders stand a fair chance of knowing clients well, and helping them to meet needs as moments arise. Families and patients are generally very grateful and show respect across generations for providers who help them. Pooling of resources is not a new thing, rural populations have always engaged in wise use of resources, sharing as indicated, and creatively addressing issues without a financial bottom line. Use of volunteers is steady, especially the elderly, who are remarkably generous with time and expertise.

CONCLUSION

United States rural psychiatric mental health and substance use has yet to come of age. Social determinants of health are intrinsically involved in this sad state of affairs and must to be addressed in a systematic manner across healthcare systems in order to dismantle inequities extending into nonmetropolitan areas. Equitable care is largely dependent upon resources, which are not distributed to areas with less funding and representation. The National Academies of Science, Engineering and Medicine Workshop Achieving Rural Health Equity and Well-Being shows the way to begin to address the convoluting variables shortchanging this abiding in rural America (National Academies of Sciences, Engineering, and Medicine, 2018).The promise of hope lies in current changes in practice include integrated care models, telemental health and digital access bridging distances, better understanding of addictions as disease processes with Medical-Assisted Treatment (MAT) availability, the burgeoning efficacious and highly portable PMHNP role, and the new vision incorporating patients as partners in care, consumer-driven care, and patient navigators. These will hopefully hold up the nation's mental health and substance use programs while rural dilemmas are untangled.

Challenges and opportunities relative to rural mental health/substance use:

1. Distance from chaos and demands of everyday can be soothing in rural settings. How do healthcare providers reconcile access to care in sleepy towns with low or no resources when health emergencies arise?
2. Adolescent screening for substance use is now expected in every encounter, including those in conservative rural communities. How does one deal manage teen interviews with conservative parents in encounters to obtain the accurate information needed?
3. A farming village receives help during planting and harvest, often, migratory workers come to town for short periods of time, for which all townspeople are thankful. You suspect an encounter you are seeing currently is with a victim of human trafficking. She has no identification, has unexplained bruises of varying stages of healing, is chaperoned by an elderly off-putting female companion, who is paying for the encounter in cash and answers all questions. They are also in a hurry. What do you do?

REFERENCES

AANP. (2019). AANP statement on Texas medical center survey on future of health care workforce. November 20, 2019. Advocacy AANP News. Retrieved from https://www.aanp.org/news-feed/aanp-statement-on-texas-medical-center-survey-on-future-of-health-care-workforce#.XdWpsxIq1SM.mailto

AANP. (2019). NP Facts. Austin, TX: AANP. Retrieved 11/19/2019 from https://www.aanp.org/about/all-about-nps/np-fact-sheet

Adams, S. M., *et al.* (2018). TeleMental Health: Standards, Reimbursement, and Interstate Practice. *JAPNA, 24*(4):295–305. Retrieved from https://doi.org/10.1177/1078390318763963

Alcoholics Anonymous. (n.d.). Big Book Sponsorship: 12 Step Recovery from any and ALL Addictions. Webpage. AA. Retrieved 11/24/2019 from https://bigbooksponsorship.org/articles-alcoholism-addiction-12-step-program-recovery/aa-history/

Alderwick, H. and L. M. Gottlieb. (2019). Meanings and misunderstandings: A social determinants of health lexicon for health care systems. *Milbank Quarterly, 97*(3) 1–13. Retrieved 11/10/2019. https://www.milbank.org/quarterly/articles/meanings-and-misunderstandings-a-social-determinants-of-health-lexicon-for-health-care-systems/?gclid=EAIaIQobChMIg-OYpd2G5gIVB8pkCh3l5AFZEAAYASAAEg-KOePD_BwE

Allen, J., *et al.* (2014). Social determinants of mental health. *International Review of Psychiatry, 26*:4, 392–407, DOI:10.3109/09540261.2014.928270. Retrieved 10/12/2019 from https://docs.google.com/document/d/0BxvP6CMrKoQGakFwdC1PT3IxaWV4Mk1oQ0RfcTFXUnhQa2NR/edit#

ANCC. (2018). American nurses credentialing center psychiatric mental health nurse practitioner role delineation study executive summary 2018. Silver Spring, MD: ANA. Retrieved 11/20/2019 from https://www.nursingworld.org/our-certifications/psychiatric-mental-health-nurse-practitioner/

American Nurses Credentialing Center. (2019). 2018 ANCC Certification Data. Silver Spring, MD: ANCC. Retrieved 11/27/2019 from https://www.nursingworld.org/~499e5e/globalassets/docs/ancc/2017-certification-data-for-website.pdf

Andermann, A. (2018). Screening for social determinants of health in clinical care: Moving from the margins to the mainstream. *Public Health Rev, 39*(2018), p. 19. Retrieved 07/23/2019 from https://scholar.google.com/scholar?hl=en&as_sdt=0%2C43&q=A.+Andermann%2C+A.+%282018%29.+Screening+for+social+determinants+of+health+in+clinical+care%3A++moving+from+the+margins+to+the+mainstream.+Public+Health+Rev%2C+39+%282018%29%2C+p.+19.&btnG=

Assari, S. (2017). Social determinants of depression: The intersections of race, gender, and socioeconomic status. *Brain Sci, 7*(12) (2017), 10.3390/brainsci7120156

Barnes, G. A., *et al.* (2015). Barriers to Mental Health Treatment in Rural Older Adults. *The American Journal of Geriatric Psychiatry. 23*(11)1172–1178. Retrieved 6/10/2019 from https://www.sciencedirect.com/science/article/abs/pii/S1064748115001876

CDC. (2018). Suicide in rural America. Web page. Retrieved 11/14/19 from https://www.cdc.gov/ruralhealth/Suicide.html

CDC. n.d. Preventing suicide in rural America. Rural Health Policy Brief. Retrieved 10/20/2019 from 18_290906-A_Turner_Policy-Brief_Suicide-002_508

Costa, C. B., *et al.* (2019). *Evidence-based care of the human trafficking patient, nursing clinics of North America: 54*(4) 569–584. ISSN 0029-6465, ISBN 9780323696586, https://doi.org/10.1016/j.cnur.2019.08.007 (http://www.sciencedirect.com/science/article/pii/S0029646519300593)

Covey, S. (1994). Law of the Farm, 7 habits of highly successful people. Webpage. Retrieved 11//4/2019 from http://www.sjsu.edu/faculty/gerstman/misc/LawOfFarm.htm

Dowell, D., T. M. Haegerich, and R. Chou. (2016). CDC guideline for prescribing opioids for chronic pain—United States. MMWR Recomm Rep 2016;65 (No. RR-1): 1–49. doi: http://dx.doi.org/10.5585/mmwr.rr6501e1

Fischer, E. P., *et al.* (2016). Overcoming barriers to sustained engagement in mental health care: Perspectives of rural veterans and providers. *The Journal of Rural Health, 32*: 429–438. doi:10.1111/jrh.12203. Retrieved 5/10/2019 from https://onlinelibrary.wiley.com/action/showCitFormats?doi=10.1111%2Fjrh.12203

Fox 13 Tampa Bay (2018). 243 first responders commit suicide last year: More than died in line of duty. Retrieved 11/20/2019 from https://www.fox13news.com/news/243-first-responders-commit-suicide-last-year-more-than-died-in-the-line-of-duty

Harvard Office of External Education. (2019). Opioid Use Disorder Education Program MAT Waiver Training for NPs and PAs Webpage. Retrieved 6/1/2019 from ttps://postgraduateeducation.hms.harvard.edu/opioid-use-disorder-education-program

Heath, S. (2017). What are healthcare navigators, patient-centered care benefits? Webpage. PatientengagementHIT. Xtelligent Healthcare Media. Retrieved 11/24/2019 from https://patientengagementhit.com/news/what-are-healthcare-navigators-patient-centered-care-benefits

Mack, K. A., C. M. Jones, and M. F. Ballesteros. (2019). Illicit drug use, illicit drug use disorders, and drug overdose deaths in metropolitan and nonmetropolitan areas United States. MMWR Surveill Summ (2017) 66 (No. SS-19):1–12. DOI: http://dx.doi.org/10.15585/mmwr.ss6619a1 Retrieved 11/14/2019 from https://www.cdc.gov/mmwr/volumes/66/ss/ss6619a1.htm

McCoy, K. T., *et al.* (2019). Anticipating Changes for Depression Management in Primary Care. *Nursing Clinics of North America: 54*(4) 457–471, ISSN 0029-6465, ISBN 9780323696586, https://doi.org/10.1016/j.cnur.2019.07.001

National Academies of Sciences, Engineering, and Medicine. (2018). Achieving rural health equity and well-being: Proceedings of a workshop. Washington, D.C.: The National Academies Press. doi: https://doi.org/10.17226/24967. Retrieved 6/01/2019 from http://nationalacademies.org/hmd/Reports/2018/achieving-rural-health-equity-and-well-being-proceedings.aspx

Quinn, M. (2019). American farmers ask for mental health help in face of economic stress. Business. Agriculture Industry. Washington Examiner. Nov. 12, 2019, 24(40)45–48. Retrieved 11/17/2019 from https://www.washingtonexaminer.com/news/american-farmers-ask-for-mental-health-help-in-face-of-economic-stress

Quinones, S. (2019). Dreamland: The true tale of America's opiate epidemic. New York, NY: Bloomsbury Press.

Ringgenberg, W., *et al.* (2018). Trends and characteristics of occupational suicide and homicide in farmers and agriculture workers, 1992–2010. *The Journal of Rural Health, 34*: 246–253. doi:10.1111/jrh.12245

Rural Health Information. (2019). Promotora de salud/lay health worker model. Webpage. Rural Health Information Hub. Retrieved 11/24/2019 from https://www.ruralhealthinfo.org/toolkits/community-health-workers/2/layhealth

SAMHSA. (2019). National survey on drug use and health (NSDUH). Retrieved 11/20/2019 from https://www.samhsa.gov/data/data-we-collect/nsduh-national-survey-drug-use-and-health

SAMHSA-HRSA. (2014). Advancing behavioral health integration within NCQA recognized patient-centered medical homes. SAMHSA-HRSA Center for Integrated Health Solutions. National Council for Behavioral Health: Washington, D.C. Retrieved 11/19/2019 from https://www.integration.samhsa.gov/integrated-care-models/Behavioral_Health_Integration_and_the_Patient_Centered_Medical_Home_FINAL.pdf

SAMHSA-HRSA. n.d. SAMHSA-HRSA Center for Integrated Health Solutions. eSolutionNewsletter. Webpage. Center of Excellence for Integrated Health Solutions. Retrieved 11/19/2019 from https://www.integration.samhsa.gov/integrated-care-models

Scheyett, A., R. Bayakly, and M. Whitaker, M (2019). Characteristics and contextual stressors in farmer and agricultural workers suicides inGeorgia from 2008–2015. *Journal of Rural Mental Health*, Vol. 43(2–3) 61–72. Retrieved 5/01/2019 from https://psycnet.apa.org/record/2019-12789-001?doi=1

Steinbeck, J. (2006). *The Grapes of Wrath*. New York City, NY: Penguin Books.

Stone, D M., *et al.* (2017). Preventing Suicide: A Technical Package of Policies, Progams and Practices. Atlanta, GA: National Center for Injury Prevention and Control, Centers for Disease Control and Prevention. Retrieved 11/14/2019 from https://www.cdc.gov/ruralhealth/Suicide.html

Sturm, T. A. and J. Varner, (2019). *Miles apart yet close to heart: Long distance caregiving. Alabama Nurse. 46* (3)12–15 Retrieved 10/7/2019 from https://alabamanurses.org/2019/10/miles-apart-yet-close-to-heart-long-distance-caregiving/

University of Michigan Behavioral Health Workforce Research Center. (2018). Estimating the Distribution of the U.S. Psychiatric Subspecialist Workforce. Ann Arbor, MI: UMSPH. Retrieved 11/19/2019 from http://www.behavioralhealthworkforce.org/wp-content/uploads/2019/02/Y3-FA2-P2-Psych-Sub_Full-Report-FINAL2.19.2019.pdf

Vance, J. D. (2016). Hillbilly elegy: A memoir of a family and culture in crisis (First edition.). New York, NY: Harper, an imprint of HarperCollinsPublishers.

Whitehead, J., J. Shaver, and R. Stephenson. (2016). Outness, stigma, and primary health care utilization among rural LGBT populations. PLoS ONE 11(1): e0146139. https://doi.org/10.1371/journal.pone.0146139. Retrieved 10/6/2019 from https://www.sciencedirect.com/science/article/abs/pii/S1064748115001876

APPENDIX A: RESOURCES

- Center for Behavioral Health Statistics and Quality. (2016). 2015 National survey on drug use and health: Methodological summary and definitions. Rockville, MD: Substance Abuse and Mental Health Services Administration. Retrieved 11/27/2019 from https://www.samhsa.gov/data/sites/default/files/NSDUH-MethodSummDefsHTML-2015/NSDUH-MethodSummDefsHTML-2015/NSDUH-MethodSummDefs-2015.htm
- Harvard Office of External Education. (2019). Opioid use disorder education program MAT waiver training for NPs and PAs webpage. ttps://postgraduateeducation.hms.harvard.edu/opioid-use-disorder-education-program
- Rural Health Information. (2019). Substance abuse in rural areas-innovations webpage. Rural Health Information Hub 11/1. Retrieved 11/24/2019 from https://www.ruralhealthinfo.org/topics/substance-abuse/project-examples
- SAMSHA. n.d. Medication-Assisted Therapy. Retrieved 10/10/2019 from https://www.samhsa.gov/medication-assisted-treatment

Tool Box of Rural Mental Health Resources

- U.S. Bureau of the Census. n.d. Rural America, a story map. Web page. Retrieved 11/14/19 from https://gis-portal.data.census.gov/arcgis/apps/MapSeries/index.html?appid=7a41374f6b03456e9d138cb014711e01

APPENDIX B: HUMAN TRAFFICKING REPORTING RESOURCES

Agencies assisting victims of human trafficking, include, but are not limited to:

- National Human Trafficking Hotline, https://humantraffickinghotline.org/ (888) 373-7888
- Trafficking in Persons and Worker Exploitation Task Force www.justice.gov/actioncenter/crime.html#trafficking Hotline: (888) 428-7581, funded by the U.S. Department of Justice; direct calls to federal law enforcement from 9:00 am to 5:00 pm EST on weekdays.

APPENDIX C: SUCCESSFUL MODELS OF DELIVERY OF MENTAL HEALTH AND SUBSTANCE USE CARE

HRSA grants to enhance the mental health workforce by training dual certified FNP and PMHNP advance practice nurses. Programs were designed to build a workforce that could serve the rural populations. Both the University of Tennessee Health Science Center, Memphis Tennessee and the University of Nebraska Medical Center, Omaha, were only two among many university Programs of Nursing recipients which successfully graduated multiple cohorts of these stellar professionals who did go forward to serve in underserved rural populations in both roles across the nation.

Suicide Prevention Programs (CDC, n.d.):

- North Dakota Sources of Strength; Rural communities and Northern Plains tribes, through adult and school engagement
- Oregon: The Rural Telemental Health program; An outreach of the Portland Veterans Administration Medical Center reaching veterans of OR, ID, and WA states through telemental access via VA outpatient clinics or "it home" if resources permit
- New Mexico: Adolescent Suicide Prevention Program; Since 1990, designed for one tribe in collaboration with the Indian Health Service, the tribal council and community, addressing suicidal risk in young people in an unconventional yet culturally appropriate manner using a strong focus on family trauma history

Helping Kids PROSPER: A program delivery system, guides communities implementing evidence-based programs to build youth competencies, improve family functioning, prevent risky behaviors, particularly substance use for youth and families in rural communities.

keepin' it REAL Rural: A drug and alcohol prevention program for middle school students specific to rural culture of Pennsylvania and Ohio to have a reduction in all substance use and less personal acceptability of substance use.

Vermont Hub-and-Spoke Model of Care for Opioid Use Disorder: Provide access to MAT for opioid use disorder in rural Vermont and effect statewide treatment capacity and care coordination.

Midcoast Maine Prescription Opioid Reduction Program: Reduce number of emergency department dental patients abusing opioid prescriptions in rural southeastern Maine by adopting an opioid prescription guideline with opioid prescribing and emergency room visits for dental pain decreased from 26 to 21 per 1,000/year.

Strong African American Families–Teen Program: Rural, locally trained leaders administered five two-hour meetings for teenagers/primary caregivers focused on reducing risks that prevent positive development, specifically sexual risk-taking leading to HIV and other STIs. Results: Reduced conduct problems, depressive symptoms, and substance abuse, families were strengthened. Better birth control adherence.

Federal Office of Rural Health Policy Madison Outreach and Services through

Telehealth (MOST) Network: Increased mental health and substance abuse prevention and treatment services in rural Texas bringing telehealth counseling services and community health workers to Brazos Valley, Texas. Results: The program improved health outcomes, increased general knowledge of the impact of SU, and raised awareness of services among Hispanic residents.

Project Lazarus: Reduction of overdose-related deaths among prescription opioid users in rural Wilkes County, North Carolina, through eEducation and tools provided for prescribers, patients, and community members to lessen drug supply/demand, and reduce harm in prescription opioid use with opioid overdose death rates have decreased in Wilkes County.

Federal Office of Rural Health Policy: Nurse Navigator and Recovery Specialist Outreach Program to address/treat patients with concurrent substance abuse/chronic healthcare issues using a referral system that utilizes community health workers (CHWs) in a drug and alcohol treatment setting. AN RN helps with provider MAT programs which reduced hospital emergency visits/ hospital readmissions for patients since inception.

Communities that Care (CTC) Coalition: A way to improve health/well-being of young people by addressing SU in rural areas of Massachusetts' Franklin County and the North Quabbin. A community-based prevention initiative reducing youth violence, delinquency, alcohol/tobacco use, promoting proper nutrition/ physical activity. Results: CTC has significant SU reductions in local youth in 30 rural towns served.

Contingency Management Smoking Cessation in Appalachia: Reduce smoking rates of pregnant women/adolescents in Appalachian regions of eastern KY and OH with web-based smoking cessation program offering monetary incentives to reducing smoking. Participants significantly reduced smoking rates or quit altogether.

Federal Office of Rural Health Policy Northern Dental Access Center Patient Support and Outreach Program: Connect low-income people in rural NW Minnesota to dental care/support services to address barriers to care. Partners work together to provide patient transportation, care coordination, insurance navigation and enrollment yielding patients accessing support services are likely to complete dental treatment. With > 1,000 people/year assisted with Medicaid enrollment, reported use of emergency department for dental pain reduced.

Federal Office of Rural Health Policy Healthy Outcomes Integration Team: Provides integrated treatment planning/coordinated healthcare services to rural residents with the Healthy Outcomes Integration Team. Treat adults with serious mental health condition s/those who have, or are at risk of developing, chronic health conditions. Coordinated care SU treatment, crisis services, and wellness planning were received with improved physical health outcomes.

Federal Office of Rural Health Policy Cross-Walk: Integrating Behavioral Health and Primary Care addressing/treating SU and depression in Upper Great Lakes region. Using "Cross-Walk", a program integrating behavioral healthcare into primary care services, was developed in Michigan's Marquette County. Collaborative efforts strengthened care management services in local healthcare facilities as primary care patients were referred to a behavioral health specialist.

Integrated Chronic Pain Treatment and Training Project (ICPTTP): To reduce NC prescription opioid misuse/overdoses. ICPTTP standardizes/streamlines chronic pain management in primary care clinics. The ICPTTP has reduced patient average morphine equivalent daily dose, and 29% of patients have successfully tapered off chronic opioid therapy.

Federal Office of Rural Health Policy 4P's Plus Pregnancy Support Project: Provision of pregnancy support services for Native American women struggling with SU use implementing an integrated behavioral health network in Lake County, California with fewer Native American neonatal exposure to alcohol, tobacco, and other drugs.

Isanti County SafeCab Program: Reduced number of deaths and injuries caused by DUI (Driving Under the Influence) in Isanti County using the SafeCab program and providing alternative transportation home for bar patrons who would otherwise drive impaired. Is credited with significant decrease in DUI arrests and lower average corresponding BAC (Blood Alcohol Content) levels in Isanti County.

Staggered Sentencing for Repeat Drunk Driving Offenders: Reduce incidences of repeat DUI by awarding staggered sentence, allowing sentence serving in segments of time, separated by several months to a year. Offenders file a motion to request a waiver for the remaining sentence period(s), if able to show sobriety maintained. Incidence of recidivism, or crime relapse, has been reduced among offenders given staggered sentences, by comparison to offenders given traditional DUI sentences, reducing average cost of jail time otherwise served with full sentence

The Mission's Pregnancy Support Center: Helps opioid-dependent/recovering pregnant women in rural TN. Women and partners can earn points to spend on essential items (bottles, diapers, and maternity clothes). Pregnancy Support Center has increased attendance.

Tobacco Use Prevention and Control (TUPAC) Program: reduces non-ceremonial use of tobacco among American Indians in NM by providing outreach, community programs, and cessation services. 139 people have received cessation services, and 7 rural communities received an award to work on cigarette/e-cigarette policy changes.

Recovery-Oriented System of Care (ROSOC): Serve adults in Mendocino County, CA with chronic SU disorders, mental health diagnoses, and/or complex medical conditions who frequently utilize emergency departments/jail services. A safety net organization works with providers/law enforcement reducing high cost of caring for frequent utilizers through intensive care coordination activities resulting in greater overall stability in clients with less utilization of low-efficacy, crisis-oriented services, hospitalizations, and incarcerations.

Morrison County Accountable Community for Health (*ACH*): Combats prescription drug misuse (rural Morrison County, Minnesota) bringing together primary care, social/support. As much as 40% reduction in number of prescribed opioids, and tapered 684 patients off opioids completely.

Health Resources Services Administration New Horizons Substance Use Recovery Network: In northern Michigan, need for an integrated approach to deliver MAT for established patients of Federally Qualified Health Centers with opioid use disorder using collaboration between one FQHC across three sites, a local waivered prescriber group, and a behavioral health organization creating an integrated treatment approach for opioid use disorder. Results included increased access to MAT/comprehensive SU disorder services leading to increased retention in treatment/ increased engagement in stable opioid/alcohol use recovery disorders.

Federal Office of Rural Health Policy: Funded by the Health Resources Services Administration Project Renew reduced opioid overdose deaths in rural SE West Virginia by training/certifying first responders/healthcare staff/lay people in naloxone administration. Project Renew provided direct education to 120 individuals, completing 173 provider education activities, and distributing 260 Narcan kits.

Project VISION: Reduced opioid use/increased quality of life in Rutland, Vermont by reducing opioid use through community engagement. Collected/disposed 550 pounds of unused medications, reduced thefts over 32%, and 50% improvement on a neighborhood quality of life survey

Seneca Strong's Certified Recovery Peer Advocates: Seneca Nation of Indians has disproportionate rates of opioid, alcohol, and substance misuse. The Seneca Nation Government and Executives founded Seneca Strong, a cultural recovery peer advocate program, to reduce substance misuse across the Nation with 300 people receiving help from recovery peer advocates with a project extension to meet the needs of Allegany and Cattaraugus territories.

Federal Office of Rural Health Policy MIST: Mothers and Infants Sober Together: Addresses the needs of pregnant women using substances and infants born into drug-positive families with the Mothers and Infants Sober Together (MIST) program assisted mothers who used substances are treated and provided a safe, drug-free home for themselves/newborn. MIST helps mothers find treatment/education and helps children grow up in safe/healthy homes.

Rehoboth McKinley Christian Healthcare Services Alcohol and Substance

Abuse Treatment Program: Provides treatment/rehabilitation in rural NM for those with alcohol and SU disorder with high rates of alcohol-related deaths. A reestablished 90-day inpatient Alcohol and Substance Abuse Treatment Program offers clients career readiness/work placement. Program growth from 3 to 69 clients enrolled in inpatient treatment and 32 in work rehabilitation programs with many clients now employed by local businesses.

School-based Drug Misuse Prevention Program: A school-based drug misuse prevention program in Appalachian OH triggered by a high school student's overdose death. Using the HOPE curriculum, in K through 12th grade drug abuse prevention program without further drug overdose deaths after age-appropriate curriculum initiated.

Federal Office of Rural Health Policy On the Move! Unlawful Narcotics Investigations, Treatment and Education (*Operation UNITE*): Illicit drug/alcohol use continues in Central Appalachian region of Kentucky, where many schools have no prevention curriculum. Using engaging simulations/presentations, project delivers SU prevention education to middle/high school students. Post-test surveys show that thousands of students are reached through the "On the Move!" project, gaining positive knowledge of SU dangers.

Federal Office of Rural Health Policy Addiction Recovery Mobile Outreach Team (*ARMOT*): Reduces number of overdoses/overdose-related deaths from opioids in rural Pennsylvania by providing (1) case management/recovery support services to those with SU disorders and (2) education/support to rural hospital staff, patients, and significant others. There were 943 referrals in the first three years of program.

Federal Office of Rural Health Policy Nevada Rural Opioid Overdose Reversal (*NROOR*): reduces number of overdoses/opioid related deaths in rural Nevada with the Nevada Rural Opioid Overdose Reversal (NROOR) Program, led by a Critical Access Hospital (CAH), furnishing naloxone/education on prescription opioid use and overdose. Training of 117 Emergency Medical Technicians (EMTs) on naloxone administration.

Foundations Family Medicine's HIV, HCV, Opioid and Substance Use Disorder Services: Austin, Indiana has seen the largest concentrated outbreak of HIV in rural America's recent history with over 200 residents diagnosed since 2015 HIV. Foundations Family Medicine offered testing/treatment services for HIV, hepatitis C, and opioid/substance use disorder with education, care coordination and behavioral health services also offered as integrated care. The HIV rate has significantly decreased, outdoing national suppression rates by 75%, compared to the national average of 49%.

Federal Office of Rural Health Policy Maine General Harm Reduction Program: Reduces deaths from opioid overdoses in rural Maine through the

Maine General Harm Reduction Program which provides community education/training for healthcare staff/first responders in rural Kennebec/Somerset counties. Maine General trained 45 deputies/246 healthcare staff/educated 60 community members during the grant.

Federal Office of Rural Health Policy SLV N.E.E.D.: Naloxone Education Empowerment Distribution Program: Growing concern in rural Colorado communities regarding prescription/illegal opioid overdoses used health worker/community education, and established a naloxone overdose reversal drug program. Almost all first responders now naloxone administration trained/participating pharmacies keep adequate naloxone stock. Ongoing service region dialogue is sustained to address opioid abuse.

Spit It Out-West Virginia: McDowell County, West Virginia, had high tobacco use rates. The Spit It Out-West Virginia program (2008–2010) was created to increase access to tobacco cessation and prevention resources with hundreds of people provided tobacco cessation efforts, five workplaces became tobacco free, and tobacco control efforts have been sustained.

The Dawn Center Intensive Outpatient Program: Treats SU in rural South Carolina avoiding expensive inpatient facilities, including a treatment aim of keeping patients in home communities offering an outpatient program for SU patients. Patients receive/treatment closer to home and are incorporated into the local recovery community.

Pathways Vermont Housing First Program: Provides housing for the chronically homeless facing mental health and/or substance abuse challenges in rural VT. Rural Housing First program provides access to permanent rental housing/numerous services to sustain housing stability. Participants report decreased undomiciled time/improvement in their standard of living.

CHAPTER 12

Turn Left at the Yellow House: Challenges of Northern, Frontier, Rural, and Remote Nursing Practice

Julianne Sanguins

Objectives:

1. Identify the health delivery needs in Northern/Frontier delivery systems.
2. Discuss legal and technical issues/conflicts that may arise in Northern/Frontier health delivery
3. Describe nursing practice in Northern/Frontier settings.

Discussion Questions:

1. What appeals to you about nursing in a northern/frontier location?
2. What challenges would you anticipate encountering if you decided to practice in a northern/frontier location?
3. How could you prepare to address these challenges?
4. Understanding their context, if you established your nursing practice in a northern/frontier location, how could you advocate for your patients?

INTRODUCTION

Imagine you step off the plane and realize that you really are above the tree line! This may be the first, but it certainly will not be the last surprise that practicing in a northern/frontier community will have in store for you. Arriving as a new staff person in a northern/frontier setting will afford you with stories to tell your grandchildren for years. This chapter provides context for northern/frontier settings as well as reflection on the rewards and challenges of nursing in non-urban locations from the perspective of nurses working in northern/frontier/rural/remote settings. Professional and personal aspects of nursing practice will be considered. While different resources and infrastructures exist depending on locale, each such practice setting has similar characteristics.

BACKGROUND

Definition of Rural/Remote/Northern

A multitude of different definitions describe northern/frontier/rural/remote settings. Definitions are determined by population density, factors of geography (distance and topography), and the availability of human and other health resources (Registered Nurses Association of Ontario, 2015), as well as by characteristics of nursing practice (Kulig *et al.*, 2008). Although remote communities may be a considerable geographic distance from urban settings, they still may have access to some resources. Typically, remote communities are accessible year-round only by air or by ice roads in the winter (Government of Canada, 2018). Frontier nursing is nursing practice in the United States in areas where health services, particularly midwifery, cannot be easily accessed (Raines *et al.*, 1996). Northern settings are communities defined by geographical location, for example above the 53′ latitude (Manitoba Health, Seniors and Active Living, n.d.). Rural settings are communities that are outside of commuting distance of towns and cities larger than 10,000 (duPlessis *et al.*, 2001; Van Hofwegen *et al.*, 2005). Clearly, there is some overlap in these definitions as, for example, a community may be remote, remote/frontier, or northern, as well as rural. For the purpose of this chapter, the term northern/frontier will be used to capture the characteristics of each of these practice settings.

Each of these settings has aspects of nursing practice in common. However, in all of these settings, there are few practitioners—you may be the only or one of a few staff, you typically will have fewer resources, and you will be far from your friends and family. Each of these aspects will influence your practice.

BENEFITS OF NORTHERN/FRONTIER NURSING PRACTICE

As a nurse or a nurse practitioner, practicing in northern/frontier settings affords a variety of professional and personal benefits. These benefits include your scope of practice and feelings of satisfaction and accomplishment in your achievements. Some professional and personal benefits of practicing in northern/frontier settings are expanded upon in the following paragraphs.

Professional Benefits

Holistic Practice

As a student, the concept of holistic practice, or viewing your patient as an entire person rather than a disease process, is typically entrenched in the curriculum. Holistic care is described as consideration of the complete person—including physical, emotional, mental, and spiritual aspects (Huljev and Pandak, 2016)—as well as the person's environment. Practice in northern/frontier communities promotes holistic practice for individual patients and provides opportunities for community development and health promotion that are holistic and grounded in community context (Van Hofwegen *et al.*, 2005).

Full Scope of Practice

Not only is practice in northern/frontier settings holistic, but it also offers practitioners the opportunity to practice within the full scope of their skill sets (MacLeod, *et al.*, 2019a). When working in urban settings, practitioners typically develop one area of expertise such as labor and delivery or public health. In northern/frontier practice, you are called upon to exercise all your assessment skills in a whole range of situations while exercising rigorous clinical judgement. You may be the emergency response, midwife, community health, and palliative care nurse in a community—all in the same day. Students who have the opportunity to engage in rural preceptorships are able to practice more skills than had they been in an urban setting (Van Hofwegen *et al.*, 2005).

Autonomy

Practice in northern/frontier settings offers an extensive opportunity for independent practice and decision making (Van Hofwegen *et al.*, 2005). Clinical practice guidelines, registration bodies' guidelines, and employers' policy and procedure manuals all provide parameters for your practice but when you are in the air in a medevac plane, or alone at the nursing station, decision making is up to you.

Interpersonal Teamwork

Another noticeable hallmark of northern/frontier practice is working together tightly as a team (Van Hofwegen *et al.*, 2005). You may be one of only a few nurses, but the other people working within your health center such as community health representatives also are integral members of your health team.

Personal Benefits

Personal Satisfaction

Coming from Generations X, Y, or Z, newly graduated nurses and soon-to-be graduated students seek to make a difference in the world (Lavoie-Tremblay *et al.*, 2010). This need to be altruistic can be readily satisfied in northern/frontier practice where continuity of care is demonstrable. Continuity of care refers to community members consistently receiving care from the same provider(s) who are familiar with them as individuals, as well as with their health history and personal context (Reid *et al.*, 2002). Continuity of care ensures that quality healthcare is being provided to patients, and also that relationships are built between care providers and patients. Continuity of care offers a source of satisfaction for northern/frontier practitioners (Bushy, 2002) who can see the difference they are making in people's lives and the results of their care.

A Bigger Fish in the Pond

As you will be well known in the community you will be offered opportunities for involvement that you might not otherwise have had. For example, you may be asked to organize or be a judge at the Science Fair or to lead a parade. You may also be asked to represent northern/frontier interests in journals or on editorial boards. These are benefits you may not have had as readily in urban centers.

Relationships

When you move to a new community to practice, you are frequently venturing out on your own. This may seem intimidating but, in reality, you will be quickly absorbed into the social life of your community. You will meet kindred spirits who also have a sense of adventure. Many of these new relationships will last well into the future.

"Travel the World"

For those with an adventurous spirit, working in northern/frontier settings offers a chance to see parts of the world and to participate in activities you may never have seen or done on your own. For some practitioners, these opportunities meet their need for work-life balance. Imagine kayaking on the Nahanni River, or mushing (dog sledding) in Juneau, Alaska, or viewing the spectacular Aurora Borealis in Nunavut, or hiking in the Weminuche Wilderness in Colorado or ...well, the choices are endless. Nurses and Nurse Practitioners are in high demand in all of these settings, so you just have to decide to go: close your eyes, point to the map, and embark on your adventure.

CHALLENGES OF NORTHERN/FRONTIER NURSING

Accompanying the benefits of norther/frontier nursing there are challenges that you can expect to encounter. These include systemic challenges as well as professional and personal challenges. Meeting and overcoming these obstacles will often necessitate that you think outside the box and be innovative.

Systemic

Equipment

When you move your practice from an urban to a northern/frontier setting the equipment you may be working with may not be as current as the equipment to which you are accustomed (Hunsberger *et al.*, 2009). For example, the incubator or IV pump may be the prototype rather than the newest 7.0 version. Accurate placement of tubes may be determined by using your assessment skills rather than by ultrasound. This aspect of your practice will require you to be innovative, creative, and resilient. To meet such systemic challenges, necessity will be the mother of invention.

Space Utilization

In most urban settings, and certainly in most contemporary hospitals and health centers, space is purpose-built. In contrast, buildings in northern/frontier settings typically have been constructed to address weather constraints and to fit within budget parameters with accessibility being a secondary consideration. Your equipment and supplies may be stowed in inconvenient places. Space utilization is a systemic challenge you are likely to encounter (Hunsberger *et al.*, 2009). Remember, if they can manage in the space station (Papali, 2016), so can you!

Technology Challenges

Technology has enhanced practice (MacLeod *et al.*, 2019a) but distribution is uneven. In many sites, access to computers and telehealth are readily accessible. In some communities, however, bandwidth is problematic. Other communities may lack cell towers and even basic telephone coverage may prove to be sketchy. Dead zones may be typical. This uneven distribution may cause practice challenges and frustration for those who are well versed with technology and accustomed to using the internet as a source of current practice information. The technological challenges faced daily by nurses and Nurse Practitioners in northern/frontier settings cannot be overstated (Hunsberger *et al.*, 2009). Technological challenges can range from connectivity issues to being able to have broken equipment repaired. You may be unable to transmit ECG tracings for a second opinion. You may not be able to receive FAXed discharge information on people returning home to your community from treatment at a tertiary hospital, or information on follow-up appointments. Accessing telehealth is not an option in many sites. On a bad day, even the landline will be down. Despite these technological challenges northern/frontier staff persevere and provide quality care for their community.

Management

Managers and policy makers who are vested with the responsibility of oversight may not understand the realities of rural and remote practice. They may not have enough experience to manage and plan using a contextual lens that is informed by their community and staff. This perspective is invaluable in the development of policies and programs (MacLeod *et al.*, 2004). To overcome the challenges such lack of knowledge can present to nurses and Nurse Practitioners in northern/frontier settings, managers and policy makers who are vested with the responsibility of oversight need to better understand the realities of rural and remote practice.

Professional

Being the Only One

In northern/frontier communities, nurses very often are the only resident provider of healthcare (Hunt *et al.*, 2016; MacLeod *et al.*, 2004; MacLeod, 1999; Zahaman *et al.*, 2016). In some settings, you may have colleagues to consult. In others, it is important to have a system in place that facilitates consultation with physicians or other Nurse Practitioners in urban centers concerning your clinical issues (MacLeod *et al.*, 2004). This resource is important to ensure that you can provide the quality of care you want to deliver. Typically, as you are not the first person to be working there, such a process will already have been established.

Assuming a Leadership Role with Little or No Experience

Practice in a community when you are working alone also means you are the person-in-charge (Luger and Ford, 2019). This presents an additional challenge when you are already negotiating many aspects of your new practice. Remember, advice is only a phone call away. You may also find the answers you need in a book or a DVD that is available in the health center. If you want to make a meaningful difference in people's lives, you will readily embrace this challenge.

Lack of Resources

The lack of resources you have at your disposal may surprise you (MacLeod *et al.*, 2019a; Osterbroek, 2017; Van Hofwegen *et al.*, 2005; Zibrik *et al.*, 2010). For example, the nurse who worked there for many months before you arrived may not have not kept the medications up-to-date and they may all have expired. Alternatively, if an order has been placed, it may not have arrived with dressing supplies or IV bags to replenish your stock.

"Jack of all Trades" or "Being a Specialist at Being a Generalist"

In your new role, you are going to be expected to have, or to develop, a wide range of skills and thereby to become a Jack of All Trades (Hunsberger *et al.*, 2009; MacLeod *et al.*, 2019a; Osterbroek, 2017; Zibrik *et al.*, 2010). To accomplish this, you will need enthusiasm, dexterity, excellent memory retention, and a great deal of patience in your tool chest.

Practice Viewed as "Lesser"

While practitioners in northern/frontier settings play a pivotal role in healthcare delivery in their communities, the role is not necessarily recognized by urban healthcare providers who may view this area of practice as less valuable than their own (MacLeod *et al.*, 2004). This attitude may be experienced as lateral violence when a northern nurse arrives in an urban emergency room after a particularly harrowing Medevac and is criticized for not having completed pristine charting or for having a rumpled "unprofessional" appearance.

Keeping Skills Current/Professional Development

Another challenge of working in northern/frontier settings is ensuring that your skills are current and that you meet the professional development requirements for your license. Staff in these settings have reported difficulties in ensuring their emergency skills are up to date (Medves *et al.*, 2015; Zibrik *et al.*, 2010) and have ascribed this situation to having inadequate or unpredictable access to educational resources (Medves *et al.*, 2015; Osterbroek, 2017).

"Who's the Boss?"

Practitioners are required to maintain active registration and to practice in accordance with nursing association standards of practice, including well-established ethical guidelines. At times there could be an inconsistency between your practice standards—what you know to be right—and your employer's expectations. This gap can be addressed by engaging in upstream information gathering. For example, do your due diligence and research potential employers prior to accepting job offers to ensure they have not previously demonstrated a habit of placing practitioners in awkward or unethical positions.

"Do You have to be Psychic?"

Nurses practicing in remote/frontier settings play a central role in natural disasters (MacLeod *et al.*, 2019a). You may be alerted by the Forest Rangers or police that a natural disaster is imminent. Predicting when an extreme weather event or forest fire will happen is beyond your control but when one happens you will be sought after to coordinate efforts to ensure the people in your community are safe. Although a disaster plan may be in place for your community, the information in it may not be current. If so, you will need to draw on any local resources you have at your disposal, such as the Community Health Representative, in order to respond. In the event that a mass evacuation is necessary, everyone in the community will need to be accounted for. This task will often fall to you. In addition, the community members will need to have enough medication to last for a few days. Eventually, the Federal Emergency Management Agency (FEMA) or the Red Cross will be available to ensure shelter and food are available, but in the first stage of a community-wide emergency, you are likely the first, and sometimes the second, responder.

Community disasters create a great deal of responsibility and occupational stress for practitioners in northern/frontier environments (Jahner *et al.*, 2019). Little has been written on the topic; however, pre-disaster preparation, such as ensuring plans are up to date and establishing strong communication channels, can help alleviate some of the chaos ensuing from community disasters. Critical incident debriefing to support nurses after disasters can be of assistance in mitigating the cumulative effects of this stress (Kulig *et al.*, 2017).

Working Beyond Scope of Practice

As previously noted, one of the benefits of northern/frontier practice is working to the full scope of your practice. In some situations, this situation may also present a challenge. Some practitioners have found that they worked beyond the full scope of their practice. Contributing factors have included working in a fly-in community, being a long distance from a tertiary care center, having lower staffing levels, and being required to be on call. All these factors have led to nurses reporting that they were working beyond their scope of practice (MacLeod *et al.*, 2019b). Consistently working beyond your scope of practice can be a source of stress for practitioners and may impact the effectiveness and quality of care you are able provide (MacLeod *et al.*, 2019b).

Personal

"Everyone Knows Your Name"

This feeling can also be referred to as "living in a fish bowl" (MacLeod *et al.*, 2019a; Zibrik *et al.*, 2010). As you are both a health professional and a community member (MacLeod *et al.*, 2019a; MacLeod *et al.*, 2004; Osterbroek *et al.*, 2019), you are under constant observation in small communities (Bushy, 2002). From the time you arrive in a community, everyone will know who you are and likely what you have been doing as well. Imagine standing in line at local store while everyone around you is looking at what you are buying as you are expected to be a role model for health and wellness.

You Are on Duty All the Time

Due to your position in the community you are on the duty all the time. All. The. Time. Even after your shift is over, or the health center is closed and you are not on call, when you are out in the community you will be approached by community members regarding their health issues (Zibrik *et al.*,

2010). Establishing boundaries is a delicate process that requires sensitivity to preclude sacrificing your developing professional relationships in the community.

Ethics

The codes of ethics under which nurses and Nurse Practitioners are bound include the principles of privacy and confidentiality (American Nurses Association, 2017; Canadian Nurses Association, 2017). Practice in northern/frontier settings places you in situations in which it is very difficult to maintain confidentiality (MacLeod, 1999; Zibrik *et al.*, 2010). Staff who work with you in the health center may want access to another community member's private health information or you may see someone you treated for an STI in the morning on the street with a different partner in the evening. From an individual perspective, knowledge of the context of the community such as spiritual beliefs may result in supporting patient and family care choices that are at odds with one's personal ethics (Cook *et al.*, 2001).

Isolation

Typically, working in northern/frontier settings means that you are far away from family or at least your extended family and friends (Hunsberger *et al.*, 2009; Van Hofwegen *et al.*, 2005). Although you will make new friends in your new community, it is not unusual to long for what you were used to. Remember to practice holistically on yourself as well. Ensure you have physical supports in the community, whatever spiritual supports you need, and emotional support by calling/videoconferencing home to talk to your family or friends.

Job Satisfaction

When you arrive and start working in your northern/frontier role, it may not exactly fit the picture you had in your head of what your new life would be. When experiencing this cognitive dissonance coupled with assuming your new responsibility, it is not unusual to feel overwhelmed and dissatisfied (Dowdle-Simmons, 2013). Satisfaction with your new job is an important factor in retention (Manahan Roberge and Lavoie, 2007; Stewart *et al.*, 2005). As you become more familiar with your role, your comfort level and job satisfaction will increase.

Self-Care

Strategies that you used to take care of yourself when you lived in urban settings may not always be available to you in your new home. Therapeutic shopping, pedicures, yoga classes, or paint ball might not accessible. This will be your opportunity to develop new self-care strategies or to adapt your old ones. For example, you could take up painting, try yoga DVDs, or enlist a walking companion from the community.

POLICY

Several policy changes could be implemented to increase the numbers of nurses prepared to practice in northern/frontier settings, and to support those who are working there to promote retention of the workforce. These policy changes could be implemented by educational institutions, employers, and governmental bodies. Policy makers must be made aware that northern/frontier nurses walk in two worlds: they are both community members and healthcare providers. When creating and implementing new policy, the northern/frontier practitioners must be included at the table.

Education

The first set of policy recommendations is related to the education of nurses and Nurse Practitioners. There is an overwhelming need for undergraduate and postgraduate education programs to prepare students to practice in northern/frontier settings (MacLeod *et al.*, 2004; Van Hofwegen *et al.*, 2005; World Health Organization [WHO], 2010), which must be addressed. Students who have had an opportunity to work in northern/frontier areas are more likely to work there upon graduation (Edwards *et al.*, 2004; Yonge *et al.*, 2006). Locating professional educational programs, especially nursing, nurse practitioner, and medical schools, in northern/frontier areas will graduate healthcare professionals, many of whom will ultimately work in northern/frontier sites. Further, the WHO (2010) advocates implementing admission policies that attract students from these areas to foster the probability of them practicing in northern/frontier areas upon graduation.

Curriculum needs to be revised to include topics that are informed by communities to ensure their needs are met (WHO, 2010). Revisions should also be informed by the experiences of health practitioners (Kulig *et al.*, 2004). To accomplish this, dedicated funding is required to develop or adapt curriculum (MacLeod *et al.*, 2004). While some programs do offer northern/frontier consolidated practice options at the end of their program, such as one-day rural clinical experiences, or online post-graduate certificate programs, these provisions are insufficient to meet the need. More nursing, nurse practitioner, and medical schools' programs should offer a northern/frontier stream in their programs in order to prepare students for practice upon graduation in these settings. Northern/frontier placements for students should be accompanied by financial incentives to offset the additional costs of the placement for the student. Many students would be more likely to embrace these opportunities if they did not have to pay out-of-pocket for transportation and accommodation.

In addition to preparing Registered Nurses and Nurse Practitioners, colleges and universities must also design programs to meet the continuing education and professional development needs of northern/frontier nurses. The content must not only be relevant but also be accessible to them in several ways (MacLeod *et al.*, 2004).

Workplace Implications

It has been established that students who experience positive northern/frontier clinical placements are more likely to seek employment in those settings (Finlayson *et al.*, 2002). Accordingly, it is incumbent on employers to ensure that placement opportunities are created and supported for students to experience practicing in that environment.

Next, incentives must be created to attract nurses to rural/remote settings (WHO, 2010). Incentives offered must extend beyond attractive employment packages and on-boarding programs. Incentives must consider the immediate and ongoing realities of the nurses, including factors such as relocation expenses, subsidized housing, access to childcare (Francis and Mills, 2011), and retention bonuses. Incentives should recognize that the three most important recruitment factors for new staff have been identified as location of community, interest in the practice setting, and income (MacLeod *et al.*, 2019a).

Once new staff assume roles in northern/frontier settings, supports need to be in place to ensure their success (Duffield *et al.*, 2002). Generally, new graduate transition programs have been effective in increasing competency and confidence in novice practitioners (Rush *et al.*, 2019). Such programs have also been identified to be beneficial for new staff in northern/frontier settings (Osterbroek, 2017), especially those that offer mentoring. Providing cultural programming such as that offered by Navajoland Nurses United for Research, Service, and Education, Inc. (Crow *et al.*, 2011) will ensure that new staff are aware of the cultural context that exists in their community, and that they are given the tools to be culturally competent in their practice.

Among the many factors related to staff retention are lack of work flexibility, stress, and demanding on-call requirements (MacLeod *et al.*, 2019a). Employers need to recognize and address their resource limitations. While it may not be possible to increase the size of the health center, or to increase bandwidth, alternative opportunities for ongoing professional development can be provided (Hunt and Hunt, 2016; MacLeod *et al.*, 2008; WHO, 2010). Dedicated time and financial support for professional development will increase retention of new staff (Mbemba *et al.*, 2013). This aspect is especially critical for northern/frontier nurses who have not always had access to the quantity and quality of professional development resources and activities as their urban counterparts (Francis *et al.*, 2011; Hunt *et al.*, 2016).

Northern and frontier populations are largely constituted in the United States by American Indian/Alaskan Inuit and in Canada by First Nations, Metis and Inuit populations along with European settlers. Nursing staff who work in predominantly Aboriginal communities need to have particular, specific, and ongoing orientation to ensure they are providing culturally appropriate care (Hunsberger *et al.*, 2009; MacLeod *et al.*, 2004). Targeted efforts to recruit Aboriginal nurses and Nurse Practitioners to these communities are also necessary to better meet the needs of culturally competent care (Zahaman *et al.*, 2016).

Governmental Considerations

Shortage of Health Professionals

There is a worldwide shortage of nurses and Nurse Practitioners (Council of State Governments, 2011). Nowhere is this situation more apparent than in northern/frontier workplaces. This shortage demands a concerted effort on the part of governmental departments to create a national rural health workforce framework. Features of this framework would include a commitment to invest in development of the workforce in terms of recruitment and retention policies (WHO, 2010).

Regarding preparation of and support for managers concomitant with the shortage of northern/frontier practitioners, there is a shortage of qualified managers who are equipped to manage in these settings. Similarly, there is a lack of resources to support these managers once they have assumed their roles. To address this shortfall, it is recommended that targeted recruitment occur for experienced managers, and that a combination of advisory boards with the local community as well regularly scheduled consultative meetings be established to support the managers.

Dedicated funding in order for colleges and universities to revise curricula, and for workplaces to bolster their onboarding and retention benefits for staff, core funding needs to be provided. Such funding would create an environment that provides room for implementation and evaluation of different approaches. Creating a loan forgiveness program would attract more students in pursuing northern/frontier practice upon graduation (Hunt *et al.*, 2016).

CONCLUSION

Whether your northern/frontier practice lasts only for the term of your contract commitment or becomes an avocation, you will have many experiences that will leave a lasting impression: an expanded skill base, increased clinical competence and confidence, babies named after you, life-long friends, and achievement of dreams few nurses will experience. Regardless of how small a role you may think you played in that community; you can be certain you have made a difference. The experience of providing cradle-to-grave care, advocating for cleaner water, or advocating for food and nutrition security, provides satisfaction that cannot be achieved in urban practice. Creating a space and a place for a northern/frontier practice in your career path will be a decision you will always remember and never regret.

REFERENCES

American Nurses Association. (2015). *The Code of Ethics for Nurses with Interpretive Statements* (*The Code*). Silver Spring, MD: American Nurses Association.

Bushy, A. (2002). International perspectives on rural nursing: Australia, Canada, USA. *Australian Journal of Rural Health, 10*, 104–111.

Canadian Nurses Association. (2013). *Code of Ethics for Registered Nurses*. Ottawa, ON: Canadian Nurses Association.

Cook, A. F., H. Hoas, and J. C. Joyner. (2001). No secrets on Main Street: Challenges to ethically sound care in the rural setting. *American Journal of Nursing, 101*(8), 67–71.

Council of State Governments. (2011). *Health Care Workforce Shortages Critical in Rural America, Capitol Facts & Figures*. Lexington, KY: The Council of State Governments. Retrieved April 27, 2020, from https://knowledgecenter.csg.org/kc/system/files/Health_Care_Workforce_Shortages_Critical_in_Rural_America.pdf.

Crow, K., M. M. Conger, and U. Knoki-Wilson. (2011). Mentorship for nursing in a rural area: A program for success for working with diverse populations. *Online Journal of Rural Nursing and Health Care, 11*(2), 43–50.

Dowdle-Simmons, S. (2013). Educational strategies for rural new graduate registered nurses. *Journal of Continuing Education in Nursing, 44*(3), 107–110. doi: 10.3928/00220124-20121217-94.

duPlessis, V., *et al.* (2001). Definitions of rural. *Rural and Small Town Canada Analysis Bulletin, 3*(3), 1–61. Retrieved April 27, 2020, from https://www150.statcan.gc.ca/n1/en/pub/21-006-x/21-006-x2001003-eng.pdf?st=yCllTyIB.

Edwards, H., *et al.* (2004). The impact of clinical placement location on nursing students' competence and preparedness for practice. *Nurse Education Today, 24*, 248–255. doi: 10.1016/j.nedt.2004.01.003

Finlayson, K., *et al.* (2002). The impact of rural clinical placement on student nurses' employment intention. *The Collegian, 9*(1), 12–18. doi: https://doi.org/10.1016/s1322-7696(08)60039-6

Francis, K. L., and J. E. Mills. (2011). Sustaining and growing the rural nursing and midwifery workforce: Understanding the issues and isolating directions for the future. *Collegian: Journal of the Royal College of Nursing, Australia, 18*, 55–60. doi: 10.1016/j.colegn.2010.08.003

Government of Canada. (2018). *Life in a Rural and/or Remote Isolated First Nations Community*. Retrieved April 27, 2020 from https://www.sac-isc.gc.ca/eng/1572875474507/1572875497971

Huljev, D., and Pandak, T. (2016). Holistic and team approach in health care. *Signa Vitae, 11*(Suppl 2), 66–69. http://dx.doi.org/10.22514/SV112.062016.1

Hunsberger, M., *et al.* (2009). Sustaining the rural workforce: Nursing perspectives on worklife challenges. *Journal of Rural Health, 25*(1), 17–25. doi:10.1111/j.1748-0361.2009.00194.x

Hunt, S., and E. Hunt. (2016). Barriers to practice of rural and remote nursing in Canada. *European Scientific Journal, 12*(36), 56–59. doi: 10.19044/esj.2016.v12n36p56

Jahner, S., K. Penz, and N. J. Stewart. (2019). Psychological impact of traumatic events in rural nursing practice: An integrative review. *Online Journal of Rural Nursing and Health Care, 19*(1), 105–135.

Kulig, J. C., *et al.* (2008). How do registered nurses define rurality? *Australian Journal of Rural Health, 16*(1), 28–32. doi: 10.1111/j.1440-1584.2007.00947.x

Kulig, J. C., *et al.* (2004). Maximizing the involvement of rural nurses in policy. *Canadian Journal of Nursing Leadership, 17*(1), 88–96.

Kulig, J. C., *et al.* (2017). Experiences of rural and remote nurses assisting with disasters. *Australasian Emergency Nursing Journal, 20*(2), 98–106. https://doi.org/10.1016/j.aenj.2017.04.003

Lavoie-Tremblay, M., *et al.* (2010). The needs and expectations of Generation Y nurses in the workplace. Journal for Nurses in Professional Development, 26(1), 2–8.

Luger, S. J., and D. J. Ford. (2019). A pilot quality improvement project facilitating clinical leadership skills in rural new graduate nurses. *Online Journal of Nursing and Health Care, 19*(1), 136–158. https://doi.org/10.14574/0jrnhc.v19i1.544

MacLeod, M. L. P., J. C. Kulig, and N. Stewart. (2019a). Lessons from 20 years of research on nursing practice in rural and remote Canada. Canadian Nurse. Retrieved April 27, 2020, from https://canadian-nurse.com/en/articles/issues/2019/may-2019/lessons-from-20-years-of-research-on-nursing-practice-in-rural-and-remote-canada

MacLeod, M. L. P., *et al.* (2019b). Rural and remote Registered Nurses' perceptions of working beyond their legislated scope of practice. *Nursing Leadership, 32*(1), 20–29.

MacLeod, M. L. P., *et al.* (2008). "I'm a different kind of nurse": Advice from rural and remote Canada. *Nursing Leadership, 21*(3), 40–53.

MacLeod, M. L. P., *et al.* (2004). *The Nature of Nursing Practice in Rural and Remote Canada. Final Report to the Canadian Health Services Research Foundation*. Retrieved April 27, 2020, from https://www.unbc.ca/sites/default/files/sections/rural-nursing/en/17-rrnfinalreport.pdf

MacLeod, M. L. P. (1999). "We're it": Issues and realities in rural nursing practice. In W. Ramp, J. Kulig, I. Townshend, and V. McGowan (Eds.). *Health in Rural Settings: Contexts for Action* (pp. 165–178). Lethbridge, AB: University of Lethbridge Press.

Manahan Roberge, C. and J. Lavoie. (2007). Who stays in rural practice? An international review of the literature on factors influencing rural nurse retention. *Online Journal of Rural Nursing and Health Care, 9*(1), 42–53. https://doi.org/10.14574/ojrnhc.v9i1.107

Manitoba Health, Seniors and Active Living. (n.d.). *Northern Patient Transportation Program*. Retrieved April 27, 2020, from https://www.gov.mb.ca/health/ems/nptp.html.

Medves, J., *et al.* (2015). Supporting rural nurses: Skills and knowledge to practice in

Ontario, Canada. *Online Journal of Rural Nursing and Health Care, 15*(1), 7–41. https://doi.org/10.14574/ojrnhc.v15i1.337

Mbemba, G., *et al.* (2013). Interventions for supporting nurse retention in rural and remote areas: An umbrella review. *Human Resources for Health, 11*(44), 1–9. doi: 10.1186/1478-4491-11-44

Osterbroek, T. A., O. Yonge, and F. Myrick. (2019). "Everybody knows your name": Experiences of belonging in rural preceptorship. *Online Journal of Rural Nursing and Health Care, 19*(1), 64–88. https://doi.org/10.14574/ojrnhc.v19i1.548

Osterbroek, T. A. (2017). *Challenges and Opportunities of Rural Nursing Preceptorship: A Photovoice Perspective*. Unpublished doctoral dissertation. Edmonton, AB: University of Alberta.

Papali, A. (2016). Providing health care in rural and remote areas: Lessons from the International Space Station. *Bulletin of the World Health Organization, 94*, 73–74.

Raines, K. H. and A. Wilson. (1996). Frontier Nursing Service: A Historical Perspective on Nurse-Managed Care. *Journal of Community Health Nursing, 13*(2), 123–127. doi: 10.1207/s15327655jchn1302_5

Reid, R., J. Haggerty, and R. McKendry. (2002). *Defusing the Confusion: Concepts and Measures of Continuity of Healthcare*. Ottawa, ON: Canadian Health Services Research Foundation. Retrieved April 27, 2020, from https://www.cfhi-fcass.ca/Migrated/PDF/ResearchReports/CommissionedResearch/cr_contcare_e.pdf.

Rush, K. L., *et al.* (2019). Best practices of formal new graduate transition programs: An integrative review. *International Journal of Nursing Studies, 94*, 139–158. doi: 10.1016/j.ijnurstu.2019.02.010.

Van Hofwegen, L., S. Kirkham, and C. Harwood. (2005). The strength of rural nursing: Implications for undergraduate nursing education. *International Journal of Nursing Education Scholarship, 2*(1), Article 27.

World Health Organization [WHO]. (2010). *Increasing Access to Health Workers in Remote and Rural Areas Through Improved Retention: Global Policy Recommendations*. Geneva, SW: World Health Organization. Retrieved April 27, 2020, from https://www.who.int/hrh/retention/guidelines/en/.

Yonge, O., L. Ferguson, and F. Myrick (2006). Preceptorship placements in western rural Canadian settings: Perceptions of nursing students and preceptors. *Online Journal of Rural Nursing and Health Care, 6*(2) [17 pp.].

Zahaman, Z., D. Holmes, and L. Chartrand (2016). An opportunity for healing and holistic care exploring the roles of health care providers working within northern Canadian Aboriginal communities. *Journal of Holistic Nursing, 20*(10), 1–13. doi: 10.1177/0898010116650773

Zibrik, K. J., M. MacLeod, and L. V. Zimmer. (2010). Professionalism in rural acute-care nursing. *Canadian Journal of Nursing Research, 42*(1), 20–36.

CHAPTER 13

Rural Veterans: Implications for Nursing Practice

Angeline Bushy

Objectives:

1. Compare and contrast rural/urban characteristics of United States veterans.
2. Discuss health-related issues confronting vulnerable veteran populations.
3. Highlight the role of the Veterans Administration/Veterans Health Administration (VA/VHA) in meeting the needs of US rural veterans.

Discussion Questions:

1. Compare and contrast characteristics of rural veterans that can impact health status.
2. Identify the health-related concerns of the most vulnerable rural veterans.
3. Highlight local, state and federal resources the nurse could access when planning care for the rural veterans and their caregivers.
4. When available, provide anecdotal information focusing on the health-related needs and concerns of veterans that you have encountered.

INTRODUCTION

Unknowingly, most nurses on a daily bases encounter veterans in their personal and professional interactions. In respect to providing quality nursing care to veterans, Dr. Pam Cipriano in *American Nurse Today* (March, 2014, https://www.americannursetoday.com/a-powerful-question-have-you-ever-served-in-the-military/) states, "Countless history and physical forms, nursing admission databases, and self-prepared health histories may be missing a critical element—the question, 'Have you ever served in the military'." If the answer is yes, the nurse is encouraged to assess a veteran's military history which could pose potential or actual health-related risk factor. This chapter highlights characteristics of rural US veterans, elaborating on vulnerable groups having military associated health risks. Challenges confronting rural veterans in accessing healthcare are discussed and resources provided by the US Department of Veterans Affairs/Veterans Health Administration (VA/VHA) are highlighted.

BACKGROUND

According to the United States (US) Veterans Administration/Veterans Health Administration (VA/VHA) of the total US adult population about 18 million are veterans; of these, nine million are enrolled in the VA/VHA (2016). Of those enrolled, about five million obtain some or all of their healthcare in the VA/VHA. Rural citizens have always been quite patriotic. For example, for the American Revolution rural citizens joined the military to fight for our nation's independence. During the Civil War the federal government instituted the first-ever military draft; overwhelmingly, rural citizens served. In World War I, World War II, the Korean Conflict, and the Viet Nam war, again there was a higher representation of rural draftees. On July 1, 1973 the US draft was eliminated and the all-volunteer force was legislated. Since 1991, the US military predominantly participated in Mideast conflicts. Significant numbers of soldiers, both active duty and those in the military reserve (Army, Air Force, Navy, Marines, Coast Guard, and National Guard) have been mobilized and deployed to serve in various capacities and regions around the world. Consequently, it is not unusual for a civilian in the military reserve to be activated and deployed multiple times within an enlistment commitment period (Gale, 2013; https://www.va.gov/vetdata/docs/Demographics/VetPop_Infographic_2019.pdf).

Of all military recruits, 44% come from rural areas. Upon discharge from active military duty, a disproportionate number of veterans with rural origins return to these communities. They return for a variety of reasons, including: having closer proximity to family, friends, and community; returning to previous employment; living in a less crowded environment with greater opportunity for outdoor activities and recreation; lower cost of living; and greater privacy with less crowded communities and schools. While veterans may enjoy the benefits of rural living, they could encounter rural healthcare access challenges which may exacerbate combat-related injuries and illnesses (Gale, 2013)

Be it patriotism or economic need, military service by rural residents has not changed much in 200 years. About 18% of the US population reside in a region designated as rural or rural remote; or approximately 25% of the population lives on 75% of the nation's land mass. Veterans comprise 30% of the US population, comprising 11% of the rural adult population. Young adults residing in the most sparsely populated zip codes (22%) are more likely to volunteer to serve in the military; an opposite trend from cities. Most enlistees come from southern (40%) and western (24%) states (VA Office of Rural Health, 2016, https://www.ruralhealth.va.gov/newsroom/background.asp). Of the 4.7 million rural and highly rural veterans, more than 2.8 million are enrolled in the VA/VHA. (Veteran enrollment criteria for the VA/VHA and definitions of military disabilities are discussed near the end of this chapter.) A greater proportion of rural veterans (58%) are enrolled in the VA/VHA compared to enrolled urban veterans (37%) (Rural Veterans Health Care Atlas 2nd edition, 2015, Accessed July 25, 2019 https://www.va.gov/vetdata https://www.va.gov/vetdata/docs/Demographics/VetPop_Infographic_2019.pdf)

RURAL VETERANS MILITARY HISTORY: AN OVERVIEW

The rural and highly rural veteran population is widely dispersed and racially, ethnically, and culturally diverse. (See Figure 13.1.) Of rural veterans, 15% self-identify as a racial or ethnic minority. The majority are Caucasian (91.7%) followed by Black/African American (4.9%), American Indian/Alaska Native

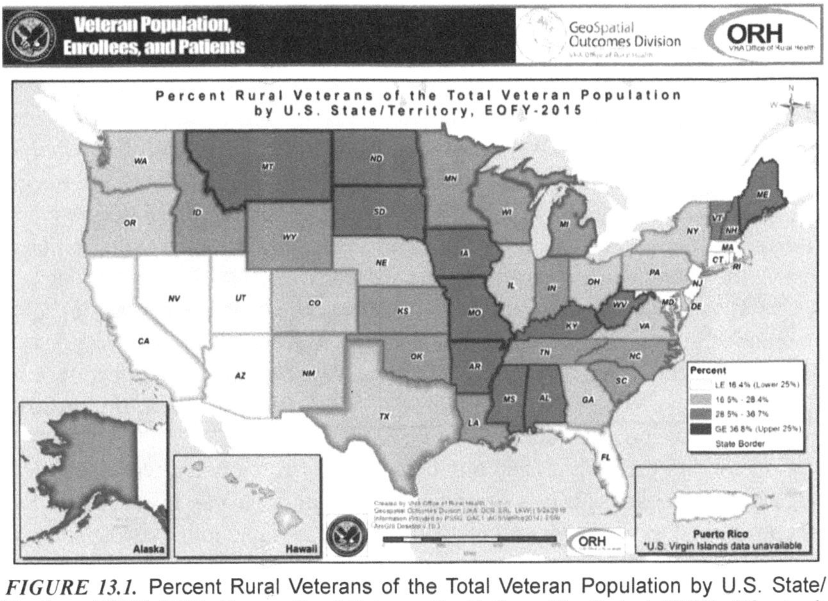

FIGURE 13.1. Percent Rural Veterans of the Total Veteran Population by U.S. State/Territory, EOFY–2015. Source. *Rural Veterans Health Care Atlas 2nd ed. (2015). (Chapter 3, P. 14). https://www.ruralhealth.va.gov/aboutus/ruralvets.asp & https://www.ruralhealth.va.gov/aboutus/rvhc_atlas_fy2015.asp*

TABLE 13.1. Overview of Rural Veterans Demographics.

Period of Service	% of Rural Veterans
Gulf War (9/2001 or later)	12.7%
Gulf War 8/1990 to 8/2001	17.4%
Vietnam Era	41.3%
Korean War	9.3%
World War II	3.8%
Gender	
Male	93.3%
Female	6.7%
Below poverty in past 12 months	7.0%
Race, Hispanic/Latino Origin	91.7
White	4.9%
Black or African American	1.1%
American Indian/Alaska Native	0.3%
Asian	0.1%
Native Hawaiian and Other Pacific Islander	2.7%

Sources: https://www.ruralhealth.va.gov/aboutus/ruralvets.asp
https://www.ruralhealth.va.gov/aboutus/rvhc_atlas_fy2015.asp
https://www.va.gov/vetdata/

(1.1%), Asian (.03%), Native Hawaiian/Other Pacific Islander (0.1%), and Hispanic/Latino (6.6%). Veterans predominantly are male (91%) compared to more than half of the non-veteran US population being female. Consistent with the military in general, there is a rapidly growing number of female veterans (10%); comprising seven percent of rural veterans. Consistent with national trends, the greatest number of living rural veterans served during the Vietnam area. With each successive year, however, here are declining numbers of rural veterans who served in World War II (3.8%), the Korean Conflict (9.3%), and during the Viet Nam era (41%). There are, however, a growing number of rural veterans who served in Mideast Gulf Wars (30%) from 1991 to the present. (https://www.va.gov/vetdata)

Considering their significant numbers in every community, when completing a health assessment, it is important for the nurse to ask if and where the veteran served as this information could provide insights into existing and potential diagnosis. Nurses are encouraged to learn historical perspectives about various US military conflicts in which veterans served as space constraints limits discussing in detail the service-associated health risks for each of these US military events.

The veteran population is significantly older than non-veterans. The median age for all US veterans is 64 years of age compared to 44 years of age for the non-veteran population. A higher proportion of rural veterans are 65 years or older (41%) compared to the rural non-veteran population (16%). More than half of rural veterans (57%) who are enrolled in VA/VHA are over 65 years of age. (https://www.va.gov/vetdata) Older veterans tend to have medically complex conditions with higher rates of chronic diseases compared to younger veterans and non-veteran populations. Veterans who live in rural areas have lower annual family incomes, and are less healthy with more disabilities. Consequently, rural veterans experience more healthcare-related disparities compared to rural non-veterans and urban dwelling veterans (Tasseff *et al.*, 2019). Nurses should be sensitive to the reality that many older war veterans never openly exhibited signs of Post-Traumatic Stress Disorder (PTSD) in their younger years. However, the VA/VHA is educating health professionals, for a number of reasons associated with aging and lifestyle changes, that PTSD may be become evident 50 or more years later in life. (https://www.ptsd.va.gov/understand/what/aging_veterans.asp)

Of VA/VHA enrolled rural veterans 65 years of age and older, nearly three-quarters have medically complex conditions along with chronic comorbidities; and 18% have at least one service-related disability. The older veteran population is more likely to be diagnosed with diabetes, obesity, high blood pressure, and heart conditions which often require frequent, ongoing, and costly care. The VA/VHA projects the "next" generation of veterans, rural and urban alike, who served in Mideast conflicts are likely to have multiple medical and combat-related conditions that require significant ongoing specialty healthcare and long-term rehabilitation. Common injuries among Gulf War veterans are associated with improvised explosive devices (IEDs) blast exposure causing mild to extremely severe Traumatic Brain Injuries (TBI), musculoskeletal trauma-related injuries, missing limbs, Post Traumatic Stress Disorders (PTSD) and various behavioral health problems (https://www.ruralhealth.va.gov/docs/ORH_Brochure_2018_v3_1_print_508.pdf).

For veterans and non-veterans alike, environmental and occupational hazards can wreak havoc on the body which often exacerbate with age and degenerative processes. In respect to a particular veteran's healthcare needs, nurses should understand that these will vary depending on military service history. However, depression, substance abuse, and sleep issues can occur regardless of when or where the veteran served. Moreover, there may be long-term physical and emotional consequences associated with environmental and chemical exposures while serving, such as pesticides, other chemicals, biological warfare agents, prophylactic drugs and vaccines, blasts, noise, radiation, smoke from oil fires and open air burn pits coupled with the lack of sleep, fatigue, and carrying excessively heavy equipment (Panangala, 2016).

SOCIAL DETERMINANTS OF HEALTH

Social determinants include the conditions in which an individual is born, lives, and works which can impact health status. In respect to socioeconomic factors, for veterans and non-veterans alike, males (compared to females), have higher incomes, are more likely to be employed, less likely to be a single parent, and less likely to live in poverty. In respect to rural veterans, more than half (52%) earn less than $35,000 annually. Likewise, there often are fewer housing, education, employment, and transportation options in small and more remote communities. Rural older veterans are more likely to be in fixed incomes with fewer financial resources, while younger rural veterans may have limited employment opportunities with higher unemployment rates compared to urban counterparts. Female veterans have higher unemployment rates compared to male counterparts and women in general. Compared to urban populations, there is a higher rate of rural residents who are uninsured or under insured. Veterans who are not enrolled in the VA/VHA often are uninsured. Of veterans who are receiving care through the VA/VHA, especially older veterans, a significant proportion have another (supplementary) health insurance (e.g., Medicare, Medicaid, and private insurance) (https://www.va.gov/vetdata/docs/QuickFacts/2017_Veterans_Profile_Fact_Sheet.PDF).

Historically, rural residents have had limited access to healthcare services across the spectrum; thus, identified as an access disparity in *Rural Healthy People*: 2020 (Bolin *et al.*, 2015). Basic levels of healthcare, preventative services, and long-term care may not be available to support rural residents across the lifespan. Large geographical regions with a low population density are associated with few(er) health-related services, and public transportation options may be limited or nonexistent. Concomitantly, there is a growing number of rural hospital closures attributable to financial insolvency. Health Professional Shortage Areas (HPSAs) are federal designations that indicate healthcare provider shortages in primary care, dental health, or mental health. These shortages may be geographic-based, population-based, or facility-based (HRSA, 2019); half of all HPSAs are located in a rural area.

It can be quite difficult for rural veterans and their caregivers to access appropriate healthcare services. Coupled with rural travel challenges and greater distances, there are fewer healthcare services and providers in general, and the VA/VHA in particular. Access to care is the most significant challenge facing rural veterans. Veterans residing in rural and rural remote areas, who rely on the VA/VHA for their healthcare, often must commute great distances in inclement weather to access healthcare. Along with poor travel conditions, the veteran and caregiver may need to take time off from work to get to and from a VA/VHA facility, coupled with costs for fuel and other travel-related expenses to commute to a quite distant VA/VHA medical appointment (Tasseff *et al.*, 2019).

For instance, VA/VHA primary care is available within a 30-minute drive for nearly all urban veterans (91%), compared to rural veterans (38%) and highly rural veterans (22%). Less than half of highly rural veterans (49%) live within 60 minutes of VA/VHA primary care services. The average commuting distance for rural veterans is 63 miles to access a VA/VHA provider. Veterans living more than 30 miles from a VA/VHA service are more likely to rely on care in an emergency department. Of all VA/VHA enrolled veterans, 25% report transportation challenges impact their ability to access care. Among all veterans, 11% do not have a valid driver license attributable either to a physical or emotional impairment or, in some cases, substance abuse restrictions (e.g., multiple DUIs, etc.). In respect to rural veterans, more than half have only one vehicle in the household (54%). Some rural veterans do not even have a vehicle (5.6%), and more than 13% must rely on family or friends for transportation (NRHA, 2019).

When available, nurses could refer a veteran to the Disabled American Veterans (DAV) Van Service. Some rural counties offer this transportation service using volunteer (veteran) drivers to transport other veterans to a VA/VHA facility for appointments. However, some rural counties to not have this service; and, sometimes, two or more counties collaborate to offer DAV transportation to area veterans. On a scheduled bases (e.g. weekly, bi-weekly, bi-monthly) the DAV van transports local veterans to the nearest VA/VHA facility (DAV, n.d.). Even when this service is available, only 11% use the DAV-sponsored transportation service. A variety of various reasons are cited by veterans and their caregivers, among others: medical appointments scheduled at times other than when DAV van service is available; having to depart from home very early in the morning sometimes in subzero temperatures; lengthy commuting times associated with picking up other veterans in the county(ies) enroute to the VA/VHA facility. Once at the facility, there often is a lengthy waiting time before departing until after all riders have been seen by their provider later in the day. Finally, another lengthy commute before being dropped off at one's home. For a veteran who is frail, elderly, disabled, or in poor health such commuting circumstances for a physician appointment can exacerbate an existing medical condition.

As alluded to above, compared to urban, rural veterans have higher prevalence of physical illness, lower health-related quality of life, and greater healthcare needs. Despite greater need, rural veterans are less likely than urban veterans to use VA/VHA or private sector health care services. Consequently, transportation challenges along with commuting distances are the most significant barrier to care, and the strongest predictor of poor treatment retention among veterans enrolled in the VA/VHA. Nurses providing care to rural veterans should take into consideration this finding may be relevant for those who are not enrolled in the VA/VHA system for care (https://www.va.gov/vetdata).

LIMITED ACCESS TO COMMUNICATION TECHNOLOGY

Millions of rural residents, including healthcare providers and healthcare facilities, lack access to electronic information and adequate communication capabilities. Especially in rural remote regions, communication technology tends to be less accessible associated with limited broadband internet capabilities and even cellular telephone connections. Depending on the geographical rural region, coupled with limited economic resources, the VA/VHA estimates that about 30% of rural veterans do not have internet access in the home. Recently (April 2019), the VA/VHA and Microsoft Corporation established a partnership in an effort to improve rural veterans access to its online resources, benefits, telehealth, and telemedicine. The goal of this partnership is to advance and improve veterans' quality of life especially in underserved electronic interconnectivity communities (NRHA, 2019; VA, 2019 https://www.va.gov/opa/pressrel/pressrelease.cfm?id=5258_).

Telemedicine and access to online resources promotes digital inclusion to support veterans, their families and caregivers. Digital inclusion will improve access to a continuum of VA/VHA health related services, enhance VA/VHA employee workflow and improve outreach efficiency, and facilitate veterans' participation in their own healthcare. The partnership with Microsoft is one step for the VA/VHA to achieve its strategic goal of providing excellent customer service and business transformation.

MENTAL AND BEHAVIORAL HEALTH SERVICES

Overall there are insufficient numbers of mental and behavioral care providers in most rural areas for both inpatient and outpatient services. Historical critical shortages of this specialty also exist in the VA/VHA, and especially for rural veterans. Rural veterans have a higher prevalence of physical and mental comorbidities compared to urban counterparts, yet they are 70% less likely to receive adequate and appropriate treatment for traumatic brain injury, PTSD, and various behavioral disorders. Associated with the suicide high rate, veterans who are screened positive for PTSD are four times more likely to report suicidal ideation compared to those who do not have this diagnosis. The VA/VHA reports suicidal ideation is 5.7 times higher among veterans screened positive for PTSD and tend to have at least two or more comorbid disorders (https://www.va.gov/vetdata).

Among all veterans substance use is the most prevalent behavioral and mental health diagnosis. Alcohol and heavy tobacco use are high among both active-duty military and veterans. Among veterans with a substance use disorder, there are higher rates of co-occurring physical and behavioral disorders, with higher mortality rates among those who have a disability. Of veterans presenting for first-time care at the VA/VHA, 11% meet the criteria for substance abuse disorders. Male veterans are more likely to have substance abuse disorders compared to female veterans. Military-related environmental and situational stressors are risk factors for beginning and exacerbating substance abuse behaviors, including deployment, combat exposure, and post-deployment civilian reintegration challenges. Substance using behaviors on active-duty end to continue post military discharge among veterans (https://www.va.gov/vetdata).

For both females and males veterans, military sexual trauma (MST) is a significant risk factor for developing PTSD. One in four women and one in 100 males report experiencing male MST. Female veterans with substance abuse disorders also had experienced a higher rate of childhood sexual abuse, MST, and domestic violence. Female veterans who have a history of MST are nine times more likely to develop PTSD compared to female veterans with no history of sexual trauma.

Use of opioids has been significant across all sectors of the healthcare system to treat and manage conditions associated with chronic pain. Consistent with national trends, misuse of prescription pain medications (i.e., opioids) has increased among veterans of all ages regardless of military history background. The VA/VHA has actively focused on this behavior through education of both providers, veterans, and their caregivers about the risks of opioid dependency and use if alternative pain management interventions (i.e., alternative prescribing practices, use of complementary therapies such as acupuncture, massage, meditation, non-addictive analgesics).

VETERANS' HOMELESSNESS

Among the total U.S. homeless population a high proportion are male veterans. Point-in-Time-Estimates ("stand down") by the VA/VHA indicate of the adult homeless population, at least 11% are veterans. However, data regarding homeless veterans in general are imprecise, and data on rural homeless veterans is derived on inferences from urban data (Statista, 2019). Compared to non-veterans, male veterans are 1.3 times more likely while female veterans are 3.6 times more likely to be homeless. Female veterans are twice as likely to be homeless compared to nonveteran females; and are more likely to be a single parent. More than half of all homeless veterans have a disability (51%) and a mental illness (49%) (i.e., PTSD, substance abuse [70%]). Of homeless veterans at least half are 51 years of age or older (50%) compared to the non-veteran population (19%), and most older homeless veterans served during the Vietnam era.

It is important to include the concept of poverty in the broader definition of homelessness. A notable link exists among poverty, security, and the lack of housing in rural areas. Sometimes rural homelessness is referred to as the "houseless" population. In other words, in small rural communities one is not likely to see homeless individuals camped under viaducts, or encounter a panhandler at a major intersection. Rather, someone who is homeless in a rural setting may temporarily move in ("bunk") with a relative or friend; assume residency ("squatter") in a vacated building; or camp in more remote and uninhabited area. Such residential choices restrict public visibility of rural homeless individuals and families; thus, the local population may lack an appreciation for the extent of the problem in the community.

FEMALE VETERANS: HEALTH CONCERNS OF A GROWING POPULATION

Females are the fastest growing veteran population. Consequently, meeting their health-related needs in a historically male dominated institution has been a challenge for the VA/VHA. For female veterans, access to appropriate VA/VHA healthcare is of utmost concern (Women Veterans Health Care, https://www.womenshealth.va.gov/). In the past decade the number of female veterans using VA/VHA services has doubled. With more than 500,000 enrolled females, the VA/VHA has focused on the growing demands for their unique healthcare needs. Efforts to serve female veterans have been ongoing for decades. However, the VA/VHA currently is focused on better understanding their healthcare needs especially female veterans who served in Mideast conflicts.

As alluded to in a previous section of this chapter, the prevalence of MST has been diagnosed in at least 25% of enrolled females. Yet, of all VA/VHA facilities, nearly one third (31%) report they are unable to provide adequate services to females who experienced MST. Traditionally, VA/VHA treatment protocols for substance abuse and other behavioral disorders focused on male veterans. Consequently, female veterans are quite uncomfortable in male-dominated therapy settings, which thereby hinders addressing their particular issues and concerns. However, it is important that nurses also understand that it is not unusual for males to also have experiences MST while serving. (VA 2015, https://www.womenshealth.va.gov/WOMENSHEALTH/docs/Womens%20Health%20Services_Barriers%20to%20Care%20Final%20Report_April2015.pdf).

Another common type of diagnosis among female veterans is various musculoskeletal injuries with persistent chronic pain. Such injuries often are associated with carrying very heavy packs, ill-fitting equipment ("gear"), issuing military uniforms (clothing, shoes, equipment, etc.) that were designed for the male physique, along with physical stress/fatigue. Subsequently, when seeking care in the VA/VHA which traditionally has had male-dominated approach, female veterans often do not receive appropriately tailored prosthetics, rehabilitation, and other essential therapies for their particular needs. In an effort to address the growing female veteran population, Congress passed Public Law 111-163, Caregivers and Veterans Omnibus Health Services Act. Section 201 (May, 2010) required the VA/VHA to examine actual and potential barriers for female veterans to access and utilize its services. The mandated systematic assessment focuses on the following areas:

- Comprehension of eligibility requirement and scope of services,
- Effect of outreach specifically addressing women's health services,
- Effect of driving distance on access to care,
- Location and hours of services,
- Childcare,
- Acceptability of integrated care,
- Gender sensitivity,
- Mental health stigma,
- Safety and comfort.

HEALTH CONCERNS OF THE LGBQT VETERAN

Within the VA/VHA system, "LGBT and related identities" is an inclusive term for sexual and gender minorities as veterans may have other ways of describing themselves. This official terminology is to inclusively recognize the full range of sexual orientation and gender identity minorities. Historically sexual and gender minority veterans encountered stigma and discrimination which impacted the health of many. The VA/VHA does not collect data on a veteran's sexual orientation or gender identity (https://www.patientcare.va.gov/LGBT/index.asp).

Best estimates suggest there are more than one million LGBT military veterans with comparable national rates reflecting urban/rural trends. Using diagnostic codes in medical record data, Blosnich *et al.* (2013) found the prevalence of transgender veterans in VA/VHA to be five times higher (22.9/100,000) compared to transgender-related diagnoses in the general population (4.3/100,000). While the findings also are somewhat dated, using a broader set of diagnostic codes, Brown and Jones (2014) identified 5,135 transgender veterans who received care in the VA/VHA. Their methodologies however did not identify transgender veterans who had not disclosed gender identity to providers, those who did not meet diagnostic criteria, or those who obtain transition-related care outside of the VA/VHA. These researchers project that if all LGBT veterans used the VA/VHA at the same rate as non-LGBT veterans, there could be more than 250,000 LGBT veterans served by VA/VHA.

Rural and urban alike, health-related concerns among the LGBTQ veteran population are varied and reflect similar trends as those of nonveterans. Interestingly, gender dysphoria was found to be higher in veterans compared to the general population. Transgender veterans' also experience higher rates of mental and physical health conditions compared to non-transgender veterans, and experience disparities in accessing appropriate healthcare services (VA/VHA, 2019, https://www.patientcare.va.gov/LGBT/index.asp; Blosnich et al., 2013; Brown and Jones, 2014). To address this healthcare deficit, every VA/VHA facility has been mandated (March 2016) to appoint a local LGBT Veteran Care Coordinator (VCC) who is responsible for promoting best practices when serving this population (https://www.va.gov/vetdata/Utilization.asp).

CONGRESSIONAL MANDATES FOCUSING ON VETERANS' HEALTHCARE NEEDS

The VA/VHA by statute is required to provide an enrolled veteran with access to timely and quality medical care. This mandate is addressed through the nation's largest integrated healthcare delivery system the VA/VHA. This massive healthcare system has more than 150 VA Medical Centers (VAMCs), 800 community-based outpatient clinics (CBOCs), and a range of other types of facilities (e.g., domiciliary, nursing homes, home health, etc.) that provide care to more than 5.5 million enrolled veterans.

Yet Congress remains concerned that some veterans are not able to access VA/VHA services. Recently, the VA/VHA implemented the Mission Act (VA Mission Act, June 6, 2019, https://missionact.va.gov/). The goal of the Mission Act is to make it easier for qualifying enrolled veterans to have additional options to access healthcare within the VA/VHA network through approved non-VA/VHA medical providers in the community (i.e., "community care providers").

For instance, if a certain healthcare service is not provided by the VA/VHA within 50 miles, a rural veteran may be able to seek care from an *approved* community care provider. Eligibility for a community care provider depends on the veteran's healthcare needs and eligibility to access an outside VA/VHA provider. If the VA/VHA Care Team determines that a veteran is eligible for community care, they send (to an approved community provider) a referral with authorization to treat the veteran. *A veteran must receive prior approval from a VA/VHA Care Team to obtain care from an approved community provider*. Health professionals in general and nurses in advance practice roles are encouraged to contact the VA/VHA for information in becoming approved *community care provider* to better serve local veterans (https://missionact.va.gov/).

Not all enrolled veterans are eligible to receive healthcare through the VA/

VHA. Eligibility for enrollment is based on specific veteran status criteria; among others, for example, the presence of a service-connected disability, or exposure, or income level, or other factors (i.e., prisoner of war, receipt of a Purple Heart). Eligibility based on exposure includes veterans who may have been exposed to Agent Orange during the Vietnam War, or who have a disease potentially related to service in the Gulf War. Veteran status is established by active-duty status in the U.S. Armed Forces, with an honorable discharge, during a specified time period. Service members discharged at any time because of service-connected disabilities are not held to these requirements. Those returning from combat operations are eligible to enroll in the VA/VHA up to five years from the date of discharge without having to satisfy the requirements for a service-connected disability. Once enrolled in the VA/VHA, a veteran remains enrolled and does not have to reapply, even if the veteran's priority group changes (e.g., income status; improved disability) (https://missionact.va.gov/). Rural veterans who are not receiving care from the VA/VHA will be obtaining healthcare from providers in their own community. Consequently, nurses probably encounter numerous veterans, across the age span, who served in various military capacities, in their day-to-day practice.

The VA/VHA, defines "service-connected disability" as "a disability that was incurred or aggravated in the line of duty in the U.S. Armed Forces" (38 U.S.C. §101 (16). The VA/VHA determines whether a veteran has a service-connected disability. For a veteran determined to have a disability, the VA assigns a rating from 0% to 100% based on the severity of the disability (38 C.F.R. §§4.1-4.31). Depending on the severity of the disability, the veteran may or may not be enrolled in the VA/VHA for receiving healthcare (https://missionact.va.gov/.)

Finally, to reiterate as part of the initial assessment, nurses should routinely include the question of all their patients, male and female alike: "Have you ever served?" Rural and urban alike, most veterans are proud of their service, and generally willing to share their story with the healthcare provider. In turn, nurse should become informed about veterans and military conflicts in which the U.S. was involved. A veteran's military history could influence the manner in which a nursing care plan is developed for this individual and his or her family.

REFERENCES

Blosnich, J., *et al.* (2013). Prevalence of gender identity disorder and suicide risk among transgender veterans utilizing Veterans Health Administration care. *American Journal of Public Health, 103*(10), e27–32. doi:10.2105/ajph.2013.301507

Bolin, J., *et al.* (2020). New decade, same challenges. *The Journal of Rural Health, 31*(3), 326–333. https://doi.org/10.1111/jrh.12116

Brown, G. and K. Jones, K. (2014). Racial Health Disparities in a Cohort of 5,135 Transgender Veterans. *Journal of Racial and Ethnic Health Disparities, 1*(4), 257–266. doi:10.1007/s40615-014-0032-4.

Cipriano, P. (2014). A powerful question: "Have you ever served in the military?" *American Nurse Today, 9*(3). (Editorial). Accessed July 25, 2019 from https://www.americannursetoday.com/a-powerful-question-have-you-ever-served-in-the-military/

Department of Veterans affairs 2019. Profile of veterans: 2017. Accessed July 25, 2019 from https://www.va.gov/vetdata/docs/SpecialReports/Profile_of_Veterans_2017.pdf

Disabled Veterans Services. DAV. (n.d). *Need a ride*? Accessed July 25, 2019 from https://www.dav.org/veterans/i-need-a-ride/

Gale, J. (2013), May/June. Rural vets: Their barriers, problems, needs. *Health Progress*. Accessed July 25, 2019 from https://www.chausa.org/docs/default-source/health-progress/rural-vets---their-barriers-problems-needs.pdf

Health Resources and Services Administration (HRSA). (2019). *Health workforce: Health professional shortage areas*. Accessed July 25, 2019 from https://bhw.hrsa.gov/shortage-designation/hpsas

Panangala, S. V. (2016, April). *CRS Report R42747, Health care for veterans: Answers to frequently asked questions*. Accessed July 25, 2019 from https://fas.org/sgp/crs/misc/R42747.pdf

National Rural Health Association (NRHA). (2019). *NRHA Rural veterans' health initiative. Veterans in rural America*. Accessed July 25, 2019 from https://www.ruralhealthweb.org/programs/rural-veterans-health-initiative

Statista. (2019). *Estimated number of homeless veterans in the United States in 2018, by state*. Accessed July 25, 2019 from https://www.statista.com/statistics/727819/number-of-homeless-veterans-in-the-us-by-state/

Tasseff, T., *et al.* (2019). Exploring perceptions of palliative care among rural dwelling veterans. *Online Journal of Nursing and Health Care, 19*(1). Accessed July 26, 2019 from https://rnojournal.binghamton.edu/index.php/RNO/article/view/528/450

US Department of Veterans Affairs. (2019). *Homeless veterans: Overview*. Accessed July 25, 2019 from https://www.va.gov/homeless/ and https://vva.org/what-we-do/outreach-programs/homeless-veterans/

US Department of Veterans Affairs. (2016). *VA research on rural health*. Accessed July 25, 2019 from https://www.research.va.gov/pubs/docs/va_factsheets/RuralHealth.pdf And https://www.research.va.gov/topics/rural_health.cfm

US Department of Veterans Affairs Website (2015). *Study of barriers for women veterans to VA health care: Final report*. Accessed on July 26, 2019 from https://www.womenshealth.va.gov/WOMENSHEALTH/docs/Womens%20Health%20Services_Barriers%20to%20Care%20Final%20Report_April2015.pdf

US Department of Veterans Affairs. (n.d.). *Aging veterans and posttraumatic stress symptoms*. Accessed on July 26, 2019 from https://www.ptsd.va.gov/understand/what/aging_veterans.asp

US Department of Veterans Affairs Website. (2019, May). *Homeless veterans*. Accessed on July 26, 2019 from https://www.va.gov/homeless/

US Department of Veterans Affairs Website (2019, June). *National Center for Veterans Analysis and Statistics*. Accessed on July 26, 2019 from https://www.va.gov/vetdata/Utilization.asp

US Department of Veterans Affairs Website. (2018). *Office of Diversity and Inclusion: LGBT*. Accessed on July 26, 2019 from https://www.diversity.va.gov/programs/lgbt.aspx

US Department of Veterans Affairs Website. (2019, May). *Office of Public and Intergovernmental Affairs. VA partners with Microsoft to improve how rural veterans access VA's online services and benefits*. Accessed on July 26, 2019 from https://www.va.gov/opa/pressrel/pressrelease.cfm?id=5258

US Department of Veterans Affairs Website 2019, June 6. *VA Mission Act: Increasing veterans access to health care*. Accessed on July 26, 2019 from https://missionact.va.gov/

US Department of Veterans Affairs Website 2019. *Veterans with lesbian, gay, bisexual and transgender (LGBT) and related identities*. Accessed on July 26, 2019 from https://www.paticntcare.va.gov/LGBT/index.asp

Veterans Health Administration. 2019, March. *National Center for Veterans Analysis and Statistics*. Accessed July 25, 2019 from https://www.va.gov/vetdata/

Veterans Health Administration—Office of Rural Health. (n.d.). *Caring for rural Veterans*. Accessed July 25, 2019 from https://www.ruralhealth.va.gov/docs/ORH_Brochure_2018_v3_1_print_508.pdf

Veterans Health Administration—Office of Rural Health. (2016). *Rural Veterans Health care atlas. FY 2015*. Accessed July 25, 2019 from https://www.ruralhealth.va.gov/aboutus/ruralvets.asp & https://www.ruralhealth.va.gov/aboutus/rvhc_atlas_fy2015.asp

CHAPTER 14

Providing Genetics/Genomics Care to Rural Communities

Tammy McKamie and Dennis J. Cheek

Objectives:

1. Define the difference between genetics and genomics.
2. Identify barriers to receiving and delivering genetic care to rural communities.
3. Discuss management strategies for appropriate identification of individuals meeting criteria for genetic counseling in rural communities.

Discussion Questions:

1. Complete a pedigree for a family member.
2. Perform a comprehensive medical history.
3. Research NCCN/ASCO cancer risk and guidelines for hereditary breast and ovarian cancer syndrome or Lynch syndrome and specific gene mutations.

INTRODUCTION

The words genetic/genomics can be very intimidating to most nurses but in reality, it is the cornerstone of our discipline. Genetics is the study of heredity and its variation. Genomics is defined as the study of genes and their functions, and related techniques National Human Genome Research Institute (NHGRI, 2019). The main difference between genetics and genomics is that genetics scrutinizes the functioning and composition of the single gene, whereas genomics addresses all genes and their interrelationships in order to identify their combined influence on the growth and development of the organism (World Health Organization, 2019). The Human Genome Project (HGP) changed the way we screen, diagnose, and treat individuals.

The HGP began in 1990. The goal was to create a map of genes as they are positioned on chromosomes. This map was completed in 2001 and it began being used to identify genes associated with particular diseases and illness. Because of this discovery, we are able to make treatment decisions tailored to the individual patient. This is known as personalized medicine. The HGP has led to reducing the risk of illness from occurring by identifying those with inherited gene mutations. It has changed the way we screen, diagnose, and treat individuals.

DELIVERY OF GENETIC INFORMATION

Genetics counselors (GC) have traditionally provided genetic counseling to individuals. They are master/doctoral-level prepared professionals trained to deliver information on genetic diseases, make recommendations for medical management, as well as to provide psychosocial support to individuals and their families. The first genetic counseling program began in the 1970s and to date there are over 4,000 licensed GCs. This estimates one GC to every 100,000 persons, putting a real strain on GC's ability to provide counseling in a timely manner, especially in rural areas (Bureau of Labor Stats, 2020).

Rural communities, by definition, are largely below the poverty level and are unable to receive services in specialty areas such as genetic counseling by a licensed GC. According to Rural Health Information Hub (RHIhub, 2020) frontier areas are sparsely populated rural areas which are isolated from population centers and services. Most rural citizens have to travel over 100 miles for services such as genetic counseling. Not only can they not afford to travel the distance, they typically do not understand the importance of genetic counseling and testing. Nurses are in a unique position to fill this void. Nurses are trained to be caregivers, educators, patient advocates, and counselors.

The nursing assessment is the first step in the nursing process. The nursing assessment includes gathering information concerning the patient's individual physiological, psychological, sociological, and spiritual needs. An accurate and comprehensive assessment is the foundation of determining patient needs and potential diagnoses.

Nurses are skillfully trained to take physical, psychosocial, and comprehensive assessments of symptoms, medical conditions, and family history. An accurate and thorough personal/ family history is the groundwork of genetic counseling and evaluation. The aim of information gathering is to determine whether genetic testing is merited. Individuals must trust the nurse taking this private information, and according to a 2017 Gallup poll, nurses are ranked number one by the public in honesty and ethics over physicians. When an individual trusts a nurse/counselor they are more willing to provide details of not only their personal history but also their family's history. Examples of a pedigree can be found through multiple resources, such as the National Comprehensive Cancer Network guidelines under Breast and/or Ovarian Cancer Genetic Assessment.

Physicians tend to be brief, problem-focused, and often hurried due to productivity burdens, whereas nurses tend to spend more time with individuals, providing crucial education and the "translation" of the physician's words into language more easily understood by the patient (Carlson, 2017).

Individuals who understand the basic importance of genetic mutations and the effects, not only on themselves but also on their family, are more likely to be compliant with medical management and risk reduction strategies. The most common concerns are: Will insurance pay? Can I be discriminated against by insurance and my employer? How will this help my family?

Cost

The average cost for genetic testing today is between $2,000 and $4,000. Ninety-seven percent of private insurance companies have coverage for hereditary cancer testing. Three out of four individuals pay zero out of pocket cost (Facing Our Risk, 2020). Medicare and Medicaid pay 100% if an individual meets the criteria. Criteria are set by the National Comprehensive Cancer Network (NCCN). NCCN is a national organization comprised of 28 leading cancer centers devoted to patient care, research, and education.

Legality

Laws are in place to prevent discrimination such as the Health Insurance Portability and Accountability Act (HIPAA) and the Genetic Information Nondiscrimination Act (GINA, 2019). GINA and laws in most states prohibit discrimination regarding employment eligibility, health benefits, or health insurance premiums solely on the basis of genetic information.

MODELS OF SUCCESSFUL DELIVERY

Due to the lack of genetic counselors, nurses must learn to fill in the gaps. There are multiple delivery systems that identify high-risk individuals with possible hereditary mutations depending on the geographical location. For example, a hereditary cancer risk program at CHRISTUS St. Michael hospital located in East Texas serves 3,580,000 individuals in a four-state region. It provides genetic counseling to those unable to travel long distances. Without this service, individuals would not be able to receive this potential lifesaving education and healthcare. The National Comprehensive Cancer Network (NCCN) is a great resource for identifying, ordering appropriate test, prevention, treatment, and follow-up recommendations.

According to the International Society of Nursing Genetics (ISONG, 2019), a genetics nurse is a licensed professional nurse with special education and training in genetics. Genetic nurses help people at risk for or those affected by diseases with a genetic component achieve and maintain health. Many common diseases are now known to have a genetic component including cancer, heart disease, diabetes, and Alzheimer's.

Genetic nurses perform a risk assessment, analyze the genetic contribution to disease risk, and discuss the impact of risk on healthcare management for individuals and families. They also provide genetic education, provide nursing care to patients and families, and conduct research in genetics.

IDENTIFY INDIVIDUALS AT RISK

In approximately 90% of patients diagnosed with cancer, the cause is related to environment, life style, and/or aging, while 5–7% is due to an inherited gene mutation found in the tumor suppressor genes (NCBI, 2019). Tumor suppressor genes control cellular growth. Although it is rare to have an inherited mutation, if identified, your siblings and children have a 50% chance of inheriting the same mutation. Some gene mutations can lead to an 87–99% risk of developing cancer in one's lifetime. This is why it is so important to learn this at an early age in order to detect cancer at an early stage or possibly prevent it all together. Knowledge is power to the individual, as well as the family. It empowers them to make life-saving decisions regarding future medical management.

Genetic mutations can be found in all specialties of medicine, e.g., cancer, cardiology, neurology, prenatal care, and many others. There are many organizations that support, educate, and guide medical providers in identifying individuals that are at risk for a genetic mutation. In the oncology arena, organizations such as Oncology Nursing Society (ONS), ISONG, and the NCCN are just a few.

The first step in a successful program is identifying those individuals at high risk. One particular program uses multiple avenues such as educating medical providers and their staff of red flags, providing questionnaires, and pathology reports. According to one study 60% of individuals meet criteria but have never been referred for genetic counseling. It is estimated that approximately 50–60% of individuals meet criteria for genetic testing but have never been identified.

COUNSELING INDIVIDUALS AT RISK

Nurses can receive training and certification in genetics through credentialing organizations, giving them the knowledge and confidence to provide genetic counseling. This training prepares nurses to:

- Obtain a detailed family history and construct a pedigree
- Assess and analyze hereditary and nonhereditary disease risk factors
- Identify potential genetic conditions or genetic predispositions to disease
- Provide genetic information and psychosocial support to individuals and families
- Provide nursing care for patients and families at risk for or affected by disease with a genetic component

Counseling consists of collecting the details of personal and family history. By collecting this data and designing a pedigree, you show the inheritance of a trait or disease through several generations. It is recommended that you take a three-generation pedigree (parents, children, siblings, grandparents, aunts, uncles, nieces, nephews, and cousins). When possible include 4th generations, which include great-grandparents, great-aunts, great-uncles, and 2nd cousins. This will assist in determining the most appropriate test to order. Testing is typically a blood draw or saliva collection.

COUNSEL INDIVIDUALS ON RESULTS

Post education to review and discuss an individual's genetic test result is just as important and pre-counseling (Table 14.1). It is imperative that they understand their results and any risk factors that maybe associated. Understanding increased risk, additional screenings, and prophylactic surgeries that may be associated with a genetic mutation can lead to early detection and ultimately save lives.

Because mutations are inherited from a parent, discussion regarding family members who may or may not need testing is important. Eliminating those who may not need testing is just as important as identifying those who do. Performing unnecessary testing can lead to increased cost to not only the individual but also the insurance providers which ultimately increases healthcare cost for all.

INFORM REFERRING MEDICAL PROVIDERS OF RESULTS AND RECOMMENDATIONS

Not all referring medical providers understand genetic results and the recommendations associated with them. Genetic counselors and genetic nurses will usually write a summary letter listing the results and any risks identified and medical management associated with the results.

TABLE 14.1. Results.

Genes	Breast	Ovarian	Colorectal	Endometrial	Melanoma	Pancreatic	Gastric	Prostate
BRCA1	X	X				X		X
BRCA2	X	X			X	X		X
MLH1		X	X	X		X	X	X
MSH2		X	X	X		X	X	X
MSH6			X	X		X	X	X
PMS2			X	X		X	X	X
EPCAM			X	X		X	X	X
APC			X			X	X	
TP53	X	X	X	X	X	X	X	X
PTEN	X		X	X	X			
PALB2	X					X		
CHEK2	X		X					
ATM	X					X		
NBN	X							X

Sources: https://www.ruralhealth.va.gov/aboutus/ruralvets.asp
https://www.ruralhealth.va.gov/aboutus/rvhc_atlas_fy2015.asp
https://www.va.gov/vetdata/

TABLE 14.2. Knowing Risk Factor-Red Flags.

Red Flags:
• Cancers diagnosed at a young age (<50)
Female Breast Cancer
Colorectal Cancer
Endometrial/Uterine
• Rare cancers diagnosed at any age
Ovarian
Male Breast Cancer
Pancreatic
• Multiple cancers on the same side of the family or in one individual
• Ashkenazi Jewish Ancestry

Referring individuals for appropriate follow-up is crucial. If the appropriate surveillance and medical management is not available in the community, it is essential that one knows where these resources can be accessed. One of the most reputable resources available is the NCCN guidelines found at NCCN.org.

Knowing the Red Flags or criteria (Table 14.2) of individuals at risk for a genetic mutation is crucial in determining who should be referred for a more in-depth evaluation. The referral should be made to a professional that has received special training in genetics/genomics. A more detailed personal and family history is taken and a pedigree is created. A pedigree is a record or drawing of a person's ancestry also called a family tree. A personal medical history is also collected in order to determine what type of genetic testing should be ordered. Individuals are educated on the possible results and medical management. Medical management can range from prevention to screening to treatment options. These can include prophylactic surgeries such as bilateral mastectomy or bilateral salpingo-oophorectomy (removal of both ovaries and Fallopian tubes). It is important to elaborate on the details of the recommended management, as well as the percentage of cancer risk reduction that can be expected. These recommendations can be overwhelming to the average lay person. Prevention and risk reduction is the key to saving lives in cancer world.

REWARDS OF HEALTH DELIVERY

Saving lives is the ultimate goal for identifying individuals with a genetic mutation. Inheriting a genetic mutation related to cancer increases a person's risk of developing cancer higher than the general population risk. Providing this information prior to developing cancer allows an individual to prepare and take steps to reduce their risk of late stage diagnoses or possibly preventing the cancer all together.

Challenges

Limited resources for genetic counseling and testing are a real challenge. This is partly due to the rapid evolving discoveries in the genetics/genomic field and lack of educators with this particular expertise. Understanding how nurses can become more knowledgeable in this unique field of nursing and provide this service to individuals within his or her community is one way to overcome this challenge. Nurses should not be afraid to extend your expertise in this fast-growing specialty. Genetics/genomics is the way of the future in modern day medicine. Prevention and risk reduction are the key to saving lives.

CASE STUDY

Kim is a 50-year-old female nursing student currently studying oncology. She was curious about her risk of developing cancer due to her family history. She decided to research the web specifically for her local hospital. She found a questionnaire designed by the hospital's cancer center titled "hereditary cancer syndrome risk assessment." This questionnaire would indicate if she met criteria for further genetic counseling and possible testing. After completing the risk assessment, she received a call from a registered nurse certified in hereditary cancer syndromes. The nurse explained that due to Kim's father being diagnosed with colorectal cancer at 44 years old, she met the NCCN criteria for hereditary cancer genetic testing. According to the NCCN, colorectal cancer diagnosed at <50 is a Red Flag or indicator for possible Lynch syndrome, as well as other syndromes.

Lynch Syndrome, also known as hereditary nonpolyposis colorectal cancer (HNPCC) syndrome, is the most common cause of hereditary colorectal cancer. It is responsible for approximately 2%–7% of all diagnosed cases of colorectal cancer. It also increases one's risk for uterine (endometrial), ovarian, stomach, small intestine, liver, gallbladder ducts (biliary tract), urinary tract, kidney, and brain (glioblastoma). Risk range from 70–80% of developing colorectal cancer by age 70 as compared to the general population of only 2%.

Kim was scheduled for face to-face counseling to review a more in depth personal and family history to determine if she was at risk for any other syndromes. During the counseling session, it was noted that Kim had other cancer diagnoses on both paternal and maternal sides. She gave the following history:

- No personal history of cancer or colorectal polyps

- Father diagnosed at 44 with colorectal cancer and expired at 47
- Paternal uncle diagnosed at 68 with lung cancer and expired at 70
- Maternal grandmother diagnosed with breast cancer at 41 and gastric cancer at 65. Now expired
- Kim has three children ages 17–26 years old.
- One brother 45 years old
- One maternal aunt and uncle both living
- Multiple paternal aunts and uncles, three living and 6 expired.

This history met the NCCN criteria for panel testing due to Red Flags noted on both paternal and maternal sides of the family. Breast cancer diagnosed at 45 or younger is an indicator for hereditary breast and ovarian cancer syndrome, as well as other syndromes. Kim was educated on the hereditary cancer syndromes, inheritance of these syndromes, and panel testing.

Panel testing consists of multiple genes called tumor suppressor genes. Tumor suppressor genes protect us from cancer by slowing down cell division, repairing DNA mistakes, or telling cells when to die. When tumor suppressor genes don't work properly, cells can grow out of control, which can lead to cancer. It is estimated that a human has over 20,000 genes that provide instructions such as the color of a person's eyes, hair, etc. A human has two of each gene passed down from each parent. When an individual develops cancer, it is estimated that 90% of the time the cancer is caused by the environment, lifestyle, and aging. Seven to ten percent of cancers are due to mutation in a tumor suppressor gene inherited or passed down from one parent. This means the individual has one functioning gene and one mutated gene from the beginning of conception. This type of inheritance is called autosomal dominant inheritance. If and when the functioning gene becomes affected through environment, lifestyle, or aging the cell no longer has the ability to prevent cancer growth (Figure 14.1).

Kim agreed to proceed with panel testing. The best people to test would have been the affected individuals with the Red Flags but they were both expired. Testing the individual affected can rule out the possibility of a genetic mutation. On the other hand, if Kim's father or grandmother had a mutation, Kim and her siblings would have a 50% risk of inheriting the same mutation.

Kim acknowledged understanding of the genetic testing and proceeded with testing. Testing consisted of a simple blood collection of 7–10 ml (one vial). This type of panel testing consisted of 35 genes and took approximately 2–3 weeks for results to return. Kim was scheduled to return for post counseling to review her results. Her results returned positive for Lynch syndrome with a mutation in the MSH6 gene. This placed her at a high risk for colorectal cancer and uterine cancer and an elevated risk for ovarian, stomach, small intestine, urinary tract/bladder/kidney, bile ducts, brain, pancreas, and sebaceous gland skin tumors. Thorough education and counseling were given to Kim during

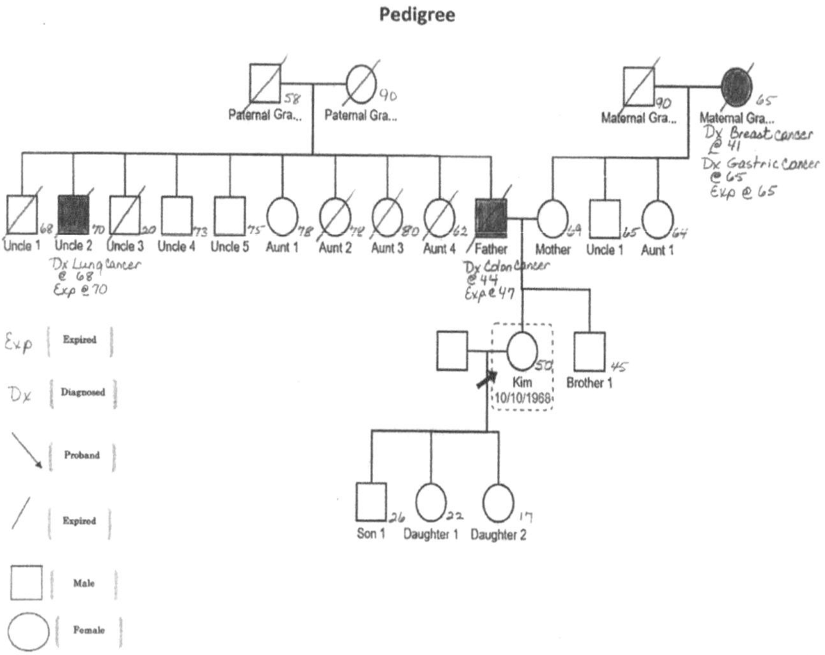

FIGURE 14.1. Pedigree.

the post session explaining in detail the estimated risk of every cancer associated with Lynch syndrome, as well as medical management recommendations indicated by the NCCN.

This particular cancer center program is located in a rural area and resources for persons identified as having a hereditary cancer syndrome with elevated risk of cancers are limited. One of the most beneficial resources is a high-risk program that staffs medical personnel educated on medical management for hereditary cancer syndromes. These particular programs follow these individuals throughout their lifetime. The nearest high-risk program was located 2.5–3 hours away. Information was also provided on high risk programs but due to the distance Kim, financially, was not able to travel the distance. Due to the lack of this resource Kim was offered an evaluation by the medical oncologist. The medical oncologist specializes in cancer care and has a more in-depth understanding of Kim's needs.

A summary letter and a copy of the results, along with medical management recommendations, were forwarded to her PCP. Kim's children and sibling have a 50% risk of having the same mutation. Single-site testing was recommended for her children, but due to the unknown possibility of another mutation or cancer syndrome related to the maternal grandmother's early onset breast cancer, full panel testing was offered to Kim's brother and mother. Single-site testing is only evaluating the specific mutation on a specific gene. Once a known mutation is discovered in a family member, typically single-site testing is recommended. Single-site testing is a fraction of the cost of panel testing. Most insurance plans cover 90–100% of the cost of both.

Kim was evaluated by the medical oncologist and medical management began. Kim's oldest two children, ages 26 and 22, agreed to have single-site testing. One was found to carry the same mutation in the same MSH6 gene and the other was negative. The 17-year-old child plans to test after she becomes 18 years old.

Kim was anxious about her risk of multiple cancers but appreciative of the knowledge she gained. She understands that increased screening can detect cancers at an earlier stage and are more likely to be cured. If she had not discovered her elevated risk of not only colorectal cancer, but multiple other cancers, screening would not have been offered as they are not recommended for the general population, i.e., radiologic scans, labs, and clinical evaluations. Knowledge is power.

GLOSSARY

Somatic mutations—Occur in a single body cell and cannot be inherited. Only tissues derived from mutated cell are affected.

Gene—The functional and physical unit of heredity passed from parent to offspring. Genes are pieces of DNA, and most genes contain the information for making a specific protein.

Germline mutations—Inherited material that comes from eggs or sperm and that offspring inherit.

Oncogene—A gene that is capable of causing the transformation of normal cells into cancer cells.

Tumor suppressor gene—A protective gene that normally limits the growth of tumors. When a tumor suppressor is mutated, it may fail to keep a cancer from growing. BRACA1 and BRCA2 are well-known tumor suppressor genes.

Sporadic—cancer caused by environmental factors, certain lifestyles, or by chance.

Familial—A phenotype or trait that occurs with greater frequency in a given family than in the general population; familial traits may have a genetic and/or nongenetic etiology.

Hereditary—Something which is inherited—passed down from parents to offspring. In biology and medicine, the word pertains to inherited genetic characteristics.

REFERENCES

American Cancer Society (2014, June 25). *Oncogenes and tumor suppressor genes.* https://www.cancer.org/cancer/cancer-causes/genetics/genes-and-cancer/oncogenes-tumor-suppressor-genes.html

Carlson, K. (2017, December 27). *Nurses ranked #1 most ethical profession by 2017 Gallup Poll.* Nurse.org. https://nurse.org/articles/gallup-ethical-standards-poll-nurses-rank-highest/

Daly *et al.* (2020, Apr). NCCN guidelines insights: genetic/familial high-risk assessment: breast, ovarian, and pancreatic. *National Comprehensive Cancer Network.* 18(4), 380–391. DOI: 10.6004/jnccn.2020.0017

Estrada *et al.* (2015). Next generation gene sequencing: looking beyond hereditary breast and ovarian cancer. *Oncology Nursing Forum, 42*(6), 691–694.

Facing Our Risk of Cancer Empowered. (2020). *Most private insurers cover genetic testing for inherited mutations.* https://www.facingourrisk.org/support/insurance-paying-for-care/genetic-services/private-insurance

International Society of Nurses in Genetics. (2019). *What is a genetics nurse*? https://www.isong.org/page-1325153

National Human Genome Research Institute. (2020), September 16. *Genetic discrimination.* https://www.genome.gov/about-genomics/policy-issues/Genetic-Discrimination

Montgomery *et al.* (2017). Genetics in clinical setting: What nurses need to know to provide the best patient care. *American Nurse Today, 12*(10), 10–16.

National Comprehensive Cancer Network. (2021). *New NCCN guidelines now available for genetic/familial high-risk assessment: colorectal.* https://www.nccn.org/about/news/ebulletin/ebulletindetail.aspx?ebulletinid=294

National Human Genome Research Institute. (2017, December 8). *Cancer genetics and comparative genomics branch.* https://www.genome.gov/about-nhgri/Division-of-Intramural-Research/Cancer-Genetics-Comparative-Genomics-Branch

Rural Health Information Hub. (2020, June 2). *Health and healthcare in frontier areas.* https://www.ruralhealthinfo.org/topics/frontier

Saletta *et al.* (2015). Genetic causes of cancer predisposition in children and adolescents. *Translational Pediatrics, 4*(2), 67–75. https://www.ncbi.nlm.nih.gov/pmc/articles/PMC4729088/

U.S. Bureau of Labor Statistics.(2020, July 6). 29-9092 *Genetic Counselors.* https://www.bls.gov/oes/current/oes299092.htm

World Health Organization. (2021). *WHO definitions of genetics and genomics.* https://www.who.int/genomics/geneticsVSgenomics/en/

CHAPTER 15

The Impact of APRN Leadership in Rural Settings

Holly Jeffreys

Objectives:

1. Understanding the disparities between urban and rural residents.
2. Reviewing historic role of nursing and the advancement of the role for Advanced Practice Nurses in Rural Health Care.
3. Overview of challenges and opportunities for APRNs in rural healthcare.

Discussion Questions:

1. Discuss the challenges and opportunities for APRNs in rural healthcare. Why would you consider taking a position in a rural community?
2. What is an APRN? How is their role different from a Registered Nurse?
3. What are the different practice opportunities for APRNs in rural communities?

INTRODUCTION

Growing up I always thought that living in the country was a healthier choice than living in a city. I believed this to be true until shortly after starting my first primary care clinic in a rural area in the Panhandle of Texas. After just a few short months of practice I realized the population I was serving not only had serious health concerns such as diabetes, hypertension, and heart failure among others, but also had become extremely comfortable neglecting health concerns as well as continued participating in unhealthy behaviors like tobacco and excessive alcohol intake.

Every day new patients would walk into the clinic with empty blood pressure and diabetes medication bottles in hand requesting refills. I encouraged patients to set appointments in advance but was told by the locals that this would never happen—patients were used to just stopping by as this is was common practice for all small towns. The patients would list the medications on their health history but would admit they hadn't filled the prescriptions in nearly three years because they hadn't been able to get to town for an appointment.

Over time we began addressing and improving health issues together—efforts at prevention would take several more years. During the first few years the most common response I heard was "if it ain't broken, don't fix it." Today, I cannot even think of the last time I have heard those words from a patient. Patients willingly come in by appointment for both routine maintenance and preventive exams and have come to understand the importance of preventive screenings such as a mammogram, colonoscopy, and flu shots, among other preventive services.

Would you believe that each time we have opened a primary care clinic in a new underserved area, we experience the same things all over again—neglected health and total lack of preventive care? I do not tell you this because I want you to think that we are really doing something special or unique, I am telling you this because I want you to know that YOU as the Nurse and Nurse practitioner can be the difference in the lives of those around you and change the future of the communities you serve.

Holly Jeffreys DNP APRN FNP-BC
Having compassion . . . Making a Difference. Jude 22

RURAL DEFINED

Over 60 million people—roughly 1 in 5 Americans—live in rural America. Rural areas are often defined by specific criteria depending on the defining organization. The federal government defines rural using two major definitions—one by the U.S. Census Bureau and the other by the Office of Management and Budget. Both definitions define urban as greater than 50,000 population and urban clusters between 2,500 to 50,000 population. The Federal Office of Rural Health Policy uses an additional method of determining rurality by using Rural-Urban Commuting Area (RUCA) codes. For purposes of this chapter, rural areas can be more simply defined as countryside that is not within or nearby urbanized areas. No matter the definition of rural, rural Americans undoubtedly experience greater disparities than residents in urbanized areas, especially with regards to health.

DISPARITIES IN RURAL AMERICA

In a pledge at the National Rural Health Association Policy Institute earlier this year, Dr. George Sigounas, Administrator of the Health Resource and Services Administration, reported a "a widening gap" of almost three years in the life expectancy between urban and rural dwellers as well as "higher rates of chronic disease . . . higher mortality and high rates of avoidable death" among rural Americans. There has been little marked improvement since this disparaging information was first published in 2013.

A study by Villapiano et al. (2017) examined hospital mortality rates in over 4 million hospitalizations from 2008–2013 and found that while urban patients mortality rate decreased from 2.51 percent in 2008 to 2.27 percent in 2013, the mortality rate for rural residents stayed constant at 2.66 percent. Another study examining rural–urban disparities in stages of diagnosis among cancer patients found that while rural populations tended to have lower rates of early stage cancers, they had higher cancer mortality rates and higher rates of distant stage cancers, including cancers with opportunities for prevention such as Human Papillomavirus–associated cancers. Additionally, a study published in the Journal of Rural Health (2018) examined screening rates for mammograms from 2008 to 2012 and found that urban areas had higher screening rates and lower rates of late-stage diagnosis of breast cancer which further pointed to the geographic disparities of accessing appropriate breast cancer screening facilities.

Rates of obesity and severe obesity were significantly more prevalent among adults living in rural areas compared to individuals in urban areas which also correlates with higher rates for hypertension, diabetes, ischemic heart disease, chronic obstructive pulmonary disease, and preventable hospital stays. Rural residents have higher infant mortality and higher mortality rates from unintentional accidents including motor vehicle accidents. Rural residents also have higher rates of suicide, increased pain and suffering and greater tooth loss (which is associated with overall higher mortality rates as well).

In addition to health disparities, rural residents are older and poorer and face additional socioeconomic disadvantages. The median age of rural residents is 51 years as compared to age 45 for urban residents. The average median income for rural U.S. residents is $40,615 compared to $51,831 for urban residents. Approximately 15.4 percent of rural U.S. residents live in poverty compared to 11.9 percent of urban residents. Rural residents tend to have fewer opportunities for employment, particularly corporate employment that includes health insurance benefits. When comparing health insurance coverage, 21.9 percent of rural residents are uninsured compared to 14.3 percent of urban residents. When rural residents do have health coverage, they often experience greater out-of-pocket expenses than that of urban residents. Spencer concludes in Health Services Research (2018), "We find that the growing urban/rural mortality gap can be more than explained by differences in the county demographics, economic, and geographic distribution at each decade from 1980 to 2010."

HISTORIC APRN ROLE

Advanced Practice Nursing may be a relatively new title, but actions constituting advanced practice nursing can be found as far back as the 1890s. In 1893 Lillian Ward a young nurse established the Henry Street Settlement in the east side of Manhattan, New York where she and her colleague provided physical care and services including ice, milk, medicines and meals to the poverty-stricken immigrants. Just seven years later, the Settlement employed 12 nurses who made over 26,600 home visits and by 1926 the visiting nurses were making over 300,000 home visits each year treating illnesses as pneumonia, polio, measles, influenza, tonsillitis, burns, and tuberculosis. Clearly these nurses were practicing to the full extent of their training and improved access to care for thousands of Americans.

Around the same time in 1926, Mary Breckenridge, a certified nurse midwife, established the Frontier Nursing Service by setting up eight decentralized clinics offering care to the poorest and most inaccessible areas of the Appalachian community in Kentucky. The Appalachian community had the highest maternal and infant mortality rates in the country and its rugged mountain territory made it only accessible by horseback. The Frontier Nursing Service nurses did whatever they had to do to treat common illnesses, deliver infants, and provide emergency care. The physicians of the time recognized that without the FNS nurses, the mortality rates would continue to soar and the Appalachian community would remain without care. The FNS nurses, much like the nurses from the Henry Street Settlement and similar nurses who provided care for the Indian Health Service on remote reservations, all practiced to the full extent of their training and improved access to care for the most rural and vulnerable populations.

NURSE PRACTITIONER ROLE FORMALIZED

It wasn't until 1965 that the advanced practice nurse role became formalized. In an effort to bridge the gap between health care needs of children and family's ability to access and afford primary care, Loretta Ford and Henry Silver, MD formalized the advanced nursing role by offering a program with specialized "certified" educational preparation with a new title of Nurse Practitioner. The role was recognized and supported not only by the public, but also by government health care leaders. In the 1970s Health Education and Welfare Secretary Elliott Richardson established a committee of health care leaders to study the role. The committee concluded that extending the scope of the nurse's role was essential to providing equal access to health care for all Americans. According to an editorial in 1971, "The kind of health care Lillian Wald began preaching and practicing in 1893 is the kind the people of this country are still crying for." The support resulted in federal support for training programs and for the preparation of several types of NPs including family, adult, pediatric, and emergency.

Finally, advanced practice nursing had received the formalized recognition the role deserved, but the new NP role was not without critics. Nursing faculty did not always appreciate the recognition and the nursing community was often split over the role until the formation of National Organization of Nurse Practitioner Faculties (NONPF) in 1974. NONPF standardized the educational program at the master's level, thus reducing interprofessional tension. In medicine, local physicians welcomed the help and collaborated well with Nurse Practitioners; however, organized medicine began to increase resistance to the role.

Despite resistance, Idaho became the first state in 1971 to recognize diagnosis and treatment as part of the scope of practice for NPs. As NPs band landmark cases began setting a precedent for Advanced Practice Nursing scope of practice. Associate Dean and Lecturer of Law at the Yale Law School Barbara Safriet called for immediate legislative reform to reduce restrictions on advanced practice nursing, particularly nurse practitioners stating:

> Although our ailing health care system presents an endless array of symptoms, the diagnosis is relatively straightforward: too few people can get good care when they need it and at a price they can afford. Any proposed cure should therefore include, at a minimum, steps to eliminate the inefficient and ineffective provision of health care...Chief among these are conflicting and restrictive state provisions governing the scope of practice and prescriptive authority of Nurse Practitioners and Certified Nurse Midwifes, as well as fragmented and parsimonious state and federal standards for their reimbursement. As a result of these provisions, NPs and CNMs are severely hampered—or disabled altogether—in their efforts to fulfill their fully proven potential to enhance our nation's health.

MODERN APRN ROLE

Three decades later the Institute of Medicine stated a nearly identical philosophy recommending that Advanced Practice Nurses should work at the full extent of their training in order to provide timely, efficient, and cost-effective care to people across the United States. The Federal Trade Commission also published its report summarizing that restrictive supervision requirements exacerbate provider shortages, increase healthcare costs, constrain innovative healthcare delivery models, potentiate competitive harm, and are not necessary to achieve benefits in coordination of care for patients. Over the last two decades research continues to support the role of the Advanced Practice Nurses and further demonstrates the need to remove restrictive barriers. On October 3, 2019 President Trump issued an executive order calling for the secretary within one year to propose reforms to the Medicare program to enable providers to spend more time with patients by: proposing a regulation that would eliminate burdensome regulatory billing requirements, conditions of participation, supervision requirements, benefit definitions, and all other licensure requirements of the Medicare program that are more stringent than applicable federal or state laws require and that limit professionals from practicing at the top of their profession (Healthcare Section 5 [a]).

Despite a plethora of research, recommendations, orders and clear evidence, many organizations throughout the U.S. continue to push back at breaking down barriers to the advanced practice nursing roles. Individual Nurse Practitioners providing primary care services across the U.S. continue to face practice barriers which further increases healthcare cost and decreases access to care as well as quality of care for patients. Despite overwhelming public support, Nurse Practitioners (even those serving in underserved areas) continue to face challenges from non-supporters in the form of harassment and unfounded allegations of "Practicing medicine without a license." Non supporters and those unwilling to support political action in favor of removing practice barriers for Nurse Practitioners are not only neglecting the overwhelming evidence, but also neglecting the needs of the American people.

APRN ROLE IN RURAL HEALTH

Supply

America is experiencing a national shortage of healthcare providers, much like the shortage that was apparent in the 1970s when the NP role was formalized. According to the American Academy of Medical Colleges, the U.S. will see a shortage of up to nearly 122,000 physicians by 2032. The primary driver of the continued demand for healthcare providers is closely associated with the expectation of the nation's population growth at 10% by 2032, with those over the age of 65 increasing by 48%. One third of all doctors will be older than 65 in the next decade and their choice of when to retire poses one of the greatest determinations on physician supply. In contrast, APRNs are projected to increase in number and become a likely means of meeting the primary care demands.

Rural Americans reside in 80 percent of the total U.S. land, but fewer than 9 percent of physicians currently practice in rural communities. Nurse practitioners comprise 25.2 percent (one in four) of clinicians practicing in rural areas, a number that increased 48% from 2008–2016. A 2017 study examined the relationship of the per capita supply of providers with county socioeconomic and health status level with regards to U.S. primary care workforce of physicians, physician assistants, nurse practitioners, and chiropractors. All roles, with the exception of the nurse practitioner role, were found to be located in areas of higher income and better health status. Nurse Practitioners were found more likely to be in counties of lower socioeconomic and health status. NPs trained in primary care continue to serve across the U.S. in areas that are rural and underserved, and care for patients who have lower socioeconomic and health status.

Demand

The population growth as well as the increasing growth of the aging population and 2010 implementation of the Patient Protection and Affordable Care Act has increased the demands for healthcare services. Nurse Practitioners are qualified health professionals ready and willing to meet the demand just as the nurses did successfully in the late 1800s and early 1900s.

The demand for healthcare providers will continue to be greatest for areas of primary care, especially in the rural and underserved areas. In the 1920s all physicians were considered primary care then by 1930, thirteen specialties were born and by 1940 76% of physicians remained in primary care. By 1969 that number had dropped to 19% and by 2013 the number of primary care physicians in the U.S. was down to 12%. A mandate was issued to increase the number of primary care physicians and despite a 28% increase in the number of medical students from 2002 to 2016, the number of primary care physicians has not increased because physicians are still entering practice with subspecialties.

The demand for primary care providers in the US is currently not being met by physicians and the future predictions of provider shortages cannot be met by physicians alone. Of the 248,000 licensed NPs in the US in 2018, 87% are trained in primary care and the number of NPs entering in primary care training programs is increasing. NPs are already meeting much of the primary care demands today, but as the future demands increase, NPs should rise to the challenge of improving the health of Americans. In order to do so, efforts should focus on working simultaneously with lawmakers to remove unwarranted barriers to practice.

REGULATORY CHALLENGES IN RURAL HEALTH

The regulatory aspects of the NP role differ from state to state. The American Academy of Nurse Practitioners (AANP) categorizes the states into the three practice types: full practice, reduced practice, and restricted practice. Sates with full practice authority permit NPs to evaluate patients, diagnose, order, and interpret diagnostic test, and initiate and manage treatments, including prescribing medications and controlled substances, under the exclusive licensure authority of the state board of nursing. This is the model recommended by the National Academy of Medicine (formerly called the Institute of Medicine) and the National Council of State Boards of Nursing. To date twenty-five states fall into the full practice criteria. Reduced practice states reduce the ability of NPs to engage in at least one element of NP practice. State laws require a career-long regulated collaborative agreement with another health provider in order for the NP to provide patient care, or it limits the setting of one or more elements of NP practice. There are nineteen states categorized as reduced practice state. Lastly, the third type of state classification is the restricted practice states where practice and licensure laws restrict the ability of NPs to engage in at least one element of NP practice. State law requires career-long supervision, delegation, or team management by another health provider in order for the NP to provide patient care. There are twelve states in the restricted category. Studies show that states with restricted scope of practice had 40% fewer NP providers than states with unrestricted practice, thus reiterating the importance of removing restrictive regulations and allowing NPs to practice to the full extent of their profession.

RURAL HEALTH CHALLENGES

Perhaps the biggest challenge in rural America is simply providing access to care. One of the most instrumental acts increasing access to healthcare in rural areas occurred in 1977 when President Jimmy Carter signed the Rural Health Clinic Act. The Rural Health Clinic Act created special reimbursement mechanisms that allow clinicians to practice in rural, underserved areas and increased the utilization of Nurse Practitioners by requiring the clinics to be staffed with either a Physician Assistant or Nurse Practitioner for at least 50% of operations. This act which is still in existence today paved the way for NPs to begin serving in the rural and underserved area. By August of 2018 there were over 4,300 RHCs across the U.S. facilitating over 35 million visits annually, ultimately increasing access to healthcare.

In addition to RHCs, many NPs practice in rural areas in non-RHC facilities. Depending on the state and type of facility, state regulatory restrictions continue to be the greatest source of practice barriers for NPs. Studies show that less restrictive practices regulations can increase primary care access and utilization. In a study of persons residing in a full practice state, the study showed 62% higher geographic accessibility to primary care clinicians, compared to only 35% accessibility in restricted practice states. Rural health priorities have changed little in the last 20 years. *Rural Healthy People 2020* continues to identify access to care as the number one health priority concern across the U.S. All efforts should focus on decreasing state and national regulatory barriers that hinder access to healthcare. This is only one of many challenges facing rural health NPs.

As NP presence in rural areas has increased, recognition reimbursement from third-party payors for NP services has struggled to keep up. Most NP services are paid anywhere from 75–85% of the same services offered by physicians. In states where restrictive practices prevent full practice, many NPs are required to pay additional fees for collaborative arrangements which increase practice overhead and negatively affect sustainability of rural health facilities. Additionally, many of the managed care organizations require credentialing of a supervising or collaborative physician in addition to the Nurse Practitioner, again increasing cost and complexity of clinic operations.

The population growth in rural areas is considerably less when compared to the growth in urban areas. Practices in urban areas have a large population to fill clinic appointments; however, rural areas have a limited population to fill appointments thus limiting clinic potential profitability. The cost associated with increased regulatory burdens for Nurse Practitioners combined with lower reimbursement and a limited population creates a serious case of questionable sustainability for rural practices.

So why should NPs even consider practicing in rural areas? Because once again, the need is so great and as demonstrated throughout history, nurses and nurse practitioners are equipped to successfully meet healthcare needs and improve the lives of millions of Americans across the country. According to the most recent Common Wealth Report Card (2018) Texas ranks 51st in the United States with regards to access and affordability of health care, yet Texas remains one of the most restrictive practice states for Nurse Practitioners. Despite a plethora of research supporting the removal of practice barriers for Nurse Practitioners, Texas politics has prevented the advancement of Nurse Practitioners at the cost of patient care. For this very reason, advocating on behalf of patients and the nursing profession should be the duty and primary responsibility of every professional nurse and nurse practitioner.

OPPORTUNITIES

While rural health has many challenges for NPs, there are so many more opportunities. Caring for rural residents provides a unique opportunity for the NP to develop a relationship with patients that goes beyond a normal patient–provider relationship. When caring for rural residents, the NP provider also cares for the parents, children, cousins, and neighbors of patients. Caring for individuals and families enables the provider to become a vested part of the community. Caring for rural communities is one of the most rewarding things an NP could ever experience. The rapport and level of trust that is gained in the close relationships enables the NP to provide better care for the patients and the patients are more responsive to the education and recommendations shared from providers.

Rural areas provide more opportunity for the NP provider to be both a leader and active participant in the community. In small communities the NP is the health expert and this expertise extends to the school and the local jail as well as the pharmacy and the senior citizens clubs. NPs serve as local role models for students and should volunteer to participate in city or county planning with regards to health initiatives like supporting smoke-free environments, developing bike or walking lanes, and organizing local health fairs. While these opportunities exist in larger urban areas as well, the NPs opportunities are unlimited, and the resulting efforts are much more visible in the smaller communities.

Lastly, rural areas provide an ideal location for NPs to focus on fulfilling a mission of improving community health through the development of a small business. Building a business is a challenge but building a business in the midst of an ever-changing healthcare environment is that much more of a challenge and not for the faint of heart. The desire for a business in a rural area has to be for the right reasons—not money or fame—but for passion and making a difference in the lives of individuals, families, and communities.

Rural health is a passion and caring for the health of hard-working people who put clothes on our back and food on our table is a priority that should never be taken for granted. NPs must continue caring for this vulnerable population and ensure health care policies do not overlook the work we are doing and difference we are making in the lives of rural Americans.

A RURAL EXPERIENCE

October 2009, the Family Care Clinic of Panhandle began offering primary care services in a small remodeled building on the corner of Main Street in a small rural town with a population of around 2,600 people. Our goal was to see at least 10 patients a day in the first month (which was a pretty lofty goal for a small community starting with no patients). Years prior the community had a town doctor who took care of everyone in the area, but when the town doctor retired, the clinic was purchased by a larger hospital about 60 miles away as has been the trend for the last few decades. The hospital continued primary care services at the clinic for a few years, utilizing the clinic as a referral source to the hospital. After several years, the hospital sold the clinic to a large group practice who also provided services for several more years then later shut the doors. The clinic had been closed for three years prior to my arrival. Upon speaking with administration from both of the previous operating facilities, I was told that a clinic in this area was just not sustainable and reopening a clinic in the area would never be worth my time or investment. Nonetheless, I ventured on and thank goodness they were both proven to be wrong. In the first month over 300 patients were seen—some affected by acute illness such as the flu (as this was the first year of the H1N1 outbreak) and others affected by chronic illness that had not been treated in several years. In just a matter of time the clinic grew in the number of patients we served as well as the number of team members we employed.

In October of 2009 I was one of the two original employees and by the end of 2010 we had a total of four employees—three sharing space in a 6x6 room and another we moved to the back of the building to office out of the tiny kitchen. By the end of 2010 the clinic was busting at the seams and unable to accommodate the number of patients that needed care. By the beginning of 2011 God had opened the door for us to purchase land and we began planning to build a new facility. I still remember the day I told my team, "I know you all may think I am crazy, but we are buying land and building a new clinic... now." Nothing like this had been done and a new facility seemed like an impossible feat and another huge leap of faith, but by January of 2012 our staff of six had relocated to a new building with 8 exam rooms, a lab, an x-ray room, and a patient education teaching area.

We have had a few growing pains over the years, but we have continued to navigate the ever-changing world of healthcare and gradually expanded our reach to three additional underserved communities in the Texas Panhandle. In 2015 CMS (Medicare) announced a set of quality measures and predicted that only 15% of independently owned healthcare facilities (like us) would ever be able to meet the measures due to expense and associated complexities. We heard what they said and determined we would be part of the 15%—again something that seemed like more than an impossible feat. We began working toward a plan that could only be possible with God and an amazing team.

As of the recently released 2018 report data, not only were we a part of the small 15% that were able to meet the quality measures, but our small yet mighty organization in conjunction with the quality measure savings within our ACO ranked 6th out of 53 ACOs in the State of Texas and in the TOP 40 out of 561 in the nation (that's the top 7% in the nation right here in the small rural areas of the Texas Panhandle)!

Ten years later we remain so very thankful, and we are still offering primary care services to underserved areas. While our team has grown from two to twenty strong, our mission has not changed. Our mission is to improve the health of individuals and communities by providing exceptional care, education, and inspiration so that people can live happier, healthier, and productive lives. I am so thankful God has allowed me and our team the opportunity to serve each of these communities and I pray that as a clinic, our light will continue to shine bright beyond the Texas Panhandle and our services will continue to be a blessing to all.

William Bradford, of Plimoth Plantation and Governor to the Pilgrims summarized it best:

Thus out of small beginnings greater things have been produced by His hand that made all things of nothing, and gives being to all things that are; and as one small candle may light a thousand, so the light here kindled hath shone to many, yea in some sort to our whole nation; let the glorious name of Jehovah have all the praise.

Going Beyond with Compassion . . . Making a Difference. Jude 22

REFERENCES

Barnes, H., *et al.* (2017). Effects of regulation and payment policies on nurse practitioners clinical practices. *Med Care Res Ref, 74*(4): 431–451.

Bolan, J. N., *et al.* (2015). Rural Health People 2020: New decade, same challenges. 31(3): 326–333.

Chandak, A., P. Najar, and G. Lin. (2017). MMWR Morbidity and mortality weekly report surveillance summaries 66(1): 1–8

Defining Rural @ the US Census Bureau. https://census.gov

Health Resources and Services Administration. Life expectancy gap illustrates disparities. https://hrsa.gov.

Heiser, S. (2019). New findings confirm predictions on physician shortage. Association of American Medical Colleges.

Henry Street Settlement. https://henrystreet.org

Hewitt, S. (2019). What does Trumps new executive order mean for nurses? https://anacapitolbeat.org/2019/10/09/what-does-trumps-new-executive-order-mean-for-nurses/

History of FNU. https://frontier.edu/about-frontier/history-of-fnu/

Institute of Medicine. (2011). *The Future of Nursing Leading Change Advancing Health.* Institute of Medicine.https://www.ncbi.nlm.nih.gov/books/NBK350160/

Ligenza, D. (2015). Loretta Ford: The mother of the nurse practitioner movement. bartonassociates.com

Long, A. S., A. L. Hanlon, and K. L. Pellergrin. Socioeconomic variables explain rural disparities in US mortality rates: Implication for rural health research and policy. *SSM Population Health* 2018, 6: 72–74.

NP Role grows to more than 270,000. Practice, AANP News. Htts://aanp.org

Policy Perspectives: Competition and the regulation of advance practice nurses. 2014. https://www.ftc.gov/reports/policy-perspectives-competition-regulation-advanced-practice-nurses

Richardson, E. (1970). Health education and welfare secretary. https://www.finance.senate.gov/imo/media/doc/Richardson1.pdf

Safriet, B. (1971). Health care dollars and regulatory sense: The role of advanced practice nursing.

Scorecard on State Health System Performance. Common wealth fund. 2018. https://interactives.commonwealthfund.org/2018/state-scorecard/state/texas/

Spencer, J. C., *et al.* Decomposing mortality disparities in urban and rural US counties. *2018 HSR, 53*(6): 4310–4331.

The National Organization of Nurse Practitioner Faculties. (1974). https://www.nonpf.org/page/1

Villapiano, N., T. Iwashyna, M. Davis. (2017). Worsening Rural Urban Gap in Hospital Mortality. *Journal of the American Board of Family Medicine. 30*(6): 816–823.

Zahnd, W. E., *et al.* (2018). Rural urban differences in cancer incidence and trends in the US. Cancer Epidemiology and Prevention Biomarkers. *AACR, 27*(11): 1265–1274.

Zahnd, W. E., A. J. Fogleman, and W. D. Jenkins. (2018). Rural Urban Differences in Stage of Diagnosis among cancer with preventive opportunity. *American Journal of Preventive Medicine, 54*(5): 688–698.

CHAPTER 16

The Rural Nurse and Social Media

Kenneth W. Lowrance

Objectives:

1. Define and identify various types of social media.
2. Describe potential impact of social media on rural populations and healthcare delivery.
3. Recognize strategies to avoid negative consequences of social media on nursing practice.

Discussion Questions:

1. Describe the history of social media.
2. What are potential benefits of social media as related to healthcare in rural settings?
3. What benefits and barriers do nurses experience in utilizing social media in rural settings?

INTRODUCTION

The term social media is well-known by the general public. By definition, social media includes "the different forms of online communication used by people to create networks, community, and collectives to share information, ideas, messages, and other content such as video" (Terrell, 2015). Popular social media applications today include Facebook, Twitter, Viber, video portals such as YouTube, Instagram, LinkedIn, and Tumblr. There are also social media applications for various disease processes, such as diabetes, cancer, etc., where individuals can participate to share their personal stories, information, and support for others. These are generally in the form of blogs. There are many others which address individuals' particular interest. Some of these are considered socially acceptable, such as Pinterest, while others may be considered appealing to prurient interests and being on the fringe or beyond of society's community standards. Such application may showcase concepts such as racism, nationalism, pedophilia, terrorism against the United States, and the occult.

Not only are social media sites used for personal socializing, but also as business marketing or professional venues. Many times, businesses, political candidates, emerging musicians, and professionals/professional organizations utilize social media sites to establish an online presence to attract more interest in their products or services. New social media sites are always being developed (Pinard, Romer, and Morley, 2017).

For younger users of social media, i.e., children and adolescents, online bullying is a major concern. Cases of youth suicide have been attributed to bullying activity on social media sites. While many believe that social media sites are safe and fun, such is not always the case. Users of social media must be cognizant of the environment and be aware of potential threats.

HISTORY OF SOCIAL MEDIA

Without the internet, social media would be nonexistent, perhaps with the exception of personal advertisements in the newspaper and/or newspaper advice columns. To understand the history of the development of social media as we know it today, it is important to understand a bit about the history of the development and spread of the internet.

In 1969, the United States Department of Defense undertook an experimental project called ARPANET, a project which got its name from the Advanced Research Projects Agency (ARPA), which sponsored its development. In the beginning ARPANET consisted of only four connected super computers. One purpose of the ARPANET project included the need to create a network where researchers located in different places had a way to communicate with one another. Another goal of the ARPANET project was to develop a system of networked computers to send and receive data over multiple pathways to ensure that communications could continue even if the network was destroyed or other technical issues occurred, such as in a nuclear attack or natural disaster (Pinard *et al.*, 2017).

Over the next several years, multiple colleges and universities connected to the ARPANET. As a result, many different types of computers were connected to the network, which required some technological adjustment to assure compatibility and interoperability of these computers to ensure that data could be sent and received by all members of the network. This growth eventually resulted in the internet that we know today (Pinard *et al.*, 2017). Currently, work is being done to develop Web 2.0, the internet version of the future.

The development of the internet was a major innovation for the world of science, education, and socialization with the potential to connect billions of people around the world. The internet and its functions were easily accepted by institutions, but for a fair period of time, the public did not embrace the concept of the internet. A few reasons contributed to the public's delay in embracing this innovation. A huge barrier was that one needed a computer. At this time, these were very expensive and difficult to acquire. In addition, computers at this time were very difficult to utilize in terms of the need to learn "how to." And, of course, having to connect to the newly developed internet was next to impossible unless one was associated with a major educational institution or governmental agency. This inability to connect to the internet is still present today in some rural areas.

According to Pinard *et al.* (2017), in 1993 professors and students at the University of Illinois National Center for Supercomputing Applications (NCSA) developed a web browser called Mosaic which allowed graphics to be displayed and was relatively easy for operators to utilize. As a result, the public became curious and engaged, and the popularity of the internet increased. Likewise, by this time, more of the public could afford computers as costs decreased. Additionally, people found that accessing the internet was not only informative, but also fun.

Today, the internet is used for multiple purposes: researching topics, email, utilization for video conferences and webinars, distance education, voice-over internet for phone calls, downloading software, music, and movies, purchasing goods and services (Amazon.com, etc.), watching TV shows in real time or streaming episodes, accessing computers remotely, and sharing files with others. The use of the internet has become a common activity for many folks due to enhancements of technology, improvements in accessibility, and affordability of computing devices and the widespread use of smart phones. Despite all these improvements, some rural areas still have tremendous access issues to the internet which creates barriers for use by individuals in these areas. Many would be lost without access to the internet, and business, commerce, and education would suffer a significant negative impact.

Social media, as a recognized concept, actually began to be developed in the 1970s as the internet became more common and accessible. The 1980s–1990s saw an expansive growth of personal computers and people who owned them. With this availability, social media began to skyrocket (Terrell, 2015).

The first two social media sites were Six Degrees and Friendster (which is no longer around). In 2004, Mark Zuckerberg founded and launched Facebook, one of the most well-known and popular social media applications with more than 2.3 billion users worldwide, just under 30% of the world's population. Another popular application is Twitter, which made its debut in 2006. Twitter currently has approximately 335 million active users. In 2010, Instagram was launched whereby users can share videos and photos. Instagram was acquired by Facebook in 2012. Another very popular social media application is Snapchat, which appeared on the scene in 2011. There are many other social media applications not mentioned here (Terrell, 2015). A Google search of "social medial applications" will yield a plethora of information in this regard.

Needless to say, social media is undoubtedly here to stay, and many new users are added to this phenomenon on a daily basis throughout the world.

SOCIAL MEDIA IN THE RURAL SETTING

Social media has enhanced the lives of many individuals in the world. At the same time, as previously noted, there is a potential dark side. To be a social media user, a connection to the internet is required. The lack of broadband internet access in some rural areas is a huge barrier, not only for engagement in social media, but also for research and multiple other functions of the internet and positive contributions to society.

The disparity of internet access between rural and urban/suburban areas is known as the "digital divide" or the "digital gap." During the last ten years, large gains have been made in acquiring digital technology in rural settings compared to previous years. Despite this, rural Americans are still less likely than their urban/suburban counterparts to have home broadband or own a smartphone. According to the Pew Research Center (2019), Americans living in rural areas are 12% less likely than Americans overall to have home broadband. In 2007, the gap was 16%, so some improvement has occurred.

Additionally, the Pew Research Center (2019) notes that mobile technology utilization among rural residents has also risen sharply. Ownership of computers, such as desktops or laptops, has only slightly risen since 2008. Thus, many rural individuals access the internet and social media via their phones. A potential barrier in this regard is whether cell service is available or not in a particular area.

The federal government is supporting efforts to expand broadband internet service to rural areas. For example, the U.S. Department of Agriculture in 2019 launched a toolkit to support the deployment of high-speed internet to rural communities. The plan to provide broadband services to rural areas is a high priority because 46 million people live in rural America, which comprises roughly 72% of the U.S. land mass. Reports from the Federal Communication Commission indicate that about 19 million of rural American households still lack reliable, affordable, high-speed internet (United States Department of Agriculture [USDA], 2019). The benefits of e-connectivity to the internet touches many facets of daily life for rural (and all) Americans such as economic development, innovation and technology, workforce issues, and quality of life. The USDA has 27 programs meant to facilitate the expansion of broadband, including grants, loans, and technical assistance from its multiple mission areas (Huba, 2019). Nurses in rural settings that lack broadband internet are in an ideal position to advocate for such by dialogue with county officials and other leaders to investigate resources to bring broadband to their areas.

Social media in rural settings many times can make this setting even see smaller when one sees coworkers, neighbors, and patients not only on social media, but also in local businesses such as the grocery store, drug store, or even in church. Given the various personalities of individuals, some people use social media to keep up with others purely out of curiosity. Thus, another reason one should be cautious in what one posts as well as make efforts to separate personal matters from professional matters.

ROLE OF SOCIAL MEDIA IN RURAL HEALTHCARE DELIVERY

There are potentially many applications of social media in the rural setting to positively affect healthcare for this underserved population. Not only can social media help to support patients, it can also support nursing professionals. A review of literature revealed a few examples of this.

Klippert and Schaper (2018) partnered with a public health department in a Western state of the U.S. to address engagement of women and men in obtaining mammograms. A tailored message mammography campaign on Facebook during Breast Cancer Awareness Month was uploaded to the public health department's Facebook page targeting women and men over age 40 in a rural area. The campaign had a duration of five weeks. Via survey and responses to a tailored advertisement on the Facebook page for the mammography campaign, the researchers aim was to identify what was the highest level of engagement with patients achieved by the Facebook campaign. The highest level of engagement was defined as an individual expression of intent to obtain a mammogram. This was determined both in Facebook comments and an anonymous survey. Eighty-two percent of survey respondents indicated the intent to obtain a mammogram within the year. Limitations existed in this study as related to demographic factors (few minority participants; few men participants), a reflected desire by participants to answer the survey question in a favorable way, and access to internet resources.

In a study by Logsdon, Mittelberg, and Myers (2014), the investigators studied the use of social media and internet by rural adolescent mothers to obtain health information. For study participants, 93% accessed the internet via cell phones and 100% utilized computers to seek health information. These results were obtained from the Pew Internet Survey during home visits with nurses from a community health agency. The take-home from this study was that technology can serve as an important resource to promote healthy behaviors and to impact the health of the adolescent mother and her baby.

The above are only two examples of how social media was used for healthcare information. Other patient-focused methodologies include blogs and specific disease-related website or blogs. Social media is a rich setting for the design and implementation of innovative ideas to address healthcare needs of the rural populations. Nurses, with their excellent assessment skills, knowledge of evidence-based practice, and skills in the translation of evidence are in an ideal situation to brainstorm, develop, and implement valuable health promotion activities for rural residents via social media venues.

Not only is social media a potential rich resource to convey messages and information regarding healthcare, but it is also a potentially significant resource to create social support networks for nurses and other professionals working in the rural setting. For example, one can search Facebook for various nursing groups and request to join. Most times, these are closed groups with the intent that only nurses can be members. In an ideal world, this would serve the profession in a potentially positive way. For social media groups of Advanced Practice Registered Nurses (APRNs), i.e., Nurse Practitioners, Clinical Nurse Specialists, Certified Registered Nurse Anesthetists, and Certified Nurse Midwives, it has been discovered that there have been incidents where physicians opposed to full practice authority have infiltrated these groups in an attempt to undermine the credibility of the APRN role. The politics of this conflict is fodder for a bigger in-depth discussion than for the content of this chapter.

Nurse leadership, of course, is another facet of professional nursing practice. Flury (2017) notes the importance of social media as a leadership tool for nurse executives. She notes the importance of the balance between "personal" information and "professional" information that one makes available on social media. Before the advent of social media, it was easier to separate personal information from professional information. Nowadays, it can be a huge challenge based on the formatting of social media sites. The networking aspect of nurse leadership is one of the most valuable benefits of social media for this nursing specialty. LinkedIn is particularly a preferred social media venue for professionals, whereas sites such as Facebook, Instagram, etc., are more appropriate for personal aspects of one's life.

The key to effective and appropriate utilization of social media outlets is to think before one posts. Once posted, it exists forever. Just because one believes he/she has deleted something, this is not true. The technology exists to retrieve deleted posts. Caution is the keyword in utilizing any form of social media whether personal or professional, and for nurses everywhere, including the rural setting.

NURSES AND SOCIAL MEDIA

As previously mentioned, there are multiple opportunities for individuals to participate in social media. In general, younger individuals are more active in social media than older individuals, although many older individuals are involved with social media as well. Social media is a way to share opinions, family activities and photos, highlights of vacations, and even bad news. Just about anything appears on social media, and sometimes one wonders that the author of a post was thinking when they posted something. Community standards play a significant part as to what the majority may consider acceptable or unacceptable in a social media post. A level of professional judgement and maturity is essential, in this author's opinion, to assure safe and effective use of social media. There has been much written in the literature about the utilization of social media by nurses, most of which deals with negative outcomes that can occur with inappropriate engagement with social media. There are some common myths and misunderstanding about social media.

CONFUSION AND MYTHS ABOUT SOCIAL MEDIA

The National Council of State Boards of Nursing (NCSBN) has published a white paper as *A Nurse's Guide to the Use of Social Media* (2018). This addresses multiple aspects of the concept of social media as it relates to professional nursing practice and can be found on the NCSBN website (https://www.ncsbn.org). Additional articles regarding social media are also archived on this website.

Patient privacy and confidentiality are of prime importance for any nurse. Sometimes nurses face negative consequences when inappropriate disclosure or posting is unintentional. These consequences could range from disciplinary actions in the employment setting to action from the State Board of Nursing to legal action against the nurse, or any combination of these. In some cases, there have been blatant issues of intentional or malicious misuse of social media which could result in similar negative consequences.

There is a mistaken belief by some that a communication or post on social media site is private and only accessible to the intended recipient. This is not true. The content could be shared and disseminated to other places. The same could occur with an email communication. As previously mentioned, many believe that once something is deleted from a site, it can no longer be accessed. This is not true. Sometimes nurses have posted a patient scenario, but have been cautious to not name the patient. However, even if referred to by a diagnosis or condition, this could be deemed as a breach of confidentiality and privacy. Particularly in a rural area where many people know one another, clues from a post, even though a name is not given, could have enough context that individuals could determine whom a nurse is speaking of.

On many nursing specialty websites, nurses are seeking the opinion of other nurses. This is particularly true on APRN sites. Sometimes a Nurse Practitioner may be presenting a case and asking for an opinion regarding management of the patient. One must be cautious before posting patient scenarios, questions, seeking advice, etc. This is a high-risk activity and could certainly lead to legal and/or disciplinary issues. Nurses should be educationally prepared to know how to seek evidence-based information without exposing themselves to criticism for questions they may ask as well as exposing themselves to breaches of confidentiality/privacy, and also possibly exposing their lack of knowledge or skills to get needed information from reliable sources. This is the basis for some of the situations that have occurred when physicians oppose full practice authority for APRNs. These anti-full practice authority physicians collect information that is posted and use it as arguments with legislators that APRNs should not be afforded full practice authority despite the fact that research demonstrates that APRNs deliver high-quality, cost-effective care. In reality, there poor APRN performers as there are poor physician performers.

CONFIDENTIALITY AND PRIVACY ISSUES

There is a difference between confidentiality and privacy. According to the NCSBN (2018), confidential information is any patient information acquired by the nurse during the course of treatment. This information must be safeguarded by the nurse and only shared to other members of the healthcare team for healthcare purposes. Certain conditions must exist before confidential information could be shared in any context other than that just described: with the patient's consent, when legally required, or where failure to disclose could result in significant harm to the patient or others. Beyond these very limited exceptions, the nurse is obligated to safeguard confidential information.

The NCSBN (2018) provides a discussion of privacy as compared to confidentiality. Privacy is related to the patient's expectation and right to be treated with respect and dignity. When nurses interact with patients, the relationship is built on trust. The patient must feel confident that his/her most personal information and basic dignity will be protected by the nurse. Unless this trust exists, the nurse-patient relationship is ineffective. If the bond of trust is broken, the patient may be reluctant to be forthcoming in reporting symptoms, private information that may have a bearing on the diagnosis and required care for fear of the information being shared with others beyond those who have a legitimate "need to know." If the trust bond is broken, even if inadvertent or by accident, this situation results in damage to the nurse-patient relationship and the general public trustworthiness of the profession of nursing. For the eighteenth year in a row, the profession of nursing has been rated by the American public as the most trustworthy profession for honesty and ethics (Gallup, 2018).

Not only is the guarding of confidential information and protection of privacy a foundational responsibility of a nurse because of the ethical implications, there are strict federal laws which mandate these protections. Privacy is further defined by the Health Insurance Portability and Accountability Act (HIPAA) (1996). HIPPA developed definitions for personal identifiable information and established how this information could be used, by whom, and under what circumstances. Individually identifiable information includes any information that relates to the past, present, or future physical or mental health of an individual, or provides enough information that leads someone to believe the information could be used to identify someone. If a HIPAA complaint is filed, and an investigation results in evidence of a violation, severe monetary fines can be applied, not to mention other licensing action.

The importance of assuring confidentiality and privacy cannot be overemphasized for nurses in all settings, including rural. For the rural nurse, it is not unusual to be asked by members of the community regarding information about a patient or family member in not only healthcare setting, but also in other settings such as local businesses, church, etc. The nurse should be aware of this possibility and realize that he/she may not divulge any information regarding a patient so as to not breach confidentiality or privacy. A good practice would be to develop a response ahead of time to use as a reply when confronted or questioned about a patient's condition by those not authorized to receive this information. And, of course, this reply should be delivered with professionalism and respect.

POTENTIAL NEGATIVE CONSEQUENCES OF SOCIAL MEDIA MISUSE

Misuse of social media could result in multiple potential consequences.

Potential Board of Nursing Implications

- Grounds on which a social media violation could trigger State Board of Nursing action:
    - —Unprofessional conduct,
    - —Unethical conduct,
    - —Moral turpitude,
    - —Mismanagement of patient records,
    - —Revealing a privileged communication, and
    - —Breach of confidentiality (NCSBN, 2018).

If after Board of Nursing investigation, allegations are proven true, the nurse may be subject to disciplinary action by the Board, to include a reprimand or sanction, assessment of a monetary penalty, or temporary or permanent loss of licensure.

Other Potential Consequences

- Civil and/or criminal penalties,
- Personal liability,
- Being sued for defamation, invasion of privacy, or harassment,
- Employment consequences, including termination,
- Bringing negative reflection on the employing agency, and
- Disrupting team work and collegiality of the nursing department if comments are posted about coworkers and considered to be "cyber bullying" (NCSBN, 2018).

Again, the importance of thinking before posting is of profound importance.

Sometimes the nurse can become the victim of social media misuse. For example, there was a case where a nurse practitioner was videoed by a pediatric patient's mother using a smart phone, but the nurse was unaware that this occurred until she saw the video posted on Facebook subsequent to the child's visit (McGill, Loveless, and McGill, 2019). In this case, the privacy and professional image of the nurse practitioner was violated. Potential issues that could result include nurse embarrassment, issues related to employee retention, unwanted legal actions, and direct and indirect nurse safety concerns. These sorts of situations are still under investigation as to what a nurse can do when such situations arise from a legal standpoint. However, from a common sense approach, the following strategies can be employed:

- *Survey the room*. Before you begin interacting with the patient, look around. Is there a family member/someone in the room with a phone or a tablet?
- *Say something*. If you notice you are being recorded, say something like, "Let me place your phone on the counter so I can communicate with (you) and the patient without distractions." Most facilities have policies regarding a no cell phone use in exam rooms or patient rooms. Remind the individual of the policy. Many places have signs posted to this effect.
- *Be familiar with social media platform processes*. If you find an unauthorized posting on a social media sight of yourself, contact the social media site describing the issue. They will be obligated to remove the post assuming your complaint is nonmalicious (McGill *et al.*, 2019).

STRATEGIES TO AVOID SOCIAL MEDIA MISUSE AND POTENTIAL NEGATIVE CONSEQUENCES

It is incumbent on every nurse who participates in social media platforms to think before posting. Is your post in good taste? Is the context of a photo you may post one in which you will not later be embarrassed about or which may result in adverse action by your employer? Have you tried to separate your personal profile from your professional profile, e.g., utilizing Facebook or another social site for your personal life and something like LinkedIn for your professional role? It is difficult to separate these, but it can be done, and would be wise to do so to avoid employment issues of Board of Nursing disciplinary issues. The key to successful navigation and utilization of social media is common sense. The question also arises: Should you friend patients? If not, how do you address these individuals when they confront you about not accepting a friend invitation? Again, a prepared response would be good to have.

Nurses in rural areas are generally well-known in the community, and like all nurses, very well-respected. As previously noted, for the eighteenth year in a row, the nursing profession has achieved the highest rating for honesty and ethics of any profession as reported by the results an annual Gallup poll. This is a prestigious recognition that professional nursing should guard and promote.

SUMMARY

The world of social media is complex and not without risks. It is a wonderful tool to stay connected with family, friends, and other professionals, but caution must be used to avoid an unintentional or intentional misuse of the platform one uses. As nurses, we have a huge accountability for trustworthiness and ethical conduct. Failure to maintain this can result in the public's deterioration of trust toward the profession.

There is significant potential for the development of innovative strategies regarding the utilization of social media for health promotion, disease prevention, and disease management in all settings, including the rural setting. It is important for those rural areas which do not have broadband internet services to get it. There are multiple programs by the U.S. Department of Agriculture for rural communities to access to make this happen. Nurses are in an ideal position to serve as advocates for this as well as multiple other positive issues in the rural community. Nurses have the respect of the community, and should take advantage of the leverage they have.

Social media is a powerful tool, and used properly, can make a significant positive difference in rural setting to supplement and assist in improving access to important health information and access to care.

REFERENCES

Flury, C. (2017). Social media as a leadership tool for nurse executives. *Nursing Economics, 35*(5): 272–275.

Gallup. (2018). Nurses again outpace other professions for honesty, ethics. Retrieved from https://news.gallup.com/poll/245597/nurses-again-outpace-professions-honesty-ethics.aspx

Health Insurance Portability and Accountability Act (HIPAA). 1996. Retrieved from https://hhs.gov/hipaa/index.html

Huba, S. (2019). New USDA "toolkit" features resources for high speed internet in rural areas. Retrieved from https://triblive.com/news/world/new-usda-toolkit-features-resources-for-high-speed-internet-in-rural-areas

Klippert, H., and A. Schaper. (2018). Using Facebook to communicate mammography messages to rural audiences. *Public Health Nurse, 36*, 164–171. doi: 10.1111/phn.12556

Logsdon, M., M. Mittelbert, and J. Myers. (2014). Use of social media and internet to obtain health information by rural adolescent mothers. *Applied Nursing Research, 28,* 55–56. Retrieved from http://dx.doi.org/10.1016/j.apnr.2014.04.006

McGill, M., B. Lovelace, and M. McGill (2019). Social media in healthcare: A 360-degree view. *American Nurse Today, 14*(10), 25–26.

National Council of State Boards of Nursing (NCSBN). (2018). *A nurse's guide to the use of social media.* Retrieved from https://www.ncsbn.org/3739.htm

Pew Research Center. (2019). Digital gap between rural and nonrural America persists. Retrieved from https://www.pewresearch.org/fact-tank/2019/05/31/digital-gap-between-rural-and nonrural-america-persists

Pinard, K., R. Romer, and D. Morley. (2017). *CMPTR^3 applications and concepts.* Boston: Cengage Learning, 146–147.

Terrell, K. (2015). The complete history of social media: From the first online network to today. Retrieved from https://historycooperative.org/the-history-of-social-media

U.S. Department of Agriculture (USDA). (2019). RDeConnectivity tool kit. Retrieved from https://www.rd.usda.gov/files/508_RDeConnectivitytoolkit12918.pdf

Afterword

Two weeks into my freshman year of college, I returned home to devastatingly bad news. My 40-year-old mother had just been diagnosed with an aggressive form of breast cancer. Her oncologist, surgeon, and radiation therapist were over an hour east of our rural Kentucky home; only the family physician and a single pharmacist lived and worked in our tiny town, and cancer was out of their scope of care "by a country mile."

Over the next three years, I made the 90-minute drive from my state university to the eastern Kentucky hospital more times than I could count, as any possible complication to cancer care one could have, my mother did have. She was a classic case of social determinants of health impacting rural patient outcomes, long before I knew what any of that meant!

If I got there early in the morning, I might catch her oncologist just in time for him to tell me she was "as well as can be expected, given the extent of her present illness." The conversations with him were always broad, brief, and anything but reassuring. Assumed poor and ignorant—and while neither was far from the truth—there was never an effort to help me or my mother's siblings who lived at her bedside and cared for her continuously alongside her nurses, to understand anything beyond what was obvious in front of us. She was dying and there was little to nothing we could do.

It was during one of Momma's long stints in the intensive care unit that I met someone who would change my life's trajectory: a brilliant advanced practice nurse. "Paula" was a Master's-prepared clinical nurse specialist (CNS) who worked almost exclusively with high acuity ICU patients, who spent "as long as it takes," she would say, to evaluate, coordinate, and plan her patients' care. From admission to discharge and every bed change in-between, Paula was there. She was far more than my mother's CNS and our go-to for answers no one else seemed to have time to answer; she was a tireless advocate until the very end. She was the first person in the hospital to ever involve me in the plans for my mother's care, even though I was barely 18 years old. She was the first person to acknowledge how real the struggle for me and my mother was during those 3 long years, as Momma begged me to go back to school and let the nurses call me if there was anything she needed. And she was the only person to ever send me a card on Momma's first "heavenly birthday," reminding me how proud she must surely be that I was about to graduate nursing school.

Paula was the reason I walked out of a pre-med organic chemistry class on a cold rainy October day, realizing that becoming a physician was not my life's calling. As I walked across the street to the nursing building, drenched in raindrops and joyful tears, I prayed they would let me change my major and join the nursing students in January. I needed to be a "Paula" in someone's life, and I needed it like I needed breath!

My mother lost her battle with cancer the week before I began my final year of nursing school. In that final year, I pledged to myself that keeping patients out of the hospital and away from ICUs would become my life's mission. Three academic degrees, over 5,000 rural Kentucky primary care patients, and 21 years later, I'm still working at exactly that, and I couldn't be happier.

Sometimes poor, sometimes stubborn, sometimes naïve, but always proud to be who (and where) they are, these patients present challenges that make every single day a new adventure. The health literacy of rural patients, and sometimes literacy in general, makes communication challenging, and advocating for the best possible care for those with extremely finite resources, is at times exhausting; yet, nothing I have ever done has ever been so rewarding.

I am not alone in my love for rural health care. Many of my colleagues in advanced practice nursing, allied health science, and medicine share my love of caring for people who call rural communities their homes. They love it so much, some of them wrote and edited a textbook about it. Whether you find it to be your calling or simply find it to be your lot in life at some point, its pages will fill you with the knowledge you need to overcome the challenges of providing care to rural populations.

Many days I leave the office feeling more like a translator, a navigator, a private investigator, a counselor, a media technologist, a policy guru, or a social media mogul—and then I realize, that's all part of being a provider in rural health. And I know, as I believe you have read and learned in this text—there's absolutely nothing better!

Wendy Fletcher, DNP, APRN, FNP-BC, FAANP
Managing Partner, The CheráWen Group, LLC
Co-Owner/APRN, Main Street Medical Associates (Morehead, KY)

Index